PUBLIC EXPECTATIONS AND HEALTH CARE

PUBLIC EXPECTATIONS AND HEALTH CARE

ESSAYS ON THE CHANGING

ORGANIZATION OF HEALTH SERVICES

DAVID MECHANIC
University of Wisconsin

WILEY-INTERSCIENCE, a Division of John Wiley & Sons, Inc.

New York • London • Sydney • Toronto

Library of Congress Cataloging in Publication Data:

Mechanic, David, 1936–
Public expectations and health care.

Includes bibliographical references.
1. Medical care—United States. 2. Medical care
—Great Britain. I. Title.

RA445.M38   362.1'0942   72-4398
ISBN 0-471-59003-7

Printed in the United States of America

10 9 8 7 6 5 4 3 2

To Edmund H. Volkart, teacher and friend

Preface

This book brings together selected papers I have written in recent years, dealing with the changing organization of medical practice in the United States and England, with some new essays. The published papers appear in a variety of sociological, medical, and law journals; together, they provide a perspective that is not clearly apparent from the individual selections. I have tried to leave the essays as originally published in order to reflect the trend of my own thinking in recent years, a period in which significant alterations in perspectives about health matters have developed.

In a sense, these essays fill a gap in two of my earlier books dealing with the broad field of medical sociology and health services. In *Medical Sociology: A Selective View* (1968) I presented a wide-ranging discussion of the field, but I very heavily emphasized a social psychological perspective. This book also devoted disproportionately little attention to the health services system as a whole, compared with the processes of defining, responding to, and dealing with illness. In *Mental Health and Social Policy* (1969) I discussed the underlying assumptions prevailing in the mental health field and the processes that lead to varying reactions to mentally ill persons. Here I gave more attention to the larger system of services, but devoted my attention exclusively to mental health. In the present book of essays, my major attention is devoted to the health care system as a whole and to the sociocultural, organizational, and technical forces that have molded it. I hope the bringing together of these essays and the integration of them into a larger perspective will contribute to a constructive discussion of the future of health care in the United States.

In the assembling of different essays, written for various audiences, a certain amount of repetition is inevitable. If all repetitious passages were eliminated, the essays would take on a disjointed and disorganized tone, and the context of an individual discussion would sometimes be lost. Here I have followed a middle course; I have tried to minimize repetitious materials without destroying the thrust of each individual essay. When I was forced to make a choice, I elected to repeat an argument instead of destroying the focus of discussion.

I thank the following journals and publishers who provided permission to reprint material previously published: *Law and Contemporary Problems*; *The Annals of the American Academy of Political and Social Science*; *New England Journal of Medicine*; J. B. Lippincott Company, publisher of *Medical Care*; the American Sociological Association, which publishes the *Journal of Health and Social Behavior*; Springer-Verlag which publishes *Social Psychiatry*; and the Pergamon Publishing Company, publisher of the *Journal of Chronic Diseases*. I am also grateful to Grune and Stratton, Inc., which provided permission to reprint my essay on "Sociological Issues in Mental Health," which appeared in *Progress in Community Mental Health*. Sections adapted from two reviews that appeared in *Science* ("Crisis in the Health Field," 1970, **168**:1563–1564, and "The Poor State of Health," 1971, **172**:701–703), copyright 1970 and 1971 by the American Association for the Advancement of Science, are integrated into the text with permission of the publisher.

The various research and other work reported in this book were assisted by Grants MH-8516, MH 14835, and MH 07413 from the National Institute of Mental Health and from Grants HS 00253 and HS 00091, National Center for Health Services Research and Development. I appreciate the assistance of Carol Tortorice who helped with the thankless task of bringing the footnotes into a standard form and with proofreading.

DAVID MECHANIC

Madison, Wisconsin
March 1972

Contents

PUBLIC EXPECTATIONS

AND HEALTH CARE

Introduction

Everyone seems to think he knows what is wrong with health care in America. Books and articles abound diagnosing the ills of the delivery of medical care, documenting the many failures to meet health needs of the poor and others, and commenting on the continuing escalation of hospital and other medical care costs. The proposed solutions that are presently in vogue are hardly original. They have been advocated for almost a half century by a small minority of persons working in the medical care field. In reading this literature, the tremendous disparity between the seemingly plausible reforms that are persistently advocated and the realities of health organization in the United States is striking.

The inconsistency between what so many people believe to be sensible and the realities produces some strain for interpretation. In seeking to explain the contradiction, some commentators argue that the failures to respond to need are the result of special interests, professional arrogance, the power of professional guilds such as the American Medical Association which serves to protect the economic interests of doctors, and prestige-seeking and empire-building. Others argue that the fault lies in poor management, rapidly changing knowledge, and the lack of appropriate incentives. The fact that all of these factors are elements in the organization of health care is indisputable; the view that they serve as an adequate explanation of the existing structure and resistance to change is dubious.

The discussion that follows is not an attempt to provide a panacea for all of our problems in the health field, although various suggestions and alternatives will be offered as the discussion develops. The major purpose of these essays is to examine the perspectives of various actors in the health sector and to explore the major issues and dilemmas from their varied orientations. Although we shall give greatest emphasis to the benefits that one or another alternative provides for the public, what is really in the public interest is not self-evident. Inevitably, resources for health, like in any other area, will be limited, and it is impossible to provide the best of worlds for all. Compromises are thus inevitable, and the proper allocations may look different from varying perspectives. It is anticipated that

1

a careful examination of conflicting perspectives as they come to terms with various issues will provide a better basis for understanding dilemmas underlying the future organization of health care and will promote more realistic and responsive reforms than are now evident.

Goal Setting in the Organization of Health Practice

It is useful to begin with a provisional statement—however inadequate —of what people appear to expect from the health care system. Such general statements are always oversimplifications, since people have differing wants, expectations, and varying social and cultural orientations. But various studies suggest that the vast majority of people have rather common notions of how they should relate to medical services. They seek to have a personal physician or a comparable source of care that is readily accessible to them and convenient to use. They want and expect their care to be competent, but they are equally concerned that those who provide it have an interest in them as people. They expect also that an adequate system of more specialized services will exist, if they should need them, and that they can obtain these services at a price that does not threaten them economically. Implicit in a system of meeting such expectations are adequate manpower and facilities properly distributed— not only socially and geographically but also in terms of various medical and other health functions—and fitted in some reasonable way to the needs of people. Similarly, such care must be structured so that it is reasonably accessible to those who are worried, ill, or otherwise in need, and sufficiently interconnected with other services so that continuity and comprehensiveness can be achieved. The best way of providing such services for the entire population at a reasonable level within realistic economic limits is the most basic issue confronting all health care systems.

Although the preceding statement provides some guidance, it contains a variety of undefined concepts: competent care, adequate manpower, proper distribution, needs of people, comprehensiveness, and the like. Although all of these words mean something to us, they mean very different things to various people; and at some point they will require translation in more specific terms. We must face the fact that there are widely varying definitions of concepts of need and competence, and that much of medical care is characterized by ambiguous guidelines and uncertain outcomes. Even though there are particular medical procedures for which there is wide agreement on the proper course to follow, much activity in the health field and the management of many of the most common diseases are characterized by considerable imprecision and disagreement.

A dramatic example challenging conventional medical wisdom was recently published in the *British Medical Journal* by Mather and his associates[1] who carried out a carefully controlled investigation in which 343 men, with episodes of acute myocardial infarction, were randomly allocated to either home care by a family doctor or hospital treatment (initially in an intensive care unit). Similar mortality experience was observed in the two contexts. Patients with a hypotensive history fared somewhat better in home treatment. This study, carried out in four British communities, provides support for the position that home care is reasonable for some patients with acute myocardial infarction and raises serious questions as to whether the vast investments in intensive coronary care units evident in the United States is the wisest way to allocate limited resources. Although this study requires replication in varying contexts, it dramatically illustrates how major resource allocations in health care rest more on convention and belief than on evidence of their social utility.

Generally, there are no clear guideposts to suggest where people with varying illnesses should be treated, how long—if hospitalized—they should spend there, or what their regimen should be. Each clinician makes judgments on the basis of his acquired knowledge, the resources available to him and the patient, and his assessment of aspects of the individual case. Whether these judgments are wise or wasteful is sometimes impossible to determine and frequently difficult to assess even under the best of circumstances. Physicians and medical scientists can define the components of quality care more precisely than they have thus far, and studies of the kind described above are of the highest priority. But we should be under no illusions. Health care is a highly intangible product, and even the most sophisticated efforts at specifying quality will have to leave much of the total effort undefined.

Recognizing the complexities of medical care and its uncertain outcome should in no sense detract from its importance to the community. The underlying basis of a society is its symbolic understandings, and these are often more persuasive than objective effects. Few of our social institutions —government, education, law and justice, the family, religion—exist because they demonstrate that they perform particular tasks well. They will continue to exist as long as men believe in them, since it is what men believe that defines social reality. If medical care is defined as vital to people's lives, and it is so defined, the magnitude of its importance is, at least partly, independent of its demonstrated effects on the maintenance of health and longevity or the control of disease. The fact that modern societies, however organized, devote such great resources to health attests to its social importance. The objective limitations of health care, however, should alert us to the probability that medicine as an institution is valued, in part, because it meets needs other than those necessarily defined as important by doctors and other providers.

Since resources are limited, we must make choices. Health care at some point must be weighed against other social preferences and commitments. Although most men value health in the abstract, the need to make choices between competing values leads varying persons and groups to allocate different importance to health investments. Choices must be made also within the health field. As one considers the various goals that health care can promote, it becomes clear that one set of goals may impede the efficient and effective implementation of other goals. In considering varying suggested criteria for the development of health delivery systems, it becomes evident that balancing them involves an extremely difficult calculus.

The problem of apportioning among priorities is more than a complex dialectic. Too frequently reform in the health field must develop in terms of administrative remedies. Administrative planning proceeds on a logic of how people will behave if they are rational, given one or another manipulation of the system. People, however, behave according to a psychological rationality which departs significantly from administrative concepts, and social policy frequently fails to influence behavior in the desired directions because people can adapt their behavior to administrative changes without significantly changing course. To structure health care or any human system on the basis of logical assumptions of how people will respond rather than inquiry as to how they do respond will lead to many serious errors. In Chapter IV we shall examine some suggested models for reform of health services and consider to what extent the assumptions made fit existing knowledge of how people behave.

It is instructive to consider briefly an example of the kinds of conflicts that arise in developing ideal targets for a health care system. It is common in medicine for doctors to believe that it is their responsibility to provide their patients with the best possible medical care they can offer, but inevitably this view has costs. For if doctors, facilities, and economic resources are limited—as they invariably are—some balance must be arrived at which weighs the value of enhancing services already provided against extending care to groups who, by any definition, are inadequately cared for. The conception of a wider and more efficient distribution— barring unlimited expansion of the resources devoted to medical care— implies some dilution of services for those using available manpower and facilities. When we consider the provision of goods and services other than medical care, it is obvious that in providing these to a mass population we compromise to some extent the highest standards of quality that would be possible if we limited the market more narrowly. In every area of social life we make compromises between ideals and possibilities realistic in economic and social terms. Victor Fuchs stated this idea nicely:

> The problem, as I see it, is that the physician's approach to medical care and health is dominated by what may be called a "technologic imperative." In other words, medical tradition emphasizes giving the best care that is technically possible; the only legitimate and explicitly recognized constraint is the state of the art. And it is more than just tradition. Medical-school training has the same emphasis as continuing education for physicians. All this sets medical care distinctly apart from most goods and services. Automobile makers do not, and are not expected to, produce the best car that engineering skills permit. They are expected to weigh potential improvement against potential cost. If they do not, they will soon be out of business. Moreover, the improvements must be those as perceived by the consumer—which may be very different from those perceived by the engineer. What is true of automobiles is true of housing, clothing, food and every other commodity.[2]

In contrast, it is not difficult to understand the unwillingness of medical schools to forego what Fuchs terms the "technologic imperative." The application of Fuchs' analysis refers to the present where decisions to move in one direction or another must be made in light of expected outcomes. Medical education, however, is ideally addressed to the future, and technical procedures that prove impractical at one point in time may become suitable at some later point. Thus most medical educators are reluctant to compromise the students' technical skills and standards because present circumstances of practice make the maintenance of such standards unreasonable investments on a mass scale.

It is not unreasonable, however, to expect medical schools to concern themselves not only with ideal standards of practice but also with the standards that are optimal under the real contingencies and constraints of community medicine. It is not at all clear that the highly expensive mode of approach to the patient that is taught is vastly superior to more modest alternatives, and some deviations from the "high standards" taught may free sufficient resources to provide services to many more people. But one set of "shortcuts" may have different consequences than another, and while some may lead to an occasional error of limited import, others may result in considerable harm. As the situation presently exists, each doctor, in reacting to the pressures of his practice, develops his own modes of handling them. It would seem more appropriate for medical education to concern itself with the types of strategies of medical practice reasonable under different conditions, so that the adaptations that inevitably occur have a more rational basis.

The establishment of priorities is more easily discussed than implemented. People are usually quite willing to specify what priorities others ought to maintain until such priorities involve some cost for themselves. Medical care involves a variety of interest groups that tend to view priorities from their own particular perspectives and interests, and it is enormously difficult to achieve a consensus. Groups are usually reluctant to yield rights and privileges that they have already exercised, and will resist significant restructuring unless it appears that there is something in it for them. New priorities, if they are to be anything but slogans, must introduce innovations and change in a fashion that does not threaten too many of the groups involved. In the following chapters I shall outline what I believe the major priorities of the system should be with the realization that it is much more difficult to implement change than to propose it.

Notes

1. Mather, H. G., N. G. Pearson, and K. L. Read (1971). "Acute Myocardial Infarction: Home and Hospital Treatment." *British Medical Journal,* 3:334–338.
2. Fuchs, V. (1968). "The Growing Demand for Medical Care." *New England Journal of Medicine,* **279**:190–195.

PART ONE

THE CONTEXT OF HEALTH CARE

CHAPTER I

Goals in Health Care

From the earliest times persons in distress have sought the aid of practitioners who offered the possibility of relief of pain and hope for recovery. Thus, healing as a social role is a product of man's dependency in times of trouble, and the healer—in offering sustenance and amelioration of distress to the sick—has proceeded on the basis of trial and error, religion, and magic. Medicine as a social role is not dependent on its scientific basis or its practical efficacy, but rather on its sustaining potentialities for people in distress. Throughout most of history healers, in pursuing their calling, have done much that in retrospect was harmful to the patient and often contributed to his early demise, but the significance of the healer lies not so much in what he did and what he accomplished in practice, but in his symbolic relationship to the distressed.

Modern medicine is a somewhat different enterprise. It relies heavily on a wide variety of basic scientific fields and continued empirical inquiry. It depends on an elaborate technology accompanied by a complex division of labor, continually growing specialization, and a highly developed educational system. It requires considerable financial and industrial input, a vast array of facilities and organizational forms, and a large manpower pool of varying skills and experience. It involves managerial problems of major proportions in bringing together, coordinating, and making effective the vast array of people and facilities that compose the health sector.

In considering the history of healing and the enormous changes that have occurred in the work of doctors and other health workers, it is instructive to inquire as to the purpose of the endeavor itself. All large systems develop a dynamic of their own, and they frequently evolve independently of clearly defined goals. The changing character of medical care is largely a response to growing scientific knowledge and developing medical technology, but these are not necessarily allied to the needs and

9

aspirations of the persons served. We can adapt blindly to technology wherever it leads, or we can attempt to make it responsive to social values and human need. To do the latter, however, requires a clear notion of what it is that we really value.

What, then, is the function of medical practice? Empirically, we can observe that at any given time in any population a certain proportion of the population suffers from a variety of symptoms and problems of functioning. Various surveys suggest that in any given month approximately 75 per cent of populations have symptoms that are sufficiently distressing to cause them to take some action with respect to them. From this population of persons with symptoms, some segment selects itself and seeks the help of a physician. This selection takes place, in part, on the basis of the degree to which the symptoms are painful, frightening, and disturbing to functioning and, in part, on the basis of other factors characteristic of the people involved, the social settings from which they come, and the characteristics of the health institutions that serve them. We know that many of the persons who seek help do not have "serious illness" by more conventional medical criteria, and others who do not seek help have conditions that doctors regard as requiring treatment.

In any case, some selection of patients presenting a variety of complaints comes into direct contact with doctors. These patients seek help mostly because they feel distress of some sort, and the complaint is the basis on which they justify or explain the request for help. Various studies of medical consultations show that a fair proportion of the patients have self-limited complaints, psychosocial or psychophysiological problems, or psychiatric difficulties. Others who present more mundane physical symptoms, when given an opportunity to "open up," make clear that their visits to the doctor were motivated by general anxieties or problems other than the ones presented on initial contact with the physician.

What, then, is the function of the physician and his proper stance as he relates to the various patients seeking his care? There is no clear or easy answer to this question, and empirically doctors behave in a variety of ways relative to the circumstances of the patient, the doctor's practice, and his attitudinal orientations. The doctor of first contact, whatever designation we give him, plays a variety of roles relative to the patients who seek his assistance. One of his major responsibilities is to identify the conditions that require specific treatment, and this kind of responsibility is particularly felt in cases where there are effective interventions and where the failure to intervene would be harmful to the patient. The doctor also must deal with the variety of less serious problems for which he can provide simple treatment or help to alleviate the patient's worry.

If the doctor is to function effectively, he must provide some support and encouragement for the many patients who consult him and who have no clearly serious physical problem, but who are anxious or disturbed about their condition or other circumstances in their lives.

However, most doctors of first contact are extremely busy and face difficulties in responding to the variety of expectations and demands made of them. To a large extent, their responses are conditioned by the pressures upon them, professional definitions of their work, and the character of the training and experience they have had in the past. Most doctors function in terms of the disease model, attempting to make clear diagnostic judgments of patients' complaints. The value of this model is clear; once the physician correctly identifies the problem underlying various complaints and attaches a name to it, he has various predictive information on which he can proceed. A diagnosis is basically a prediction; once it is made, it usually provides a point of reference for viewing the etiology of the problem, its likely course, useful treatment approaches, and probable outcome. The physician who diagnoses his patient's problem as appendicitis obviously proceeds differently than if he decides the patient has tuberculosis.

No matter how valuable the disease model is under many circumstances, its limitations in general practice result from the fact that many of the problems and complaints presented by patients do not readily fall fruitfully within this framework. To the extent that the primary physician relies almost exclusively on the application of this model to his patients' complaints, he will feel frustration in coping with many of them. If he overemphasizes the disease approach in dealing with his patients, he is likely to be unresponsive to many of their needs and worries. At the same time, there are many pressures to rely on the disease model because of its usefulness and relative clarity, the doctor's concern that he may fail to recognize a clear-cut disease condition and thus fail to provide adequate therapy to the patient, and his more general orientations which may involve the expectations of his medical colleagues, fear of a malpractice suit, and the like. The doctor knows that the failure to diagnose a treatable physical condition will bring greater disapproval from his colleagues than his failure to manage the patient whose symptoms fall into no clear-cut pattern. Thus, despite the doctor's realization that the disease model is often irrelevant to many of the concerns of his patients, he frequently feels that he must proceed in a manner that maximizes his opportunities for effectively screening treatable physical conditions.

Discussions of primary medical care involve much loose talk, and suggestions for change often fail to take into account the real social, moral, and medical dilemmas in which the physician finds himself. A good primary care physician has to sensitively balance a variety of functions that demand somewhat different approaches, and he must make difficult decisions on how to weigh various risks. How should he weigh an untested but reasonable approach to a patient whom he believes to have tension headaches and to be overconcerned with her own complaints against the real possibility that the headaches are indicative of a "serious physical problem" that requires early treatment? To the extent that he pursues the diagnostic workup conscientiously he risks reinforcing what may turn out to be a "hypochondriacal pattern," while if he minimizes the medical workup he may miss a significant medical problem. The clinical qualities that allow doctors to pursue the appropriate course are not easily defined or taught.

Yet, medicine is an activity that has responsibilities beyond the recognition and treatment of clear-cut disease. Indeed, it is usually contended that medicine or health care must be oriented toward health maintenance. To understand the concept of maintaining health, we must be clear on the relevant dimensions of the concept. If we think of health as well-being in its largest sense, then it is clear that health is dependent on social values and social definitions, and that men are unlikely to agree on the priorities in weighing one dimension against another. Moreover, health in the sense of overall well-being is dependent on the quality of living and the environment generally, and any contribution from the medical sector will be relatively small in comparison to other factors amenable to political and social control. Thus, while overall well-being is a goal and an aspiration for doctors to have in mind, the realities of their intervention potential do not make this a very useful concept on which to devise strategies of care.

An ambitious but somewhat more modest concept of health is concerned with the ability of the patient to function without undue suffering or limitation of function. This concept incorporates not only the absence of disease but the more positive view that it is necessary for the doctor to be concerned with the ability of the patient to perform his social roles —at work, in the family, and in the community. It also makes clear that it is the physician's responsibility to weigh his interventions in human problems not only in terms of the effects of his actions upon the body but also in terms of how his treatment affects the ability of the patient to retain his function in the community. Stated more concretely, the doctor must be aware that the drugs he uses, the diagnostic labels he applies, and the alternative treatments he adopts have a differential impact on the patient's ability to perform his job, to maintain his status in the family, and to obtain satisfaction from his life. In choosing therapeutic interventions he must balance the risks and gains of the medical value of one treatment or another against its social value for the patient and his family.

Thinking of the general problem in paradigm form, we can visualize two general dimensions that bring people to seek help from physicians: human suffering and problems in functioning.

| | *Suffering* | |
	Yes	No
Yes *Functioning*	1 "Sufferers"	2 Healthy
No	3 Clear-cut Sick	4 Other— Defined Problems

These are highly complicated and multifaceted dimensions, and the paradigm is, of course, a vast oversimplification. But nevertheless it is useful in defining a number of relevant issues. In Cell 1 are the patients who manifest no clear-cut evidence of either physical illness or social disruption, but who experience pain, anxiety, dissatisfaction. These patients are self-referred and are often extremely frustrating for the average physician. They constitute a large proportion of the patients treated in psychotherapy and outpatient psychiatry, but these treated groups are only a small proportion of the total number of patients with such complaints. Most bring their problems to physicians who frequently are unprepared to deal with them. Cell 2 contains the patients who fall within the normal range on both functioning and feelings of well-being. They do not feel sufficiently troubled to seek help, and their behavior is not sufficiently disturbing to others to cause them to insist that these patients get care except perhaps for preventive and routine services. Cell 3 includes the more conventional concept of the patient who has complaints, and on examination a clear basis for the complaint is evident. Cell 4 includes patients who do not report great distress but who perform in such a way that others in their family or community identify them as having difficulties. Cell 4 might also include patients who feel well but are found, on screening examinations, to have illness conditions requiring intervention.

The categories have been very broadly described so that they pertain to psychiatric as well as nonpsychiatric problems and social functioning as well as bodily functioning. In defining the dimensions, however, I have not specified who it is that defines them, and it should be clear that there may be various definers applying different criteria and having different motives. Suffering, for example, is experienced and reacted to differently by persons in varying social groups and, thus, individuals who seek help for their suffering are not necessarily those in the population who are most disturbed or pained. Similarly, definitions of social functioning depend on the application of varying norms that may differ by age, sex, and social circumstances.

The multiplicity and complexity of definitions of functioning—and the extent to which they may vary from one person, group, or social setting to another—make tremendous demands for judgment and sensitivity on the physician. He must not only apply increasingly complex concepts of disease and intervention, and show awareness of the patient's psychological and social functioning, but he must be able to apply such concepts in terms of norms characterizing the individual patient's functioning and background. This involves knowledge of and familiarity with the patient that is extremely difficult to sustain, in view of the current demands on the doctor and the existing organization of medical practice. To complicate matters further, the doctor performs a variety of social and organizational functions that go beyond the ordinary care of the patient, but that serve other needs such as employment and disability certification, insurance appraisal, and the like.

Illness remains one of the few legitimate justifications for reducing role activities and absolving oneself from ordinary social responsibilities. Patients, therefore, naturally come to use illness as a way of explaining difficulties they encounter and in seeking to reduce social pressures that they face. Given the context in which illness comes to be viewed, medical consultations become a means of coping with human dilemmas and, similarly, the physician can be used as an instrument by society to attempt to contain the extent to which patients gain release from social responsibilities. It is in this context that the organizational auspices of medical care take on some significance, since definitions of health are sufficiently pliable that they may be used to enforce conformity or to encourage escape. Thus physicians with similar technical training can serve the patient and defend his interests against the society or can defend organizational interests that may be in opposition to the patient. In the ordinary course of events, doctors may find that they face pressures from both spheres and may develop in some way their own resolution of such pressures. The doctor, under present forms of organization, is sufficiently autonomous so that he has considerable latitude to form his own idea of his role and to determine for whom he is an agent. These matters are neither trivial nor theoretical, for as medicine develops a more organized form—and this is inevitable—conflicts between patients and other agencies will become more sharply defined, and resolutions of conflicting interests will become more difficult. This is most apparent at present in the area of financial controls where third parties, in attempting to control costs, are suggesting various mechanisms that will make it personally costly for physicians to use public resources for their patients. These mechanisms are motivated by a desire to develop incentives to avoid inefficiencies and unnecessary use of expensive services, but they do have potential for making the physician's interest compete against the patient's. Today, many analysts believe that existing incentives encourage both physicians and patients to waste expensive facilities and resources at public expense, since there are few economic incentives to avoid such waste.

Thus far, I have discussed primarily the doctor of first contact, and I have focused mainly on the patient with an acute complaint. An adequate health care system involves a variety of other facilities not only for the acute patient requiring more complicated diagnosis and care but also for patients with chronic disorders and patients with handicaps such as the blind, the crippled, and the mentally retarded. Similarly we must deal with the components of the health care system that are oriented to preventing illness and to maintaining community health as well as those geared to providing services to the sick and the disabled.

Well-organized primary health care units, staffed by physicians assisted by other health workers, can handle the vast majority of all health problems, but a relatively limited proportion of all patients will require more complicated and intensive services that demand more comprehensive facilities. On the basis of general surveys, in any given month approximately 9 persons in 1000 use some hospital care. This level of use may reflect the manner in which services are organized in contrast to "real need," but it is nevertheless true that an effectively organized health system must have sufficient hospital beds to meet the existing need, however defined, and the hospital must be organized to provide a wide array of services involving a spectrum of medical expertise and technical and ancillary assistance. Such services may vary from simple obstetrics to complicated care for patients with serious chronic illness involving specialized technical facilities and personnel. To effectively organize hospital services, priorities must be balanced so as to deal with varying needs for staffing, proper allocation of beds and space, and the like. Ideally, the organization of the hospital should be based on some reasonable prediction of the prevalence of varying kinds of needs in the community the hospital serves, and the staff should be distributed in some reasonable relationship to demand. The actual variations in the availability of hospital beds and supporting services from one community to another suggest how difficult it is to establish realistic guidelines. The availability of hospitals and physicians generates demand, and the criteria for specifying the appropriate mix of facilities and manpower are somewhat arbitrary. Providers of medical care tend to generate work in relation to their own priorities. This is facilitated by the fact that most of the major decisions concerning necessary medical care are made by providers of care rather than by consumers. In short, the types of medical work performed do not flow naturally from the prevalence of patients' needs but also reflect the way medical activities are organized.

Some illnesses require facilities and forms of organization that the usual hospital is ill-suited to provide at reasonable cost. There is a variety of alternatives that can meet certain needs more effectively than either outpatient care or the usual intensity of hospital inpatient care. These facilities might include minimal nursing units, nursing homes, rehabilitation units, home care services, and the like. An effective system grades the level of service to the level of need, and the specialized expertise of the health worker to the complexity of the task at hand. Our system of medical care has not been particularly successful in organizing around such considerations, and there are many organizational and legal barriers to developing a wide spectrum of services.

Health systems, like any other large-scale institutions, must face certain organizational dilemmas. If the system is organized optimally to take advantage of gains in scientific knowledge and technology, then it will become increasingly specialized and elaborated. We have suggested that both facilities and personnel be graded to the ordinary level of the tasks they perform, and that specialized services and facilities are necessary to deal with specific problems that patients may have. But such elaboration itself and the process of accommodating and responding to changing knowledge and technology bring about new problems in organizing and coordinating the various specialized services and facilities that are most optimal in dealing with specific tasks. Unless such coordination can be effectively organized, the system—which is now more sensitive to breakdowns and disruptions—may perform at a lower level of service than if it were less specialized. For the units of service are people and not tasks, and if the needs of people are forgotten in performing tasks, the outcomes may be poor despite high levels of technical efficiency and performance.

Coordination is probably the most profound problem in the organization of health services, particularly within a system of services like our own, which has no central direction. It is often easier to develop expertise in a specialized task, however complicated, than it is to coordinate in a meaningful way a wide variety of units and personnel under varying management, in different locations, and with diverse perspectives. Indeed, there is a point where the problem of coordination may become so great that it is more effective to sacrifice technical efficiency and competence than to further elaborate the distribution of tasks and facilities. One cannot continue to elaborate organizational tasks without trading off other values, and how far one is willing to go will depend on how priorities are established and on the relative emphasis given to varying facets of the medical task.

Most people in the health field agree that difficult tasks should be done by persons best trained to perform them, but knowing the patient in detail and continuity of care are similarly important. However, these are to some extent competing values in that continuity of care is best assured when a small number of people provides care to a patient over time, but highest technical performance is achieved with a highly specialized division of labor and an elaborate referral system. Both values cannot be simultaneously optimized, and some decision must be made concerning their relative priorities.

The provision of health care must be seen as functioning through time and cannot be evaluated solely in terms of performance at specific points. For health care systems must balance short-term and long-range goals, and these too may be competing. It has become fashionable in certain circles to be extremely critical of research and medical education, and some observers have maintained that these functions have debased patient care. Commentators often complain that tasks are performed by medical students and interns rather than by better trained personnel, and that patients are used as guinea pigs for medical education. It is probably true that the patient will be more comfortable if his care is confined to fewer participants, and that the needs of medical education not infrequently inconvenience patients. But the quality of future doctors will depend on the assumption of responsibility during training, and thus a medical system that shelters its patients from health personnel in training must pay some price in later generations. Although medical education must be structured so as to deal with patients responsibly and with consideration, health personnel to be effective must learn through the gradual assumption of responsibility. Since all patients benefit from good medical education, all patients should be equally available for such training. Medical schools, too frequently, have maintained a double standard in their teaching hospitals where the poor have served as their "learning material" and those well-off have gained many of the benefits.

A similar situation exists in the research area. Health institutions must not only attempt to optimize the results of existing knowledge but must also continue to develop innovations in care and new and more effective forms of intervention. Medical interventions are relatively limited, and it is necessary to balance efforts to do what we can with those already available against using our resources to increase the future potentialities of medical care. The allocations between research and other aspects of health or between different fields of research may not always be balanced, but global criticism of research efforts hardly directs itself to this type of problem. The subjects of research often do not benefit directly from their participation just as the blood donor may receive no future return from his benevolence. But as Titmuss[1] has so nicely argued, such gift giving serves society in a major way and, in addition, many persons receive substantial gratification from helping others. Optimizing such benevolence is constructive not only for medical care but also for society as a whole. At times, some medical researchers have failed in their responsibilities and have seriously violated the doctrine of informed consent; but it is both shortsighted and destructive to confuse individual abuses that can be corrected with the overall value and contribution of research.

Some Specific Goals in Delivering Health Care Services

I have already suggested the importance of a well-organized primary health service, adequate hospital facilities, a coordinated system for providing more specialized services than those most frequently provided in hospitals, and other preventive and rehabilitation services. Now, let me state more specific priorities from the point of view of the consuming public, quite independently from those that may be endorsed by providers or those that are seen as optimizing certain professional and technical interests. Later I shall discuss the problems and conflicts in implementing such priorities and the kinds of resistances to change that can be anticipated. Here the intention is to state goals quite independently of the political realities or estimation of the strength of various interest groups.

The highest priority, in my judgment, is a commitment to provide a minimal standard of health care to all Americans who require such care regardless of their ability to pay or their geographic location. Implicit in implementing this priority is a program to distribute manpower and facilities so as to insure that those in need have accessible services and can receive assistance. It is also implicit that health care, at least at the levels indicated, should be organized so as to eliminate other barriers to access, as well as economic ones, which are within the control of health service delivery systems such as location, modes of functioning, and attitude toward patients. These barriers are not always easy to define but involve the kinds of care that are humiliating and offensive to people and that retard their ability or desire to benefit from it.

The most difficult concept to define in the above statement is the notion of benefit. Benefits can be objective or subjective and conceivably can include any aspect of the health endeavor. In the economy, in general, benefits are frequently defined by the willingness of a consumer to expend his resources for one rather than another product in terms of perceived value and price. Health care usually deviates from this model in that the consumer finds it difficult or impossible to measure when he needs a service, the quality and characteristics of the service he is acquiring, its likely impact, or even its cost. For the most part, medical practice in the United States is organized so that it is the professional rather than the patient who makes most decisions on necessary action, and the patient frequently has no concept of the price until the service is already rendered. The usual economic model based on market decisions might have some applicability to medical care under certain theoretical conditions, but medical care is characterized by professional monopolies, severe restrictions on the flow of information and competition, and regulation of supply and the conditions of provision. These circumstances have developed under the aegis of protecting the consumer, which they do in part, but they even more powerfully protect the interests of the provider and make it virtually impossible for the consumer to make an informed choice even if this was deemed desirable.

If the market is not a satisfactory mechanism for determining the nature of benefits to the consumer, either because it is assumed that consumers cannot make such weighty decisions on technical issues or because providers will vigorously protect their autonomy and control and thus infringe on the conditions necessary to make intelligent consumer choice possible, then other means must be developed for defining what constitutes reasonable benefits. One means would involve defining a minimum floor of services to which all persons would be insured access because of their centrality to health maintenance. Within this definition I include ready access to primary health services which relieve worry and promote peace of mind, and which provide a potential for preventive practice, treatment of many existing conditions, and screening for necessary referral and further treatment. Such primary services are relatively inexpensive in comparison to other more specialized services and could be provided to all without straining existing resources. The price of primary care, as it is presently organized in the United States, is inflated by the organization of medical care and the values and priorities emphasized by physicians. The cost of making the physician or health team accessible is small compared to the costs generated by the physician's decisions once the patient has entered the health care system. Beyond primary health care services, I believe that it is necessary to review all facets of medical work in terms of known efficacy, and to insure coverage to all for medical work judged efficacious in limiting disease, disability, or defect, or in primary prevention. Implicit in this statement is my firm belief that much of medical care, which has been sanctified because it is performed by physicians, is of limited import and dangerous as well, and that it is necessary to promote more serious evaluation which separates the worthy and the worthless in medical work more clearly than at present. Medicine, of course, can never be a fully exact science, and it is necessary to leave room for experimentation and innovation. Thus I approve of relatively liberal notions of medical worth and there is not much chance, in any case, of very strict limitations. But it cannot be contested that much publicly supported and subsidized medical work is of little benefit to the consumer. Although there are numerous examples (some will be given later), I emphasize here the need for a national or even an international effort to ferret out diagnostic and therapeutic practices that clearly do not contribute to human welfare and those that, on the whole, do more harm than good. Although biomedical and clinical medical research is highly developed, practicing doctors have been exceedingly reluctant to examine their own work.

Let me illustrate the point. It is increasingly clear that prenatal and postnatal care of pregnant women and their newborn children can, under some circumstances, prevent prematurity, birth defects, infant death, mental retardation, brain damage, and a variety of other problems that take a great toll of human suffering and involve great costs to society. The continuing failure to provide these services to many high-risk women —services that are relatively inexpensive to deliver—has a great impact on society and on individuals. In contrast, the failure to provide tonsillectomies (a more expensive service performed at the rate in excess of 600 per 100,000 in 1965),* except under very specialized circumstances, is likely to contribute generally to the health and welfare of children, since there is clear-cut evidence that medical harm resulting from this procedure exceeds its benefits. The number of such procedures performed is better explained by the high prevalence of surgeons relative to needed surgical work and by existing forms of reimbursement than by the con-

* A recent report based on the *Hospital Discharge Survey of the National Center for Health Statistics* notes that tonsillectomy was the single most frequently reported operation for inpatients discharged in 1965, followed by repair of inguinal hernia and hysterectomy. The rates of discharges per 100,000 population for males were 636 for tonsillectomy and 507 for inguinal hernia; females had a rate of 641 for tonsillectomy, 52 for inguinal hernia, and 517 for hysterectomy. Tonsillectomy is the most important of all causes of hospitalization of children, despite its dubious value. See National Center for Health Statistics, April, 1971, *Surgical Operations in Short-Stay Hospitals for Discharged Patients: United States-1965*. PHS Series 13, No. 7. Washington: U. S. Government Printing Office.

ditions necessary to maintain the health of children.* A prudent social policy would attempt to significantly reduce the number of tonsillectomies rather than to provide blanket government payments that include incentives for increasing the prevalence of this procedure.

The difficulties of ferreting out the worthless procedures that doctors and other health professionals perform as part of their overall efforts should not be underestimated. I emphasize, however, that such a task is justified—indeed, it is mandatory—in a society that invests more than $75 billion a year in health services and devotes in excess of 7 per cent of its gross national product to health care. I am not advocating that nonphysicians interfere in medical practice. I share the view of many others that health care is too important to be left to doctors alone, and that the public has both the right and responsibility to promote its priorities in determining the structure of health services. But in the realm of determinations of medical efficacy, such judgments must be made by scientifically qualified physicians and other medical scientists who represent the highest levels of competence available. Individual doctors are not qualified by their training, skills, or vantage point to be the final arbiters on scientific questions concerning the efficacy of various therapeutic interventions and forms of management, and the pitfalls and failures of the clinical perspective in making such determinations in contrast to carefully designed studies are well known. But there is little doubt that physicians constitute a large segment of the persons who are most prepared and qualified to make these kinds of judgments.

In considering how benefit will be defined, priorities must be ordered in terms of the functioning of the whole man. A medical technique that successfully fulfills a very limited medical function but results in the social incapacitation of the patient is of questionable benefit. There have been occasions when physicians have confused technical success with human benefit, and therefore I believe that benefits must be conceptualized in terms of reducing suffering, limiting disability, and enhancing the individual's ability to fulfill his goals. I am not oblivious to the human and moral dilemmas implicit in such judgments, but in an arena of scarce resources I cannot understand how one can justify actions like those that keep the hopeless alive for a few more days while patients with more hope die because of the unavailability of health care services. These matters obviously must be considered with the greatest care and seriousness, and with humility; but we deceive ourselves if we believe

---

* There has been growing evidence that general surgeons are having difficulty in keeping sufficiently busy (See E. Hughes, V. Fuchs, J. Jacoby, and E. Lewit, 1972, "Surgical Work Loads in a Community Practice." *Surgery,* **71:**315–327).

that the failure to face these issues resolves them. The failure to make decisions is a form of decision, and it has consequences that may be far more damaging than even uncertain choices. Broad demarcations can be established in developing priorities and directions for investing our resources, and it is remarkable how little serious concern the health sector has given, until recently, to either the implications of its performance, its effectiveness, or its total impact on the health and welfare of the population.

Another major priority is that the system of care should be so organized that the response to various needs for service will be coordinated and that reasonable continuity will be provided for the patient among various services provided at any point in time as well as through time.[2] It is implicit in this statement that each patient has a sponsor, whether his care is provided by an individual physician, a clinic, a health center, or a hospital. The sponsor would know the patient, his history, and his needs, and would be responsible for the proper management and coordination of care rendered to that patient from whatever source. One of the greatest failures of the present system of care for many Americans is its episodic nature, its lack of coordination and continuity, and its segmentation. High quality care that makes use of advances in knowledge and technology will require a division of functions and specialized services, but it, in no sense, will relieve health care units of responsibility for bringing these together in some meaningful way for successful management of the patient's problems. Whether these functions are best performed by a physician or some other type of health worker is subject to debate, and it is likely that varied patterns of response will evolve to deal with these needs. Later, I shall discuss the relative merits of physicians or other health workers performing such functions.

Assuming that a reasonable level of care is accessible at both primary care levels and in hospitals, and that associated with these are various intermediate care facilities and rehabilitation services, then another important priority is to provide services reasonably fitted not only to more traditional medical needs but also to the variety of medically relevant pathologies that persons have that affect their vitality and functioning. Since many types of human problems are presented within the context of medical care, it is reasonable to use health facilities as a location to focus and coordinate a variety of human services. Associated with this concern is the pressing need to better train primary physicians to deal with depression, anxiety, and varying types of social disabilities. Despite much lip service to the mental health area, a great separation persists between the provision of primary medical care and the delivery of mental health services. Although a great deal of attention has been devoted to discussions of prepaid group practice and to notions of comprehensive care, the psychiatric component has been badly neglected. The danger exists that, despite an emphasis on comprehensive care, the integration of more general medical and mental health services may be no more advanced than in the existing situation. This would be an unfortunate failure, indeed.

In sum, patients desire reasonable access to health services and competence and interest in them from physicians and other health workers. They want such services at a price they can afford and with protection against the risk that a serious episode of illness or disability, or a chronic condition requiring continuing care, will not undermine their economic viability. These are not unreasonable expectations, and the inability of our health care system to meet them—despite vast infusions of funds from the federal government—requires detailed examination and analysis. For, despite large public investments in health care and high competence among health workers and a high level of technology, all is not well in American medical care. This book examines the reasons why the vast health sector has been unresponsive to particular social needs and expectations. It also considers the alternatives that might be available to shift persistent trends in the health field, which threaten an even more profound crisis in the future than already exists.

Notes

1. Titmuss, R. (1971). *The Gift Relationship: From Human Blood to Social Policy.* New York: Pantheon.
2. Brook, R. H., F. A. Appel, C. Avery, M. Orman, and R. L. Stevenson (1971). "Effectiveness of Inpatient Follow-up Care." *New England Journal of Medicine,* 285:1509–1514.

CHAPTER II

Physicians, Hospitals, and the
Health Care System: An Overview

It is not easy to sketch out the broad outline of the health care system in the United States. The health sector is extremely large, complex, and varied; and there are few studies that provide broad descriptive information on even one locality, much less the vast range of variations in different geographic areas. Thus the sketch offered here is a preliminary one. It is intended to provide a context within which major issues may be viewed, instead of a comprehensive view that describes the system in any detailed way.

The three major components of the health services system are manpower, facilities, and technologies. About 3.5 million people work in the health sector, encompassing a wide range of skill levels and competence. Although the most attention is given to physicians and nurses, they are only a minority of all health workers and, in recent decades, there has been a great proliferation of new technical jobs relevant to the delivery of health services. The vast majority of such positions are based in hospitals where the components of medical care technology are best organized and integrated, but an increasing number of health workers are also found in other community contexts. The organization of manpower in the health field involves such issues as the forms of organization of health workers, their selection, training, and career structures, licensure and responsibilities relative to other health occupations, and, most important, how an optimal allocation and use of such manpower can be achieved and how barriers to more rational forms of organization of the health labor pool can be overcome.

Facilities refer to all physical locations in which patients are treated or which provide ancillary assistance or support in their treatment. The most basic facility, of course, is the hospital; but also included within this concept are physicians' premises, research and clinical laboratories, nursing and convalescent homes, locations for the training of health manpower, and the like. Among the issues relevant to a consideration of facilities are the kinds of facilities necessary for different levels of service, forms of financing, and how facilities are best organized in relation to one another, and under what auspices.

The concept of technology—perhaps the most difficult and most important of the three components—refers to any set of operations that is believed to be instrumental in the recognition, treatment, or prevention of disease or disability. These operations may be encompassed within a set of technical facilities such as computers, laboratory tests, diagnostic instruments, or drugs. But technologies also include physical, psychological, and social theories that direct the approach of health workers toward their clients. Technologies thus include such varied operations as x-ray, prescription of insulin, psychotherapy, the social organization of the hospital ward, and so on. In considering technology we shall examine the way that approaches to recognition of disease, treatment and rehabilitation have developed and changed over time, the forces affecting such evolution, the social and medical impact of changes, and the alternative structures developed to organize and make use of new technologies. Here we shall be concerned not only with the objective consequences of changes in technology but also with belief systems and values and their effect on how facilities and manpower come to be organized and applied.

The health care sector, of course, is not a tight little island; it is closely interwoven with other aspects of the economy and social life, and these relationships must be grasped to appreciate the whole picture. A fantastic array of federal, state, and local legislation affects the financing, operation, and further development of health facilities and manpower. The health sphere also depends on the industrial sector for drugs, equipment, and a host of other products necessary to carry out its work. It relies on universities and vocational schools to prepare the large numbers of health workers and for much of the research that leads to further development of knowledge and technology. It depends on a variety of fiscal intermediaries to administer the range of insurance programs through which various facets of health needs are covered for different segments of the population. It requires not only personnel to provide services but considerable managerial skills to administer the complex development and operation of facilities, programs, and forms of insurance. Almost every major aspect of our society impinges, in one way or another, on the organization and workings of the health care system.

The Context of Health Care in America

Economic factors profoundly affect the organization and functioning of health services systems. It is impossible to understand American health care, or that in any other country, outside the context of the socioeconomic system and how it functions. The variations in American health care are enhanced by the fact that there is a large number of decision points where major directions are determined. Power in the health care system is highly decentralized, and the development and expansion of health facilities, the establishment of new medical practices, the evolution of particular technical services and most other matters are the product of thousands of individual decisions made by physicians, government groups, universities, industrial firms, hospital boards, and the like. This does not mean that government units, which now contribute about 40 per cent of all health care expenditures, do not attempt to direct in various ways the manner in which the system evolves, but even these programs do not have any consistent underlying policies, since they are distributed among multiple agencies with different functions, goals, and orientations. Moreover, their technique has been the carrot and not the stick, and even if they attempted to produce change more forcefully, the outcome would in no sense be predetermined. For the various interest groups in health care are active in the political arena, producing a forceful and influential form of feedback to governmental units. Governmental policy in health clearly encompasses contradictions that reflect the many interest groups that come to influence it.

It is evident that a large part of the health sector is organized around the concept of profit. Although this does not technically apply to nonprofit voluntary hospitals, it applies to most other providers such as physician groups, nursing homes, medical-industrial product firms, pharmaceutical houses, and proprietary hospitals. Many of the nonprofit forms of organization are also profit-oriented in that they frequently engage in aggressive investment policies that increase their capital holdings. The issue, of course, is not whether profits exist, and to what extent, but the consequences of profit-oriented motives on the workings of the system. Here we are confronted basically with a repetition of all of the arguments and counterarguments heard in many other sectors of the economy. Persons who seek government control argue that the profit motive debases the system, distorts priorities, leads to exploitation of the poor and the powerless, and encourages unnecessary proliferation of technology and resources. Persons supporting the existing system, and some who feel that the profit-orientation should be developed even further in health care affairs, argue that the profit motive and competition lead to efficiency, more incentive to provide attractive services, more active research and development, effort and incentive on the part of health personnel, and responsiveness to the consumer. Some of these advocates have argued that the failures in American medical care, and particularly in the hospitals, are the product of a lack of incentive for efficiency produced by the non-profit status of hospitals. They maintain that reimbursement, which makes payments to hospitals on the basis of their costs, produces no incentives for efficiency, the establishment of priorities, or careful expenditure patterns.

It is not particularly productive to frontally attack the question of the role of profits in health affairs, for it is a morass from which extrication is impossible and one where polemics rule; and we can be no more successful than those who have debated this issue in other areas. It is more productive, in my opinion, to describe how the health system operates and its major problems, thus examining how profit motivation (or the lack of it) has consequences of one sort or another from area to area. I think that there are some spheres where profit motivation is a significant barrier to meeting needs adequately, such as in the case of profit-run blood banks where blood is acquired and distributed without proper controls leading to high rates of hepatitis transmission; while in other spheres profits may produce necessary incentives or innovations. Moreover, it is useful to distinguish between the profit status of organizations and the motivation of its personnel and incentives affecting their behavior. Strong "profit orientations" frequently exist among personnel in non-profit organizations, and these organizations often follow remuneration practices that are substantially the same as those evident in the profit sector. Behavior occurs within particular value contexts; changing the character of incentives without also changing more fundamentally the basic value structures within which they are embedded may be a futile endeavor. The issue is not whether profits stimulate abuse and exploitative behavior, since they inevitably do; it is necessary, however, to weigh these abuses against anticipated gains that may result from profit incentives.[1,2]* Examining the matter in relation to specific issues is more fruitful than ideological discussion on a global level.

Clearly, the major health care decisions in the United States are determined through the political process and, more specifically, through the ability to influence the enactment and forms of administration of legislative mandates. As with other political decisions, the strength and or-

---

* For a contrary view, see Barbara and John Ehrenreich, 1970, *The American Health Empire: Power, Profits, and Politics*. New York: Random House.

ganization of particular interests become central, and those groups that have less relative power have considerably less influence on the outcome of political debate or the administrative process. As we consider the emerging power confrontations in the health sector, we find a considerable dispersion of political influence aligned around various major groups. The notion that any particular political group, like the AMA or the AFL-CIO, dominates health policy in the United States is not consistent with the history of recent social legislation in health; and as new interest groups such as senior citizens have emerged, the Congress has paid more attention to their needs and wishes. This does not imply that such groups as the AMA do not wield disproportionate influence because of their organization, financing, and access to important decision makers. Generally, the clash of strong interests in the political field do not lead to the domination of one or the other but, instead, to compromises that protect the major interests of varying groups. Thus, although organized medicine lost its battle to stop major legislation in the health field (such as Medicare and the Regional Medical Program) and is likely to lose more battles in the future, there is little doubt that the final character of the legislation that passed Congress and the development of administrative procedures took the objections of the AMA into account and provided protections for the major interests of its members. The current cost crisis in health care is partially the result of political policies that grant new benefits without attempting to force a redistribution within the health sector itself. Thus new money must be found from outside the health sector to support new programs. A more efficient approach is one in which priorities and the distribution of benefits would be reorganized significantly, but the political difficulties of bringing about this change are evident. Although interest groups can accept changes that may not be consistent with their best interests, they bitterly resent and fiercely fight the loss of privileges and rights that already exist. Thus the government tends to attack problems and needs by establishing new programs and bureaucracies alongside those that already exist, and although some shifts in funding and support may develop, they tend to occur in stages that do not dramatically challenge major interest groups.

In describing the perspectives of various groups, there is this final qualification: they do not necessarily seek their self-interest in a crass or selfish fashion. Although one can say from the outside that a particular group has adopted a political stance that promotes its own profits and comforts, it is frequently apparent that such persons sincerely believe that their motives are not selfish and that the policies they advocate are in the interests of the country. The system of health care is sufficiently complicated—and its products sufficiently intangible—that persons can hold contradictory viewpoints, each consistent with his own self-interest, yet each sincerely believing that his viewpoint is in the interest of the public good. While we should not underestimate man's capacities for self-deception, we should be aware that many of the desirable public policies in health care are not self-evident, and that there is considerable room for disagreement among honorable men. The fact that there are dishonorable men in the health sector requires no elaboration; the evidence of deception and fraud on the part of a small segment of providers within the Medicaid program attests to this.[3,4] Villains, however, are no more common in medicine than in other areas, and a problem we face is how to control this small minority, capable of destroying public programs by their greed and deceptions, without handicapping the optimal conditions for care among the vast majority of professionals who are basically honorable. Most people pursue self-interest in one way or another; we should try to separate the pursuits that fall within the bounds of reason from the pursuits that are clearly destructive to the public welfare. It is one thing to allow persons a decent reward for useful efforts; it is quite another to encourage or condone profit-making, which distorts the system of care and promotes activities that enrich the persons who perform them but not the persons who pay for them.

The Special Position of the Physician

Although physicians constitute less than 10 per cent of total health care manpower in the United States, they control and determine the basic organization of care. Physicians owe their position and power to the fact that they control not only the conditions of their own work but the conditions of work of most of the other health occupations as well. Most other health care personnel are clearly ancillary to the medical function, and in a clinical context they take orders from physicians.

It is difficult to understand the perspectives of physicians without considering the manner in which they are selected, educated, and initiated into the world of medical care. An understanding of this requires some appreciation of the development of medical education in the United States. In early America, physicians received their training largely through apprenticeship with another physician and very limited formal teaching. As medical schools developed during the 1800's, they varied substantially in their academic programs and the degree of scientific training they required. At the beginning of the present century, considerable competition developed between the American Medical Association, representing the interests of practicing physicians, and medical educators as to who would control medical education and, related to this, the output of physicians. In the first decade of this century Abraham Flexner, a nonphysician, was commissioned by the Carnegie Foundation to make a study of medical education. This study, using as a model of excellence the Johns Hopkins Medical School, attacked the structure of medical education as it existed, and encouraged a standard scientific curriculum for medical education involving anatomy, biochemistry, physiology, microbiology, pathology, and pharmacology in the first two years, and supervised clinical contact in the final two years. This training pattern, suggested by Flexner, was incorporated into many state laws governing the qualifications for licensure for medical practice. A consequence of the report and the attitudes crystallized by it was a reduction of medical schools from 162 in 1906 to 69 in 1944, with an associated decline in the number of medical graduates produced. Until very recently, students in medical schools, regardless of where they were educated, were initiated into medicine through a lock-step rigid curriculum that allowed little variation or experimentation in training. The development of licensure standards and accreditation procedures for medical schools, no doubt, increased the scientific training and qualifications of medical students, but it also encouraged a very limited view of the responsibilities and education of a physician and set the stage for the existing shortage of physicians in the United States. Although the contention is usually made that the major motivation for the changes in medical education and the imposition of strict licensure was to protect the consumer, Kessel[5] makes a strong case against this interpretation. He illustrates in detail that attempts to raise standards were made largely when better standards were in the interests of medical practitioners, but similar standards were neglected in other areas where the standards did not similarly serve their goals. Nevertheless, the objective consequences of the changes that followed the Flexner report were a more adequately scientifically trained practitioner, a more homogeneous product, a more limited conception of the physician's role, and a smaller output of physicians from American medical schools.

The conception of the physician's role as a scientist received considerable impetus following the Second World War when the National Institutes of Health were established and vast infusions of research funds to the medical schools occurred. This transfusion of funds allowed medical schools to recruit faculty, to develop laboratories, and to significantly increase their operations without major interference and opposition. Although it was clear by this time that serious problems existed in the organization and provision of medical care in the community relative to scientific developments and the expansion of technology, the medical schools were not anxious to come into conflict with the powerful interests of private medicine and the local medical societies by interfering in the community practice of medicine. They found that emphasis on the development of their technological and research capacities was a smoother course to follow with considerable support from the entire medical community and rich subsidy from the federal government.

As the gap between what was taught in medical schools and what constituted medical practice in the community widened, medical educators encouraged their students to specialize in smaller and smaller aspects of medical activity; and during this period there was a large growth in specialization and subspecialization within medicine itself. Although large proportions of students entered medical school with the intention of engaging in general practice upon graduation, relatively few of them retained this intention by the time they completed four years of medical school. Promising students were encouraged by medical school faculty to specialize, and the students themselves realized the difficulties of practicing at the level of their training if they entered the existing structure of medical activities in the community as general practitioners. Therefore, students oriented themselves toward specialty practice with the result that primary care physicians have become a smaller and smaller proportion of the total medical manpower pool.

Medical education also has had other important influences on the perspectives of developing physicians. Since the physician's education was focused on the work carried out within the teaching hospital and dealt with a highly selected population of patients that hardly represented the patients seen in a typical medical practice, he tended to develop modes of working that were far from optimal in handling ordinary patients. Hospital training placed great emphasis on a precise differential diagnosis, on the use of advanced technical aids, on exploring in detail remote possibilities, and on doing all that was technologically possible to manage the case in an optimal fashion. In emphasizing these values, insufficient attention was given to a scientific approach to behavioral factors affecting patient response, to the costs and benefits of adopting one or another technical procedure, to the proper and improper use of the hospital and its supporting facilities, and to the consequences of managing the patient in one way or another relative to family, work, and other social consequences. This approach to medical education had both purpose and value in training a scientifically oriented physician but it generally failed to teach the type of optimal management of the patient which weighs medical against psychological and social factors affecting outcomes. This failure was reflected in the fact that physicians learned to devote great effort and time to making an adequate diagnosis and prescribing a proper course of treatment but, in contrast, relatively little attention was given to understanding why such large proportions of patients failed to conform adequately to medical advice. In short, medical education was process-oriented rather than goal-oriented, and it failed to sufficiently alert the emerging physician to the larger social consequences of his decisions and actions for patients and society.

The hospital orientation involves learning to depend heavily on laboratory and other technical diagnostic facilities in contrast to greater reliance on the medical history, physical diagnosis, and clinical judgment. Good scientific medicine obviously depends on taking advantage of available technology. But too many doctors have developed a promiscuous approach to the hospital bed, the clinical laboratory, and a variety of gadgets, which frequently fails to take into account the cost-benefit outcomes of adopting various procedures.

Young physicians tend to learn that it is part of their medical responsibility to do all they can for their patient and, unlike most other areas of endeavor, doctors develop little consciousness of cost effectiveness. The orientation learned within the context of the teaching hospital, as noted in the previous chapter, is to depend on expensive diagnostic evaluation—whatever the problem—and this has lasting consequences for lack of economies in the work of physicians generally. There is a danger in commenting on this problem in too brief a fashion, for it is likely that the course encouraged by medical schools contributes something to the practice of a high level of scientific medicine, and such care is expensive. But the approach within the teaching hospital, where many patients tend to have serious and complicated medical conditions, is one thing; and the same approach practiced within the context of ordinary medical practice, where patients commonly bring their troubles, is quite another. We have already noted that a large proportion of the consultations characteristic of general medical practice involves psychological difficulties and self-limited complaints. Many of these cases require sympathetic and supportive management, and an alertness to the consequences of social stress, rather than a technical approach that subjects the patient to an array of diagnostic work but pays little attention to the major motives that brought him to a physician in the first place.

As doctors have become more specialized and have moved away in their orientations (if not in fact, from the more routine management of common difficulties), they not only use many more diagnostic aids but also tend to make greater use of the hospital for diagnostic and treatment purposes. The hospital has become a convenient and preferred workplace for the doctor to perform many of the diagnostic and treatment features of his role, and thus there is a strong tendency for physicians to readily hospitalize patients. Since insurance has covered a larger proportion of the inhospital costs of patient care, there has been little barrier to both physician and patient in using the hospital in this fashion and, indeed, in some cases the character of the insurance policy, which frequently pays for inpatient care but not for outpatient diagnostic procedures, provides a further incentive for working the patient up in this way. Furthermore, within the context of the hospital, physicians have shown little appreciation of or incentive to concern themselves with the tremendous costs resulting from their patterns of work. They have come to regard the manner in which they use the hospital as part of their professional prerogatives, and they resent interference from nonphysicians in such matters. Where beds are not scarce and hospitals have relatively high vacancy rates, the hospital also has little incentive to discourage an inefficient use of its facilities because its financial status depends partly on its ability to keep its beds occupied. Under these circumstances, hospitals become highly dependent on physicians; they want their facilities used in preference to possible alternative ones in the community. This dependence gives physicians considerable power vis-à-vis the hospital and creates pressures for the hospitals to accommodate to unreasonable physician demands. One of the most serious consequences of this power balance is the tendency for community hospitals to unnecessarily duplicate extremely expensive facilities and equipment, to keep on hand specialized personnel to operate such facilities, and generally to provide the tools of medical work that physicians insist on. The reason why physicians make such demands—the consequences of which may be unreasonable and inefficient—is a product of a variety of factors.

Because of the manner in which medicine is organized educationally and in terms of its practice, physicians are judged mainly in terms of their expert knowledge and technical abilities. Prestige is not gained from doing the mundane tasks that any doctor or an ancillary can perform, but from perfecting more specialized skills. Physicians, like other scientifically oriented professionals, develop such skills and acquire prestige by being on the forefront of new technical medical activities and by using the newest methods of practice. Surgeons, for example, want the hospital in which they do their work to have facilities for relatively rare and complicated procedures so that they, too, have an opportunity to engage in this type of practice, even if the duplication of these facilities is uneconomic and not particularly conducive to good care. Many physicians insist on such facilities, also, because they believe that if their hospital does not have specialized facilities that are available elsewhere in the community they may lose patients and possibly referrals as well. Patients do become aware, for example, that one hospital has a special coronary care unit, while another does not; and it is possible that some patients are influenced in their choices by these matters. More serious from the physician's point of view, however, is the referral of certain cases in his area of concern to other hospitals because they have specialized facilities not available to him. In cases of this kind, he comes to perceive an economic disadvantage and may put heavy pressure on his hospital to equip itself equally. Doctors may even threaten to take their patients elsewhere if the hospital does not make the desired facilities available. Hospitals tend to have relatively little counterpower under these circumstances unless a clear shortage of hospital beds exists in the community. Whether planning agencies can restrain such developments in the future, and whether hospitals can insulate themselves from unnecessary costs through mergers of various sorts, will depend importantly on the nature of the incentives developed by government programs.

It is now apparent that a key problem in the health field is the doctor's control over hospital affairs without financial or administrative responsibility to the institution itself. Physicians require the hospital to perform their work, and they control the decisions affecting the ultimate costs of medical care for the patient and the community, but they have no economic stake in controlling costs or expenditures. Indeed, the existing incentive is to build and expand, since this can only result in an improvement of their private economic interests. The result is well known—a growing escalation of the price of hospital care, needless elaboration and duplication of facilities, resistance to planning and control, and an enormous maldistribution of facilities relative to the needs of the community.

Obviously, there are many other factors affecting the costs of hospital care, and I do not suggest that the total trend is a product of physician behavior. As knowledge and technology have developed in the hospital field, so have the costs of providing the facilities and specialized personnel necessary to practice modern medicine. Labor costs constitute a large proportion of hospital expenditures, and increasingly organized labor is demanding better wages for the vast numbers of hospital employees who have been poorly paid over the years. Unquestionably, a large component of increases in the costs of medical care are inflationary and provide no comparable increment of new services. But one of the many relevant factors—perhaps most serious and also most remediable—has been the growing tendency of physicians to depend on the hospital as a workplace for the care of their patients, thus requiring the maintenance of more facilities and manpower to care for cases that could be handled more economically in other ways. The variations in the use of hospitals are enormous from one area to another, and it is reasonably clear that great economies are possible at this particular locus of the health care system.

Much of the emphasis in various proposals for new health legislation incorporates incentives for the physician not to depend so heavily on hospital facilities when they are not really necessary. The definition of what is necessary, however, is one that does not yield easy agreement.

Many of the problems evident in primary medical care are related to the issues we have already discussed relative to the hospital. Since medical training and the medical division of labor are based around the needs of the hospital, these come to affect the character of primary health care in the community. Physicians are trained to believe that they cannot practice medicine without a hospital close by, a variety of specialized facilities and personnel, and the various components of a highly specialized division of labor. Having been trained primarily within a hospital context, they have become unfitted to perform the more ordinary and mundane tasks that many patients need and want. Their dependence on specialized facilities, in conjunction with other factors, leads doctors to distribute themselves relative to such facilities leaving great gaps of untended areas in the inner core of cities and in rural areas. Their orientation to the hospital and the kinds of values emphasized there make them unwilling to carry on many of the very general functions of the physician, thus contributing to an impersonal and unresponsive orientation to care. Since a comprehensive pattern of care, under existing conditions, comes to depend on an array of referrals to doctors and facilities, the care of patients often lacks coordination and coherence, and patients are increasingly dissatisfied. Moreover, the nature of the division of labor itself, with its dependence on referrals, and the use of various specialized personnel, cause even the most simple of medical services to become extremely expensive.

There is a growing view that more organized group practices and health centers would have the capacity to provide a more effective and efficient pattern of medical care. Certainly such organized practices provide opportunities to take advantage of economies of scale in the use of facilities, equipment, and personnel. Although economies can be worked out in other ways without more organized groups, such practice appears to facilitate these potentialities. Group practice also can more effectively use and supervise specialized nonmedical personnel who take on various health tasks typically performed by doctors or nonmedical tasks that doctors who work by themselves often have to perform. In short, well-organized group practices, it is maintained, constitute a compromise between the supertechnology of the hospital, which is more than is needed in most cases, and the underdeveloped character of the existing pattern of medical care in solo or partnership practices.

Although group practice has certain assets, it also has certain potential disadvantages. Indeed, one of the major advantages believed to be associated with group practice, and which makes it popular with reformers, is the belief that it can be used as an instrument to limit the use of the hospital and the resulting costs of medical care. Incentives to limit use of the hospital need not necessarily be tied to group practice, and thus such potentialities do not really constitute a unique advantage. Also, a possible disadvantage of large group practices is that they can become bureaucratic and less personal than smaller units of care. There is reason to believe that salaried group practitioners are somewhat less responsive to their patients than private fee-for-service physicians, and that the efficient organization of such practices can stimulate bureaucratic barriers that undermine a sympathetic approach to the patient. Such problems are in no sense insurmountable but require organizational mechanisms that insure the quality of responsive care. These mechanisms become costly and begin to consume some of the savings that result from more efficient organization. In short, although organized group practice appears to offer possible advantages for high quality care which surpass those available under existing conditions, it is not at all evident that such care, if it is to be effective and conform to high expectations of preventive and responsive care, can be provided at significantly reduced cost. We will return to a discussion of prepaid care later.

This chapter by its very nature has been sketchy. It has introduced a variety of issues that will be elaborated on in various ways in the remainder of this volume. The basic point, which deserves emphasis here, is that existing problems in the health care sector are the product of a variety of social, economic, political, and technological factors. These problems are ingrained in the perspectives, interests, and orientations of key groups who have adapted to changing conditions in terms of their own needs and professional cultures. New legislation oriented toward changing the basic structure of health care delivery has little potentiality for success unless it can come to terms with these adaptations and the underlying factors that have molded them.

Notes

1. Havighurst, C. (1970). "Health Maintenance Organizations and the Market for Health Services." *Law and Contemporary Problems, 35:*716–795.

2. Steinwell, B., and D. Neuhauser (1970). "The Role of the Proprietary Hospital." *Law and Contemporary Problems, 35:*817–838.

3. Stevens, Rosemary, and Robert Stevens (1970). "Medicaid: Anatomy of a Dilemma." *Law and Contemporary Problems, 35:*348–425.

4. Bellin, L. E., and F. Kavaler (1971). "Medicaid Practitioner Abuses and Excuses vs. Counterstrategy of the New York Health Department." *American Journal of Public Health,* **61**:2201–2210.

5. Kessel, R. (1970). "The AMA and the Supply of Physicians." *Law and Contemporary Problems,* **35**:267–283.

CHAPTER III

The Changing Structure of Medical Practice*

Although medical practice has been continuously adapting to social and technological changes, American medicine will be confronted in the coming years with social, economic, and ideological challenges of a magnitude it has never before experienced. In almost every area of medical activity—in the distribution of services, allocation of costs, assessments of quality, recruitment into medical work, organization of care, ethics of practice—the traditional medical view that these matters are to be decided solely by doctors will be under scrutiny and reevaluation. For it is increasingly recognized among public officials and the educated public—if not among doctors themselves—that medicine is most basically a social enterprise, and although doctors have the technical competence for treating the sick, they have no monopoly on wisdom in matters concerning the organization, distribution, and economics of medical care. Already the rumblings from such conflicts are evident, and in the coming years the various interested parties will require great patience and understanding if acrimony is to be minimized. Given the expected clashes between ideologies and perspectives in the medical field, it is important that we attempt to isolate those issues which are most basic to the organization of medical practice so that our attention is not diverted in the rhetoric of controversy.

Varying Perspectives Relevant to the Organization of Care

Medical practice in the United States is one of the last bulwarks of an individualized, entrepreneurial tradition. In comparison with the other

---

* Adapted from a paper published in *Law and Contemporary Problems*, **32**:707–730 (1967), which appeared in the Symposium on Medical Progress and the Law.

professions and occupations, the ability of medicine to resist group organization to the extent that it has, despite the enormous complexity of medical technology, is in itself an extraordinary phenomenon. Despite the tremendous influences encouraging group organization, the persistence of the solo practitioner or partnership as modal forms of practice attests to the strength of the entrepreneurial ideology and its importance in molding the doctor's view of medical care. This ideology makes it all the more difficult to attract doctors to new organizational forms for meeting changing social conditions and developing technological and economic demands on medicine.

The pattern of medicine that continues to persist in the United States has a distinctive character. Although early American developments in medicine, as well as the development of the hospital, followed European patterns, they took on some unique features.[1] By the nineteenth century the European countries with the greatest influence on the colonies were already highly urbanized, and medical education and practice had taken on a specialized character with a growing separation of general practitioners from hospital doctors and clear distinctions between physicians, surgeons, and apothecaries.[2] But America was frontier country and largely rural, and such distinctions were inappropriate for a population scattered over a vast land area with a low population density.[3] Doctors functioned for the most part as generalists, doing whatever they thought was necessary to meet their responsibilities, and the jealousies and distinctions so important in European medicine did not take root. When the idea of the general voluntary hospital, borrowed from Great Britain, was implemented first in Philadelphia and later in other cities,[4] the doctors who offered their services free to the indigent obtained the privilege of using the hospital to treat their own private patients as well. This pattern, first established under conditions very different from those that now exist, has persisted as the dominant one to this very day and carries along with it certain merits, but also some important diadvantages. For example, despite the far-reaching trend toward specialized medical functions, access to the hospital and complexity of work undertaken by the individual doctor have only a very limited relationship to the length of his training and competence. Even today a vast bulk of the total surgical work in the United States is undertaken by doctors regarded as "nonqualified surgeons" by the American College of Surgeons.[5] In short, even in this most basic area—the specification of qualifications to undertake work graded in its complexity and difficulty—doctors who have met minimal qualifications for licensure are left for the most part to make their own individual decisions as to their competence and capacity to function in various medical spheres.

Understanding doctors' views of medical care requires awareness of the perspectives from which they perceive the medical scene—orientations which conceptualize the problems of medical practice from a personal rather than an organizational perspective. Unlike the organizational theorist, the doctor asks how medicine should be organized so that he can provide his patients with a high standard of care and also maximize his personal and professional satisfactions. The solutions thus obtained might look very different from those posed by medical care experts, who phrase the question in terms of how medical practice might be most effectively and efficiently organized so as to provide a high level of care through maximal use of health resources and personnel. Indeed, the optimal organization of medical resources may require a degree of control and surveillance over the doctor's work which is threatening and unattractive to him. One needs no theory of professional conspiracy to explain conflicts between the health professions and other groups; conflict is a natural product of the different perspectives from which they view the medical context.

The Elements of Medical Care

The concept of medical care applies not only to the care received by individual patients but also to the manner in which medical resources are provided and distributed to the population at large. Even if every patient treated received optimal patient care, the medical care system itself would be inadequate if a close congruency did not exist between need and the distribution of services. Thus, systems of medical care must be measured not only in terms of individual care but also in terms of the adequacy of personnel and facilities and the distribution of services among various economic strata and geographic areas. Persons of sufficient ability and motivation must be recruited into the health professions and trained, and the conditions for continuing innovation and adaptation to change must be maintained.

Given the growing demand for medical services[6]—inflated by an increasing rate of utilization for the average person, a growing population, a larger number of persons in age groups that require more concentrated medical attention, and greater health coverage stimulated by new government programs—the number of physicians available to the population in coming years will be inadequate.[7,8] At the end of 1964 there were 297,200 physicians and osteopaths (active and inactive) who were listed as part of the American health manpower pool. Although the number of doctors relative to the population has been maintained, a much larger part of the total medical work force is involved in nonclinical activities, such as medical research and administration, leaving relatively fewer doctors to meet the growing demands for medical services.[9] In comparing 1950 and 1964, there were more general practitioners in the early period than general practitioners, internists, and pediatricians combined in 1964.[10]* There are basically two ways to respond to the situation: we can continue to stimulate the development and growth of medical schools to a much greater extent than has yet been attempted; or the resources available can be concentrated into programs and forms of organization designed to increase the doctor's productivity.† Although it is necessary to take steps in both directions, it is not clear that these remedies will have much impact on the vast maldistribution of medical manpower and facilities throughout the United States.[9–11] Thus far, we have not been extremely bold in considering the development of incentives and subsidies that might stimulate a more adequate distribution of medical manpower.

There are few areas in medical care that can compete successfully with the manpower problem in evoking platitudinous comment. The manner in which we attempt to meet medical demands and the types of responses we evoke in meeting manpower problems will have a vast influence not only on the amount of medical care available but also in its patterning and structure. If we, indeed, decide that major emphasis should be given to increasing the doctor's productivity, then we must be cognizant of the fact that this is likely to change the nature of the physician's role itself with possible dangers of destroying the sustenance aspect of medical practice. The failure to tangle with the real analytical issues in the structuring of medical care is exemplified by the report to the President from the National Commission on Community Health Services. Compare, for example, the two following notions suggested by the Commission:

It is critically important to make full use of available medical manpower. The physician is neither nurse, social worker, nor physical therapist. He is a physician. His training and talents as a physician must not be dissipated by employing them—except in crisis situations—in any tangential, nonmedical discipline.

* As of the end of 1969, there were a total of 339,000 physicians and osteopaths, approximately 163 per 100,000 population. Approximately two-thirds provide patient care in office-based practice. (National Center for Health Statistics, 1971, *Health Resource Statistics: Health Manpower and Health Facilities, 1970.* Public Health Service. Washington: U.S. Government Printing Office.) Medical school places have increased rapidly in recent years. For example, first year places have expanded from 8,173 in 1959–60 to 11,348 in 1970–71. See W. F. Dube, F. T. Stritter, and B. C. Nelson, 1971, "Study of U. S. Medical School Applicants, 1970–71," *Journal of Medical Education,* **46:**837–857.

† In defense of the latter argument, see E. Ginzberg, 1966, "Physician Shortage Reconsidered," *New England Journal of Medicine* **275:**85–87.

There are not enough of him in the United States today to warrant wasting a minute of his education and experience on jobs others can do as well. Because it is necessary to face up to this fact squarely, and make the most efficient use of limited physician manpower, health care functions not requiring medical training should be delegated by the physician to other members of the health care team to the maximum extent practical (p. 22).

The physician should be aware of the many and varied social, emotional, and environmental factors that influence the health of his patient and his patient's family. He will either render, or direct the patient to, whatever services best suit his needs. His concern will be for the patient as a whole and his relationship with the patient must be a continuing one. In order to carry out his coordinating role, it is essential that all pertinent health information be channeled through him regardless of what institution, agency, or individual renders the service. He will have knowledge of the access to all health resources of the community—social, preventive, diagnostic, therapeutic, and rehabilitative—and will mobilize them for the patient (p. 21).[12]

To all but the most rampant optimists the goals defined in the two statements above will appear inconsistent. Continuing relationships with patients and concern for the patient as a whole by necessity require doctors to engage in tangential, nonmedical functions that do not require his technical medical education. Indeed, the kind of medical stance that maximizes technical forms of productivity is incompatible with the definition of the doctor's role as a coordinator of services and an attendant to the social and emotional welfare of patients. Since this issue is central to future decisions concerning the organization of medical practice, I turn now to a more complete discussion of the consequences of varying forms of practice organization.

Medical Practice and Bureaucracy

As the needs for greater efficiency and productivity in the provision of medical care grow, and as increasing developments in medical technology demand greater organization and coordination, the arguments toward the bureaucratization of medicine are compelling. Many technical-scientific aspects of medicine can be efficiently organized within bureaucratic forms, thus making it possible to reach more people and to facilitate a more adequate pattern of distribution of medical services. Moreover, bureaucratic contexts facilitate the imposition of quality controls (for example, routine auditing of medical care) and enhance the possibilities for continuing education in a situation of rapid social and technological change. The trend toward greater bureaucratization of medical practice is not only a certainty because of the forces within medical practice, but it is also being encouraged through the growing involvement in medical affairs of other organizational forces; government agencies, labor unions, and other major purchasers of medical care are increasingly conscious of the value received for their investments and are concerned that their constituencies enjoy a standard of medical care at least equal to that of the individual consumer who purchases his own services.[13]

The solutions to some problems usually create others, and it is of the greatest importance that thought and energy be devoted to considering bureaucratic mechanisms and alternatives that counteract some of the more noxious side effects of the growing bureaucratization of medical practice. The great variety of life problems brought to doctors indicates that from the patient's perspective the nontechnical aspects of the doctor's role are important. Indeed, it seems apparent that the physician has to a great extent occupied a sustaining role in Western society, handling a wide range of problems outside the sphere of his technical-scientific expertise. The continuing importance of the social aspects of medical practice is attested to by the increase of utilization of medical resources despite the fact that the level of the population's health is probably higher than ever before. Certainly, the growing demand for medical services is in part a product of general affluence, increased consumer spending power, innovations in medical care, and the expanding provision of medical resources resulting from new medical and government developments. But the nature of medical demand and the wide-reaching character of problems brought to the physician suggest that increased utilization may also be a product partially of the changing organization of social life itself.[14]

As opportunities for intimate personal contacts diminish and as the American population becomes increasingly mobile, problems that have been previously handled in familial, social, and religious contexts may be transferred to formal sustaining professionals (doctors, lawyers, social workers, and the like). Although a wide variety of professionals deal with problems which in previous decades were handled by informal sources of help, it is generally believed that physicians appear to have experienced the most substantial part of this additional consumer demand. Because the formal structure and definition of the doctor-patient relationship provide a legitimate way for expressing intimacy and requesting help, it is only natural that various psychosocial problems and other problems in living should be brought to the physician.

There is little reason to believe that doctors presently deal adequately with the sustaining aspects of their role. But the continuing bureaucratization of medicine threatens even further danger in this sphere, as evidenced by the growing clamor over the contraction of general practice despite the fact that the average consumer of medical care receives better technical services than ever before. One possible source of such dissatisfaction is the commonly held feeling that it is necessary to have someone to rely on during times of trouble. And it is expected that such a relationship would allow an opportunity for expressing deeply felt attitudes, doubts, and uncertainties. Thus, if the sustaining professions are to be effective in responding to many patients' needs and expectations, these professions must be organized to insure some opportunity for the expression of intimacy and for the provision of close personal supports. It is essential that the patient feel that the person to whom he allows access to the private regions of his "self" be truly interested in him and his welfare, and not regard him as one more item on an assembly line.[15] Yet at the same time that societies and their various institutions become more bureaucratized, making the sustaining professions more important than ever before, these professions themselves are becoming more formalized. As already noted, there are many excellent reasons for formalizing medical care, but it is not clear to what extent such relationships can be bureaucratized without seriously damaging the potential emotional sustenance functions of the helping professions.

When we think of bureaucratizing medical practice, we usually conceive of medicine in its more narrow perspective—that is, as an applied science rather than as a sustaining profession. As doctors become more capable technically, they tend to think of medicine in its more restricted medical aspects. And increasingly doctors trained in modern, hospital-based, scientifically oriented medical schools, operating with heavy patient loads and faced with severe time pressures, resist rendering some of the services the "old family practitioner" saw as an integral part of his role. Moreover, in organizing the technical-scientific components of the doctor's role so that the same facilities reach more people, opportunities for the emotional aspects of medical practice diminish. As Freidson[16] has illustrated, bureaucratic roles facilitate high quality care in a technical-scientific sense, but a certain degree of inflexibility in dealing with patient definitions, expectations, and desires also results from such organizational forms.

Just as it is unnecessary that medical care be organized to fit every personal wish of the physician, so is it equally unnecessary to respond to every whim of the patient. Since medical resources are substantially limited, it is likely that the optimal pattern of medical care from a national perspective will require some compromises on all fronts. There is little point in encouraging a continued pattern of solo, entrepreneurial practice, as it will increasingly become as inappropriate to the dimensions of medical demand and technology as the individual tutor is to modern education and scientific development. However, the character of the particular bureaucratic forms we develop deserves very serious study since the future offers abundant opportunity for the exercise of administrative stupidity.

On a simple logical basis it would appear reasonable to attempt to separate the technical-scientific aspects of medical practice from the more amorphous sustaining function. Presumably large group clinics could provide separate professionals to deal with the needs of different kinds of patients, and some experiments along these lines have been attempted. For example, within the Health Insurance Plan of New York a demonstration program was attempted in which families were assigned to health teams including nurses and social workers as well as medical men.[17] Although many more such experiments need to be attempted, it appears that many patients are reluctant to deal with emotional problems outside the medical context, and they are clearly partial to the physician.[18] Thus, regardless of whether physicians agree to allocate certain problems of patients to other professionals, it is not unlikely that patients will continue to bring emotional problems to physicians despite the availability of other channels of help. Given such a tendency, it appears expedient to develop other social services around general medical services.[19]

The coordination of the doctor's work in conjunction with the work of other professionals and related health workers raises certain difficulties. For example, if we are to take seriously the notion that work that does not require a medical education be delegated to other practitioners, then the reinstitution of midwifery appears reasonable. Experience in other developed countries suggests that well-trained midwives can provide a level of obstetrical care comparable to the care provided by physicians. But since medical care is largely private, patients may very well choose to receive such care from physicians; and individual doctors, making their own choices, would be agreeable to providing this service. There is danger, however, that even a more highly stratified medical care system than presently exists may develop where those with means buy the services they wish, while those who are less well-off receive what is socially defined as inferior care. Indeed, the social definition of midwifery under such circumstances may discourage the recruitment of competent personnel to this work, resulting, in fact, in inferior care. Midwifery is only offered as an example; it is the general issue to which I wish to draw attention. In a medical market which is largely private, persons with adequate income will be able to buy services from the practitioners of their choice, thus leaving the new physician-substitutes to provide similar services to those with lesser purchasing power. Given this threat of a highly stratified medical care system, as well as the unwillingness of the physician to share control over his work with "lesser specialties," it seems more appropriate to think in terms of new supporting specialties that facilitate the doctor's performance and efficiency but which do not operate in competition with him. In areas where there are, in fact, competing specialties (that is, professionals having a clearly defined sphere of activity), we should encourage independent practice which offers the consumer an alternative to the doctor. But even in such areas as social work, psychological counseling, and the like, there are compelling reasons for providing opportunities for help at the settings where the client is most likely to appear.

The future of medicine is faced with a dilemma common in organization life. Bureaucracy allows a more efficient and effective standard of medical practice and facilitates the use of available resources so that more people benefit. But bureaucracies also develop certain rigidities and inflexibilities in dealing with specific unique problems in that there is a tendency toward standardization of modes of professional practice. The dilemma we face is that the bureaucratic form most appropriate for the efficient organization of scientific medical work is not the best form to deal with the emotional sustenance aspects of medicine, nor does it encourage the flexibility and variation which are so useful in dealing with social and emotional problems.

There is a vast range of possible bureaucratic forms, and it is a serious error to assume that the most typical bureaucratic forms characteristic of government agencies are those best suited to medical practice.[20] Nor is it necessarily correct to assume that bureaucracies need give priority to quantity over quality or to technical aspects of medicine over emotional and social sustenance. It is not difficult, for example, to conceive of a medical bureaucracy that defines its main goals in terms of the social and emotional needs of patients and gears its activities and procedures toward this end. The difficulty in modern medicine, however, is that although medical bureaucracies often give lip service to the social and emotional needs of patients, the bureaucratic organization of medicine continues to reflect the priority—and it may be a correct one—attached to the technical-scientific aspects of the medical role. Although medical bureaucracies can be organized so that they give emphasis to the patient's education, his social and emotional needs, and comprehensive care, few medical bureaucracies are truly committed to these ideas and willing to assume the necessary economic costs.

While bureaucratic forms may vary, thus fulfilling needs differently, bureaucratic organization regardless of its type poses certain problems from a social viewpoint. Bureaucracy encourages specialized activity, routinized procedures and modes of operation, formalized methods of requisition, and standardized modes of training and evaluating personnel, and there is a strong tendency for bureaucracies to limit client control.[21] On the assumption that professionals know best what is good for the client, patients are usually given little power or formal channels through which to express their dissatisfaction or influence the type of care they receive. Unless known channels for patient influence are available and used, doctor-patient relationships can take on a stereotyped form resulting in the medical staff's giving highest priority to organizational needs and values rather than to those of patients. As clinical settings become larger and more impersonal, the patient finds it difficult to contact his doctor without first dealing with a variety of intermediaries who may try to deflect the patient's request. Since the organization is unlikely to make the patient aware of its staff rotation policies, it is not unusual that he does not see the doctor he expected or wanted to see, and, indeed, the patient may have difficulty finding someone who assumes major responsibility for his care. Moreover, as medical bureaucracies not only develop in size but spread out in space, it is not uncommon for the patient to be sent on a wild-goose chase in attempting to complete some facet of his care. All of these problems, of course, are not unique to bureaucracy, but there is a strong tendency for them to be exacerbated in such organizational contexts.

Assuming that bureaucratic organization is essential in medicine—and I for one would take this position—there continue to be alternative choices open to us. Bureaucracies can be structured so that they offer flexibility and choice to patients with different needs and inclinations.* They can also be structured so that they provide patients with power in those areas where critical patient scrutiny and evaluation are likely to improve the quality of services while, at the same time, protecting doctors from frivolous and trivial demands that detract from the overall quality of medical care. It is not too farfetched to suggest that just as students are demanding some role in decisions at universities that concern their welfare, patients, too, ought to demand some voice in the structure, organization, and provision of services which they pay for directly and indirectly. Although such demands can be excessive, medical care—like education—has not been as responsive as it should be to the many legitimate criticisms of its clients.

In organizing new forms of medical practice, caution is required so that as we eliminate economic barriers to medical care, we do not substitute in their place a variety of other social barriers.[22,23] The success of new forms of organization in medical care will depend in large part on the

---

* For a provocative discussion of the issue of choice within welfare bureaucracies, see B. Abel-Smith, 1964, *Freedom in the Welfare State*. London: Fabian Society.

flexibility, alternatives, and control mechanisms that are devised to mold bureaucratic processes in a direction which enhances choice and meets needs conducive to the health and welfare of patients as individuals.

The Principle of Countervailing Forces in Medicine

One of the most important social changes in medical care in recent decades has been the development of collective power among consumers of medical care. As labor unions moved into the medical care field, patients' interests were consolidated into powerful bargaining forces for the kinds of medical programs deemed desirable. These new attempts on the part of the consumer to structure care alternatives were frequently resisted, of course, but, having banded together, patients' interests were now consolidated into an effective bargaining framework. If the medical profession was not prepared to bargain in a reasonable fashion, the unions were in a position to build and develop their own facilities and disregard local practitioners; when these practitioners placed obstacles in the path of such developments, the vast legal resources available to major labor unions allowed them to carry the battle to the courts.* It was clear that public policy concerning health care would never again be the unique province of the medical profession.

The substantial and continually growing involvements of the federal and state governments as purchasers of medical care provide very powerful countervailing forces in the medical care field, and new programs such as Medicare, Medicaid, and the medical programs of the Office of Economic Opportunity afford tremendous opportunities to affect organization of medical care, controls over standards of medical practice, and the qualifications of providers of medical services. For example, in its first year of operation it is estimated that the Medicare program covered five million hospital admissions at a cost of almost two and one-half billion dollars.[24] Under the voluntary part of the Medicare program, it is estimated that payments were made for twenty-five million bills covering physician and other services, at a cost of approximately seven hundred million dollars. Between 1966 and 1967, the proportion of personal health care expenditures involving public funds increased by ten percentage points—from twenty-two to thirty-two per cent—largely due to

---

* For an example, see *Group Health Cooperative* v. *King County Medical Society*, 39 Wash. 2d 586, 237 P.2d 737, 1951. See also *American Medical Association* v. *United States*, 317 U. S. 519, 1943. See generally R. Munts, 1967, *Bargaining for Health*. Madison, Wis.: University of Wisconsin Press.

Medicare. In short, the magnitude and scope of such a program cannot help but have a deep impact on medical care, especially if government administrators have some clear notion as to the directions in which medical care should be moving.

In contrast, the community of physicians is very powerful not only by virtue of its tight and effective organization[25] and unity of sentiments but also because of the nature of the medical care market. Since there is a scarcity of physicians relative to medical demand and a growing scope of utilization stimulated by general affluence, doctors are in a position to boycott effectively new programs without excessive economic hardship, and thus they are in a position to bargain for conditions of service which are favorable in terms of their perspective. The federal government, appreciating the power of the medical community and the state of the medical market, has moved carefully and conservatively in attempting to protect the success of its new programs. In its Medicare program, for example, an exceedingly cautious position has been taken on such central concerns to the medical profession as fees. The willingness of the government to accept direct billing to the patient under the Medicare program and its agreement to accept the doctor's "customary charge" without insuring the concept of a "customary service" (which can be defined as the provision of a service comparable to that provided to fee-for-service patients in the same locality) reflect the caution with which the federal government has approached the sensitive area of bargaining with the medical profession. And there is little question but that the Medicare program has added some increment to the average doctor's income.* A panel study of a sample of physicians in New York State[26] found that prior to Medicare only thirty-eight per cent of doctors favored the bill. Following the enactment of Medicare seventy per cent reported approval, and six months later the endorsement rate went up to eighty-one per cent. After the passage of the bill and also six months later, ninety-three per cent of the doctors interviewed indicated that they had planned or were planning to treat Medicare patients.

In contrast, the Medicaid program in New York State has had a much more stormy entrance. Six months following its enactment only forty-two per cent of a sample of New York State physicians favored the program,

---

* There has been a continuing debate as to whether the 7.8 per cent increase in physicians' fees in 1966—the largest annual increase since 1927—was in part a response to the acceptance of the "customary fee" criterion within the Medicare program. For a conservative review of the question, see U. S. Department of Health, Education, and Welfare, 1967, *A Report to the President on Medical Care Prices;* for a less conservative view, see L. T. Smedley, September, 1967, "Medicare." *The American Federationist* (AFL-CIO).

and a substantial number of doctors are alleged to be boycotting the program. Compared to Medicare, title 19 appears to be less popular among doctors, and although there are many explanations for their reactions, it is very likely that an important element involves a dispute over controls. Unlike Medicare, New York State's title 19 program has attempted to impose regulations dealing with the quality and costs of medical care by specifying criteria concerning who can render specialist care and by attempting to provide a fixed fee schedule rather than using the "customary fee" criterion. In this dispute one can see the clash of powerful countervailing forces, and one begins to get some view of what medical care politics will look like in the future.

As government programs in the medical care field expand in their coverage and as inclusion rules become more liberal over time, concern with costs and quality becomes inevitable. Such new programs provide the government with considerable opportunity to upgrade medical education and levels of medical skill at the same time that they encourage efficient practices. Such pressures obviously frighten professionals who are accustomed to unquestioned independence, and they disenfranchise others with lesser qualifications. If, for example, the government requires that providers of particular services be board-eligible or board-certified in the relevant specialties, such requirements arouse the opposition of many doctors who do not meet these qualifications but ordinarily undertake similar work. In the long run specification of such criteria will upgrade medical practice, but in the short range confrontations are inevitable.

One of the major problems in such confrontations is that the rhetoric of dispute is rarely in terms of the issues at hand. Doctors who are fearful of government regulations concerning the quality auditing of medical care find it more expedient to attack the government's alleged intrusion in the doctor-patient relationship rather than to bargain for a fair and reasonable auditing system that protects both sides from abuse. And the false rhetoric does little to refine and resolve such pertinent issues as what constitutes a fair auditing system, how penalties and authority will be administered, how reviews will be undertaken, how auditors will be selected, and the role doctors will have in their selection. Despite the pervasive paranoia among the medical profession concerning government, there are realistic problems resulting from growing government involvement in medicine, and negotiated safeguards for both doctor and patient are required. The obnoxious attachment of a loyalty provision to the original enactment of title 18 is symptomatic of possible dangers to the patient's privacy* and to the worthy ethics of the Hippocratic oath. Al-

---

* The Justice Department has conceded in response to ACLU's objections that the Medicare loyalty oath is unconstitutional. ACLU Annual Report, 1967, **46**:31–32.

though such problems can be exaggerated, it remains important to insure that government's role in medicine is structured so as to protect the integrity of patients and those aspects of independence which are necessary among professionals. Despite one's attitudes toward the degree of benevolence exercised by the medical profession, it is too much to expect doctors to passively await developments while the structure of their work situation is so radically changing. We can, however, attempt to channel the discourse into more pertinent and constructive areas of discussion.

Just as the medical profession chooses its own rhetoric, so do government officials. Although they may promise "equal access to quality care" to all persons covered by their programs, the powers of implementation are frequently insufficient to induce the appropriate organizational changes. Making medical care a right rather than a dole does not necessarily change the organization of clinics and how they operate, the attitudes of physicians toward their clients, and the liberties medical organizations take with patients of differing social status. Indeed, the increased provision of medical services to underprivileged groups faces problems in many respects identical to those involved in welfare administration generally.[27] If the government pays medical bills directly, they have better opportunity to control the quality and costs of care and to influence the structure of medical practice. In contrast, if the patient pays his own fees, he has greater opportunity to escape the stigma of receiving a welfare service and whatever consequences flow from such a definition. But in the latter circumstance the government has no way of using its influence to insure that the patient receives a good value for his money. Moreover, under the direct billing scheme recommended by the American Medical Association, there is no protection to the Medicare patient that the doctor will not charge an exorbitant fee in excess of the reimbursement possible under the government program. Furthermore, requirements to pay bills before reimbursement can produce difficulties for elderly patients on limited incomes.

In my opinion direct billing would be desirable and conducive to good quality care only if local medical societies would protect the patient against exorbitant fees by accepting a standardized fee schedule within the limits of government reimbursement. Under such conditions patients would have greater freedom in seeking sources of medical care without being labeled as welfare recipients and would, at the same time, have assurance that they would not be held for expenditures beyond those allowable by the government. From the government's standpoint, if there is a predetermined agreement on medical fees reimbursement could be expedited, thus protecting the patient from incurring unnecessary loans to pay medical expenses and negating the need for such obnoxious mechanisms as promissory notes used by some physicians. Here, it appears, is an opportunity to substantially improve the patient's position in the medical care structure, if only the medical societies were willing to undertake action consonant with their verbalized philosophy concerning the freedom of patient choice of doctor and if the federal bureaucracy was able to overcome the inefficiencies of its reimbursement mechanisms.

The field of medical care administration in the United States is complicated by the fact that doctors function in a "seller's market." Unlike England and Wales, where government medicine is used by the mass of the population[28] and where nearly all doctors must depend on the Health Service for their livelihood, doctors in the United States, as noted earlier, are sufficiently busy so that if necessary they can work outside of government schemes. This allows the medical profession a powerful bargaining position, one which permits it to resist to a considerable extent government pressures for change. But there is also evidence that the power of the medical profession is becoming more fragmented as the changing technology and structure of medical practice produce within the health professions new pressure groups who come into conflict with the policies of the American Medical Association. Doctors can no longer work effectively without the availability of the hospital, but hospitals are faced with their own problems and increasingly are looking toward the government for financial support and are showing a willingness to accommodate to administrative pressures from the government. Similarly, medical educational institutions and particular medical specialties are to a greater extent identifying with their own particular problems and spheres of concern, and when their interests are at stake they are willing to form coalitions with the government against the American Medical Association. In the past few years we have had the opportunity to see several such instances: the American Hospital Association supporting the government on Medicare; the medical schools supporting regional government-supported clinics for chronic disease; and the American Psychiatric Association supporting government investments in staffing community mental health centers. The changing political and social climate in the country at large and the growing ferment among the young also have not failed to penetrate the medical schools, where there is a growing consciousness of the social responsibilities of the medical profession.

The Changing Contexts of Medical Practice

The greatest problem in health care evident in the United States involves the lack of congruency between the need for medical care and its distribution. Those groups in the United States with the most abundant health problems and need for adequate medical attention use proportionately the smallest share of health services.[6,15,29,30] Whatever the defects of nationalized systems of care—and there are many—they have made impressive progress in closing the gap between the need for services and their availability.* In comparison to the United States there are few developed countries in the Western world that have such great discrepancies in access to care and health status between the rich and the poor.† Much of the problem in the United States stems from large pockets of "impoverished health" in underprivileged areas which have not been reached effectively by medical programs already available.‡

At the same time it is apparent that in recent years the government has made major strides in attacking the morbidity problem among the poor. Through the Medicaid program the states were offered an excellent incentive to increase the scope of health coverage among those with limited incomes, and, although the criteria vary among the states which have thus far enacted programs, the potential scope of such programs can be observed in the liberal requirements specified in New York State.** But even Medicaid tends to benefit those areas of the country that have comparatively good state services, and such programs do not do enough to overcome health problems in many of the most impoverished areas of the United States.‡‡

Despite short-run setbacks, it appears evident that when the war in

---

* For example, recent studies in Britain show no clear relationship between social status and medical care utilization. The studies available suggest somewhat more utilization among the working class who probably need medical services more. See, for example, A. Cartwright, 1967, *Patients and Their Doctors: A Study of General Practice*. London: Routledge and Kegan Paul.

† Although health and longevity are related to various aspects of culture and society more than to the availability of medical care, it is important to note that despite the affluence of the American health sector, American adult mortality and infant mortality far exceed such indices in many other developed Western nations. See, for example, National Center for Health Statistics, *International Comparison of Perinatal and Infant Mortality*, 1967. Public Health Service Publication No. 1000, Series 3, No. 6. Washington: U. S. Government Printing Office.

‡ The high infant mortality rate in the United States is largely a product of the great excess of deaths among nonwhite infants. See, for example, National Center for Health Statistics, *Infant and Perinatal Mortality in the United States*, 1965, Public Health Service Publication No. 1000, Series 3. No. 4. Washington: U. S. Government Printing Office. Also, the excess in nonwhite deaths at all ages, except among the very old where data are particularly unreliable, reflect such discrepancies in access to medical care. See D. Mechanic, 1968, *Medical Sociology: A Selective View*. New York: Free Press.

** Since this was written, Medicaid eligibility was made more stringent in New York as well as in other states, and federal matching funds were limited by a Congressional amendment.

‡‡ The most "liberal" Medicaid programs are available in the following states: California, Connecticut, Massachusetts, Maryland, Minnesota, New Hampshire, New York, Rhode Island and Wisconsin.

Vietnam ends* and abundant funds are once again available for a variety of domestic programs, medical benefits through government support will be increasingly liberalized. Since government's role in providing and organizing health care is really only beginning, it is important that we consider various alternatives for structuring care and attempt to learn what we can from other countries concerning the consequences of different forms of organization. I therefore wish to use the remaining space to consider the relevance of the British experience for developing trends in the United States.

Some Comparisons Between British and American Medicine

The major goals of any medical system are to provide and distribute health services to those who need them and to use the resources, knowledge, and technology available to prevent and alleviate disease, disability, and suffering to the extent possible under prevailing conditions. There are many alternative ways in which these goals may be pursued, and the form that health institutions take is inevitably related to the form of other societal institutions and to the economic, organizational, and value context of which they are a part.

Most medical structures, as in the case of other social institutions, have not been organized to fit a plan of maximal efficiency. Instead, they are "hammered out" in the politics of compromise, responding as well to tradition, societal need, and changing technology. The organization of the English National Health Service illustrates this point since it was clearly part of a long evolution of social services, and it expressed values and embodied traditions that were in no sense new.[2,31,32] By the second half of the nineteenth century the poor in England had gained the right to institutionalized care when they were sick. In the Metropolitan Poor Act of 1867 it was explicitly acknowledged that it was the obligation of the state to provide hospitals for the poor. The National Health Insurance Act of 1911 provided wage earners with a general practitioner service not so different from the one available today. Thus, the formation of the National Health Service in 1948 served to extend guarantees of access to care and to organize the nation's hospitals into a national scheme, but the Service itself was of an old and traditional cloth, embodying many of the irrationalities and organizational absurdities that existed prior to the National Health Service. We, too, are in this position as we

---

* It appears that my optimism was unwarranted, and the statement in retrospect strikes me as naïve!

forge ahead in developing new programs. For as we compromise with the medical profession and other groups to facilitate the implementation of particular organizational forms, we allow various absurdities to persist which will plague us in the future. I believe that the billing arrangements under the Medicare Act constitute one such example.

Essentially, the English National Health Service was organized in three parts. Hospitals were organized on a regional basis to assure greater rationality, thus improving to some extent the very poor distribution of beds and facilities. General practice was, for the most part, organized separately from the hospital system, very much extending the form of the medical panel as it existed under the National Health Insurance Act of 1911. The general practitioners, slow to accept the inevitability of the new National Health Service and weak in their prestige and bargaining position, found themselves with little power but to grumble as the government pushed through a "deal" with the more prestigeful hospital doctors—a deal that won their support and cooperation.* Previous to 1948 many general practitioners took on work in hospitals that could not support a full-time hospital doctor, but the new organization of hospital regions allowed assignment of consultants to these institutions, thus more completely disenfranchising the general practitioner from hospital work. Moreover, the salaried hospital doctors were no longer in any sense beholden to the general practitioner for private referrals, and this perhaps has led to an attitude that more readily allows expression of the status distinction between the general practitioner and the hospital consultant— a distinction that has become in recent years more pronounced than ever before with the growing technological sophistication of specialized medical work. Although it was anticipated that the conditions of general practice would be improved through the establishment of general practice centers supplied with ample diagnostic facilities and ancillary help, neither the practitioners themselves nor successive governments were particularly enthusiastic about the idea. The doctors coveted their independence, distrusted both the central and local governments, and were wary about working under the gaze of their medical colleagues. The government, preoccupied with other problems of some magnitude, was probably reluctant to expend the substantial sums necessary to improve the conditions of general practice.

Although conditions in Great Britain and the United States are not comparable, I believe that American doctors have an important lesson

* For a brilliant analysis of the bargaining relationships between the British Medical Association and Ministry of Health, see generally H. Eckstein, 1960, *Pressure Group Politics: The Case of the British Medical Association*. Stanford, Calif.: Stanford University Press.

to learn from the British experience. British general practitioners have done so poorly in part because they have taken a negativistic and unconstructive stance in opposing inevitable social changes. Had they taken a more constructive view toward social conditions, they might have done much not only to enhance medical practice but to elevate their own position within the structure of the National Health Service. Organized medicine in the United States has also been characterized by stubborn and unconstructive responses to government attempts to attack pressing social problems in the medical field.* Although the American Medical Association is no doubt successful in delaying and deflecting programs of change in the short run, they may have a lesser role in structuring future solutions. For example, instead of fighting government subsidy of medical students, thus having a detrimental impact on the quality and range of manpower attracted to the medical profession, the American Medical Association could play an impressive role in insuring that government fellowships would not infringe on the choices made by the student and the integrity of medical practice. Indeed, as the image of the American Medical Association becomes more tainted, its ability to provide leadership among informed and respected medical men is undermined. I have little doubt that leading medical figures will to a larger extent participate in *ad hoc* policy-making groups outside the committee sphere of organized medicine itself.

In one major sense, the situation of general practice in England and Wales portrays in vivid form a dilemma increasingly characteristic of the United States and other Western countries—that is, the dilemma concerning the organization of general practice services within the overall structure of medical practice. As medical practice becomes more specialized and more dependent on laboratory aids and technical diagnostic approaches, there has been growing concern in defining the relevance and appropriateness of the general practitioner in the overall scheme of services. In the United States the noticeable departure of doctors from the general practice role poses the important issue of whether or not vast effort should be devoted to reviving or restructuring such services. In England it is believed that the general practitioner has a unique role in dealing with the social and psychological problems of patients as well as serving as a "first line of defence in times of illness, disability, and

* In recent years, there has been a significant shift in the responses of many medical organizations and particularly the local medical societies as evidenced by the development and growth of medical foundations and sponsored prepaid programs. To a large extent these changes reflect attempts to offer alternatives to more forceful government controls and more extensive changes, but they also reflect a sincere interest on the part of many physicians in improving the quality and distribution of medical services.

distress."[33] However, such definitions of the role are rarely accompanied by an explanation of how such a stance might be effectively communicated to the doctor except in the grossest generalities. Since medical education in Britain is extremely conservative and based predominantly on hospital practice, the average doctor does not always assimilate such socially benevolent views.[34] He, too, frequently identifies with the values of the medical school, which places greatest emphasis on the diagnosis and treatment of less common disorders and not on those most frequently seen in general practice. Even more important, however, is the fact that the stance the doctor takes toward his patients is determined as much by the conditions under which he practices as it is by his own motives and values. To the extent that the doctor is faced by a large panel of patients and an exceedingly heavy work load, it becomes difficult for him to practice in a manner which gives high priority to psychological and social needs of the patient.[35] The average general practitioner is far too busy to provide a high standard of social medicine and emotional sustenance.

We are now in a situation in the United States where we are being urged to restimulate general practice and to institute comprehensive medicine at the same time that we are encouraged to meet growing medical demands by increasing the doctor's productivity. But the social changes required to increase the doctor's productivity are contrary to the gains we anticipate would result from a revitalized general practice. To the extent that the doctor's time is organized to provide a maximum of technical services in a particular period of time, it becomes difficult indeed to enhance those aspects of the doctor's role that nourish emotional and social health.

The question of general practice also brings out in sharp focus some of the economic issues underlying health care, although they take a somewhat different form in the United States and Great Britain. Although the impression is often given in both countries that patients receive the best medical care that money can buy, the kind and quality of medical care depend very largely on the funds invested in health care and health resources. In spite of the fact that the National Health Service tries to make access to medical care more equitable, its presence does not insure the availability of a high standard of care to the average patient. The typical doctor sees far too many patients to assess their problems carefully, and he devotes far too little time to each patient. In a study of a random sample of general practitioners in England and Wales,[36,37] more than half of the doctors studied reported that under present conditions of organization it was not reasonable to expect general practitioners to provide a high standard of medical care or to practice good social or preventive care. More than two-fifths of the doctors felt it was not even realistic to expect the general practitioner to adequately screen out patients with serious physical disorders, to keep informed of new knowledge in medicine, or to provide a high quality doctor-patient relationship. Although we do not have comparable data relevant to medical practice in North America, there are indications that the situation is not much better.* To the extent that medical practice affects mortality and morbidity—and this may be a dubious assumption—there is little basis for assuming American superiority.[38,39]

Economic issues affect medicine in other ways as well. Because such high economic valuation is placed on the doctor's technical services, certain aspects of medicine which may still be desirable become relatively uneconomical. Doctors are increasingly unwilling to make house calls because of the loss of time and money intrinsic to such inefficient forms of practice; patients as well would be unwilling to pay the cost of such house calls as measured against a comparable value received in office practice for a given time unit. The unwillingness to make house calls is highly developed in the United States where doctors, for the most part, work on a fee-for-service basis; but the proportion of the doctor's time spent in home care is decreasing in developed medical systems throughout the world.

Finally, it is important to consider the relevance of general practice to modern technical medical care. The general practitioner is a doctor of first contact. Ideally, he is sufficiently trained, technically speaking, to deal with most of the common disease conditions and to recognize those less common situations which require specialized attention. Moreover, he is a kind of medical ombudsman in that he is expected to make assessments of the quality of specialized services available, to channel his patients into those routes most likely to offer a high quality of care, and to survey and, if necessary, intervene in the medical care provided to his patients so that their interests are best served. He is an educator in that his role is partially concerned with instructing the patient in health care, advising him on general medical problems, and encouraging his understanding and cooperation in treatment. Also it is assumed that he is sufficiently conversant with the personal and social history of the patient so that he can provide a meaningful kind of emotional sustenance and can consider social and personal factors in managing the patient and his illness in an optimal manner. Finally, it is assumed that taking into account the social and psychological dimensions of medical care enhances

---

* For a picture of the quality of work of general practitioners, see K. Clute, 1963, *The General Practitioner, Study of Medical Education and Practice in Ontario and Nova Scotia*. Toronto: University of Toronto Press.

treatment decisions in that social facts and attitudes affect the course of illness and the range of disability.

It is reasonable to inquire as to what structural and organizational factors would allow such a role to be implemented and what social features would interfere with its success. Obviously the doctor must be reasonably competent in a technical sense, and conditions must be conducive to allowing him to maintain and upgrade his skills. Also he must be in a position to assess realistically the qualifications of specialists in the community and the quality of care they are able to provide. Moreover, he must have real alternative choices among such specialists, and this assumes access to a large specialist pool. Furthermore, he must be in a position to provide continuing care to his patients and be sufficiently aware of their histories and needs to instruct and advise them intelligently. It is also assumed that his relationship with the patient is a continuing one and that his practice is characterized by a relatively low degree of mobility. Finally, it is assumed that he is sufficiently in contact with other doctors providing care to his patients so that he can bring important facts concerning their health and personal histories to these doctors' attention and, in general, can look out for his patients' interests when they are placed within particular referral routes. Using these structural prerequisites, it is instructive to evaluate the role of general practitioners as they most commonly function in Britain and the United States.

England is an interesting country to assess since practitioners and officials frequently express pride in their ability to resist the trend toward specialization and impersonal medicine. The average general practitioner there is as well trained as his American counterpart, although the scope of his responsibility for caring for patients is much more limited because of his exclusion from hospital practice. He practices, for the most part, in isolation from other doctors who can scrutinize his practice and can help correct his mistakes, and he usually does not experience situations where medical problems are intensively discussed and skills sharpened. Moreover, his busy practice, largely devoted to common and uncomplicated medical problems, provides little incentive to maintain and develop new skills in dealing with less common disease entities. Although efforts are made to encourage continued postgraduate involvement, the doctor's investment in continuing education is less than ideal.* Although the general practitioner may know specialists by reputation, because he has little

* Since this was written, the NHS has increased substantially the extent of postgraduate education of general practitioners by linking postgraduate education to remuneration. In 1969–1970, 16,356 general practitioners attended 44,242 refresher courses arranged by universities in England (Department of Health and Social Security, 1971, *1970 Annual Report.* Cmnd. 4714. London: Her Majesty's Stationery Office).

place in the hospital he rarely has a personal opportunity to scrutinize the quality of the consultants' work, and even if he did he would have little power to affect the hospital situation. Finally, unless he is located in a major medical center such as London, he may have few real alternatives for referral, and his major role may involve scheduling an appointment for the patient or arranging for a hospital bed. Frequently patients are referred to the hospital without designating a consultant at all.

The continuity of general care in Britain is very much disrupted because the doctor has no place or responsibility in his patient's care once the patient is sent to the hospital. Sometimes the hospital report on the patient is so late that the doctor is not in a position to follow up treatment when the patient returns to him. Moreover, the separation of the general practitioner from hospital care usually means that his knowledge of the patient will not be used at a time when it might be most relevant. Furthermore, the general practitioner has no controls or sanctions to exercise in relation to the hospital or the consultant if he feels his patient is not receiving optimal care. Even if his contribution were valued by the hospital, his own feeling of lack of welcome and his lower prestige relative to the consultant make him reticent to interfere in hospital work. In short, despite the high ideals with which general practice is often described within the National Health Service, the location of general practice within the structure of care does much to negate the possibilities of the general practitioner's role.

General practice in Britain, however, has some assets more obviously lacking in general practice in the United States. British populations are less geographically mobile, and individual practices are more likely to be organized so that they correspond with neighborhood and family patterns. Moreover, the typical British general practitioner seems to know his community and patients better than does his American counterpart, and he spends much more time visiting their homes. He appears to have a better appreciation of the social problems existing in the community and how these problems impinge on the life and health difficulties of his patient. Indeed, the British general practitioner seems more concerned with the social aspects of medicine, although the organization of general practice does much to interfere with the success of a social viewpoint.*

The role of the American general practitioner is more difficult to describe since it is less patterned and more variable. The American situation provides opportunities for both better and poorer general care than is available in Great Britain in that it provides the general practitioner a greater chance to use his influence to encourage and stimulate a high level

---

* Despite the concern of the British G.P. with family and community, he is relatively intolerant of more marginal consultations as a result of his heavy work load.

of medical care, but it also provides greater incentive to exploit the patient for economic gain and greater need to protect himself from competition with other community practitioners.

Although the typical American practitioner is no better trained than his English counterpart, he undertakes a wider variety of work because of his access to the hospital. Although this increases the risk of errors in the management of a serious disease, it also provides incentives for the doctor to maintain his skills, and it encourages greater contact with other doctors. Moreover, in such situations the doctor's work is more visible to his colleagues since much of his activity takes place in the more open atmosphere of the hospital where others obtain some opportunity to observe how he manages his cases. However, because of the economic structure of general practice in America, there is greater incentive for a doctor to keep his patients and treat them himself than to refer them to outside practitioners. The American doctor is frequently faced with the threat of losing his referred patients not only because of the competitiveness of private practice, but also because of patients' increasing sophistication concerning the qualifications of doctors. If the doctor is in group practice, he can protect himself by restricting referrals within the group, but this severely restricts the range of care he can provide his patients. In other situations he may seek to avoid loss of his patients by referring patients to specialists outside his immediate locality. The convenience factor is thus likely to bring the patient back to his original doctor. In short, it is reasonable to believe that doctors will develop solutions to protect themselves and their practices which may not be conducive to the highest level of care. Therefore it is necessary to encourage organizational forms which are conducive to practicing a high level of care in the patients' best interests.

In contrast to his English counterpart, the American general practitioner has a better opportunity to assess the competence of his colleagues since he may come into closer contact with them through hospital work and consultations. But the extent of his awareness can be very much exaggerated, and it is often based on hearsay rather than on a serious opportunity to evaluate colleagues' work. Since the American specialist, however, is dependent on general practitioner referrals to a large extent, he is more susceptible to the general practitioner's influence. Thus, in this respect, the American general practitioner is in a much stronger position to play the role of a medical ombudsman and to influence the specialist in directions conducive to his patient's well-being.

The same conditions and scope of flexibility that provide the American general practitioner with an opportunity to promote the interests of the patient also promote a variety of abuses. The incentive to maximize income and, therefore, to retain one's patients encourages the doctor—perhaps not consciously—to undertake work beyond his capacity, and it may bring about unnecessary and harmful medical procedures.[5,40] Moreover, the referral system itself encourages trading relationships, some regarded as clearly unethical such as fee splitting, others more ambiguous from an ethical point of view but probably not conducive to a high level of medical care. With the studies available, it is impossible to ascertain to what extent the greater flexibility of referral in the United States serves to maximize patients' care as opposed to benefiting the doctor; the optimal interests of the patient and his doctor are not always compatible, however.

In contrast to the British general practitioner, the American doctor is less likely to have his patient population concentrated in one small area, and his patients are more likely to be geographically mobile. Thus the costs of home care are greater, and it is more difficult for the doctor to know his patient and his family situation well. Also, like the British general practitioner, his work load under present conditions of demand is sufficiently large to make it difficult to provide the time and attention necessary to deal with emotional and psychosocial problems of patients.

Some Final Notes on Medical Practice in the Future

Although it is possible to construct ideal models of what medical care should be, the types of medical care programs that will evolve in the future will be of the same cloth that presently exists. Despite the rhetoric and enunciation of high ideals, we should be aware that medicine will accommodate to the community forces that affect it, and the community will have little impact on the overall structure of medical services unless it can modify the community conditions, resources, and demands that compel medical adaptations. Ultimately, the condition of medical practice will depend on who controls the organization and structure of medical work, and this is the basic key to the growing confrontations between government and the medical profession.

With medical care in a state of crisis and medical thinking in a state of ferment, and with vast federal and state funds flowing into the medical care area, there is a great opportunity for constructive government action that provides the incentives for the restructuring of medical care so that the distribution of services is more equitable, the delivery of services is more effective, and the organization of medical care is geared more closely to the medical and social needs of the population. We must constantly be aware that the various facets of the medical care area—the financing of medicine, medical education, building of hospitals, development of new specialties, and so forth—are intertwined in a complicated net, and that decisions made in any sphere have consequences throughout the entire medical structure. We must attempt to use the growing government influence in medical care not only to increase the scope and quality of medical care, but also to insure that new medical structures provide a range of choice and a scope of action that facilitate serving man not only as a biological entity but also as a person.

Notes

1. Shryock, R. H. (1960). *Medicine and Society in America: 1660–1860.* New York: New York University Press.

2. Abel-Smith, B. (1964). *The Hospitals: 1800–1948.* London: Heinemann.

3. Stern, B. J. (1945). *American Medical Practice.* New York: Commonwealth Fund.

4. Shryock, R. H. (1966). *Medicine in America: Historical Essays.* Baltimore: Johns Hopkins Press.

5. Roemer, I. (1962). "On Paying the Doctor and the Implications of Different Methods." *Journal of Health and Human Behavior,* 3:4–14.

6. Somers, H., and A. Somers (1962). *Doctors, Patients, and Health Insurance.* Washington: Brookings Institution.

7. U. S. Surgeon General's Consultant Group on Medical Education (1959). *Physicians for a Growing America.* PHS Publication No. 709. Washington: U. S. Government Printing Office.

8. Fein, R. (1967). *The Doctor Shortage: An Economic Diagnosis.* Washington, D. C.: The Brookings Institution.

9. *The New York Times* (1967). September 28, page 53, col. 2.

10. National Commission on Community Health Services (1967). Report of the Task Force on Health Manpower. Washington: Public Affairs Press.

11. Darley, W., and A. Somers (1967). "Medicine, Money and Manpower: The Challenge to Professional Education." *New England Journal of Medicine,* 276:1414–1417.

12. National Commission on Community Health Services (1967). *Health is a Community Affair.* Cambridge: Harvard University Press.

13. Munts, R. (1967). *Bargaining for Health.* Madison, Wis.: University of Wisconsin Press.

14. Balint, M. (1957). *The Doctor, His Patient, and the Illness.* New York: International Universities Press.

15. Mechanic, D. (1968). *Medical Sociology: A Selective View.* New York: Free Press.

16. Freidson, E. (1963). "Medical Care and the Public: Case Study of a Medical Group." *Annals of the American Academy of Political and Social Science,* **346:** 57–66.

17. Silver, G. (1963). *Family Medical Care.* Cambridge: Harvard University Press.

18. Freidson, E. (1959). "Specialties Without Roots: The Utilization of New Services." *Human Organization,* 18:112–116.

19. Jefferys, M. (1965). *An Anatomy of Social Welfare Services.* London: Michael Joseph.

20. Goss, M. (1963). "Patterns of Bureaucracy Among Hospital Staff Physicians." In E. Freidson (ed.), *The Hospital In Modern Society.* New York: Free Press.

21. Freidson, E. (1961). *Patient's View of Medical Practice.* New York: Russell Sage Foundation.

22. Rosenstock, I. M. (1969). "Prevention of Illness and Maintenance of Health." In J. Kosa, et al. (eds.), *Poverty and Health: A Sociological Analysis.* Cambridge: Harvard University Press.

23. Mechanic, D. (1966). "Response Factors in Illness." *Social Psychiatry,* 1:11–20.

24. U. S. Social Security Administration (1967). *Health Insurance Statistics,* November 20. Washington: U. S. Government Printing Office.

25. Hyde, D., et al. (1954). "The American Medical Association: Power, Purpose and Politics in Organized Medicine." *Yale Law Journal,* 63:937–1022.

26. Colombotos, J. (1969). "Physicians and Medicare: A Before-After Study of the Effects of Legislation on Attitudes." *American Sociological Review,* 34:318–334.

27. Handler, J., and M. K. Rosenheim (1966). "Privacy in Welfare: Public Assistance and Juvenile Justice." *Law and Contemporary Problems,* 31:377–412.

28. Cartwright, A. (1967). *Patients and Their Doctors: A Study of General Practice.* London: Routledge & Kegan Paul.

29. National Center for Health Statistics (1964). *Medical Care, Health Status, and Family Income.* PHS Publication No. 1000, Series 10, No. 9. Washington: U. S. Government Printing Office.

30. Sheps, C. G., and D. L. Drosness (1961). "Prepayment for Medical Care, Parts 1–3." *New England Journal of Medicine,* 264:390–396; 444–448; 494–499.

31. Eckstein, H. (1964). *The English Health Service.* Cambridge: Harvard University Press.

32. Stevens, R. (1966). *Medical Practice in Modern England.* New Haven: Yale University Press.

33. British Ministry of Health (1963). *The Field Work of the Family Doctor.* Report of the Subcommittee of the Standing Medical Advisory Committee. London: Her Majesty's Stationery Office.

34. McKeown, T. (1965). *Medicine in Modern Society.* London: George Allen and Unwin.

35. Mechanic, D. (1970). "Doctors in Revolt: The Crisis in the British National Health Service." *Medical Care,* 8:442–455.

36. Mechanic, D. (1968). "General Practice in England and Wales: A Report on a Survey of a National Sample of General Practitioners." Mimeo, Department of Sociology, University of Wisconsin.

37. Mechanic, D. (1968). "General Practice in England and Wales." *Medical Care,* 6:245–259.

38. Peterson, O., et al. (1967). "What is Value for Money in Medical Care?" *The Lancet,* 1:771–776.

39. Moriyama, I. M., and L. Guralnick (1956). "Occupational and Social Class Differences in Mortality." In *Trends and Differentials in Mortality.* New York: Milbank Memorial Fund.

40. Columbia University School of Public Health and Administrative Medicine (1960). *The Quantity, Quality, and Costs of Medicine and Hospital Care Secured by a Sample of Teamster Families in the New York Area.* New York: Columbia Univ. Press.

PART TWO

THE CHARACTER
AND DISTRIBUTION
OF HEALTH SERVICES

CHAPTER IV

Human Problems and the Organization of Health Care*

In recent decades there have been important developments in scientific medicine, and although medical care, as we usually conceive of it, has relatively limited impact on the occurrence of disease or death in modern society, few men doubt that medical care can make a difference in particular circumstances. With such recognition, there is a growing feeling that medical care is a right and not a privilege, and that it ought to be available to all in need regardless of their position in society.

The growing demand for medical care and the increasing scientific complexity of modern medicine have made the provision of medical care an expensive venture. With increased affluence and education, people demand more rather than less medical services; and as the patient becomes more sophisticated, he insists on better care. This growing demand and its associated costs have contributed to the current crisis in the delivery of modern health care, and in recent years abundant reforms have been advocated, culminating in a variety of proposals on National Health Insurance now before the Congress.

A pervasive theme in discussions of medical care concerns the profound inefficiencies and irrationalities in the provision of health care. Medical care in the community is provided for the most part by individual practitioners or partnerships from private offices with limited paramedical assistance. Even existing group practices tend to be small and utilize very limited ancillary assistance.[1] As a consequence, doctors practice a level of medicine inferior to that in which they have been trained, or they attempt to meet the standards of their training by restricting their efforts to a narrow set of problems. In neither case does the consumer get a

---

* Adapted from a paper published in the *Annals of The American Academy of Political and Social Science,* **399:**1–11 (1972).

well-coordinated or efficient service. The problems of hospitals are even more profound. Poorly coordinated with primary care in the community, hospital care is largely unplanned, extremely expensive, and plagued by duplication of facilities, underutilization of beds, and persistent labor problems. The complex technology and utilization pattern of the hospital and the growing unionization of the health occupations, with the resulting growth in wage demands, increase costs and inflate the medical care dollar. Each hospital tends to be an island to itself, oblivious to developments in other community hospitals, poorly coordinated with general primary care in the community, and suffering from a vacuum of power or leadership. Major operating control thus resides in the doctors who use the hospital as their workplace but who are not financially responsible to it. The hospital is frequently used for the economic and social convenience of both patient and doctor under circumstances in which other health care arrangements might be more economical.

It is not surprising, then, that the concept of efficiency is the mainstay of medical reformers.[2] More efficient operation would presumably provide more services for more people, would limit the costs of third parties, and similarly would limit the costs of medical insurance for consumers. Greater efficiency further would retard the erosion of inflation, and this is particularly appealing to government, which now contributes two-fifths of the nation's medical care costs.[3] The advantages of efficiency have also been described as a boon for the doctor. By increasing his productivity, he can see more patients, respond to growing patient criticism of the unavailability of doctors, increase his earnings, and help more people. Some economists have even suggested that we face no doctor shortage.[4,5] They argue that doctors can work more efficiently than they now do, that they are poorly distributed, and that through the adoption of the efficient practices of big business the crisis in medical care can be contained.

No serious observer of the American scene can take issue with the need for correcting the appalling inefficiencies characteristic of American medicine. Moreover, the maldistribution of doctors, of other health manpower, and of medical facilities has been appreciated for some time. The patient pays more for medical care than he should because of the lack of receptivity among leaders in the health professions for planning and coordination, and the persistence of prestige competition or special interest among hospitals, doctors, and other health facilities. These are not easy problems to deal with, nor will they be easily corrected, but they merit persistent effort. The argument, however, that we do not face a significant doctor shortage is faulty, in that our system of care is not likely to develop the kind of efficient distribution or organization that will allow maximal use of the doctors' efforts, nor is this particularly desirable, as I will argue later. Although a rapid increase in the pool of physicians will not necessarily insure adequate access to care, it is a prerequisite for any serious solution to the problems in health care that we presently face.[6]

In their enthusiasm, too many of the new critics of medical care have lost a sense of what medical care is all about. For the cult of efficiency prescribes an elaborate division of labor characterized by various specialties, each performing tasks graded to its special skills. To achieve maximal output, time is organized in terms of the performance of discrete technical skills, providing the doctor with an opportunity to serve more patients than before. Although such organization has obvious value and is useful under some conditions, there is the implicit assumption that medicine as an activity can be separated into discrete functions and the application of specific technical skills. Although such organization is well suited to a variety of specific aspects of medical care, it is inappropriate for patients whose problems are complicated by psychosocial and emotional difficulties or whose treatment requires understanding them as people.[7]

The efficiency experts fail to appreciate that much of the demand for medical care is motivated by people's personal problems, which affect their health and vitality. Others suffer from psychological difficulties and chronic problems for which the physician primarily provides understanding and support. Still others suffer from profound disabilities that require sustained educational and rehabilitative efforts. Those items of medical practice that can be organized in the manner of the assembly of an automobile constitute only a small fraction of contemporary medical care.

Indeed, if the role of psychological and social distress was an aspect of the illness of only a handful of patients, there would be no real problem, but this is clearly not the case. Many doctors recognize that many patients seeking their advice are motivated by psychosocial problems, and a variety of medical researchers has shown how the failure to take such factors into account leads to routinized and ineffectual medical care.[8,9] Other doctors bitterly protest that a large proportion of the patients who seek their help present complaints that are trivial, unnecessary, or inappropriate. What they mean to say is that many of the human problems of their patients do not fit into the definition of medical care as a technical endeavor, efficiently organized for maximal doctor productivity. It is interesting to note that under many medical circumstances doctors do not agree on the proper management of the patient, or even on appropriate guidelines for treatment, and this has been a continuing barrier to developing quality controls in medical practice.*

* For some examples of such significant disagreements, see F. Ingelfinger, A. Relman, and M. Finland (eds.), 1968. *Controversy in Internal Medicine.* Philadelphia: W. B. Saunders.

It is significant that complaints of triviality in presenting symptoms are in part a result of how doctors practice and of their orientations to medicine. It is primarily the extremely busy doctors who find it difficult to relate to patients' human problems in a helpful manner, and who become frustrated in trying to deal with such difficulties while in their offices the waiting patients become more numerous.* Thus as the pressures for greater personal productivity develop, the doctor comes to demand that his patients' illnesses fall more within the narrow limits of the medical disease model. It is not surprising that patients who require assistance with profound personal problems that contribute to their illnesses come away feeling frustrated and dissatisfied, and that they may go from one doctor to another.

So this is the dilemma: how can medical services be made available to more people in a more efficient way and still retain what in traditional times was referred to as the "art of medicine"? Obviously, one answer to this question is that we need many more doctors, better trained to understand and cope with the human difficulties that patients bring to them. But this suggestion must face certain realities. It is extremely difficult and expensive to expand rapidly the pool of physicians, and it is particularly complex in a period where funds for the expansion of medical schools are not available in abundance. Although various programs might help to stimulate a growing pool of physicians in the next decade, and such efforts are already evident, the current problem will be with us for a long time.[10]

What, then, are the alternatives? One view is that the wealthy will continue, as always, to buy preferred services, whether in health, housing, or education, and those with lesser means will have to settle for what they can get.[2] However "practical" this view may appear, the complacency it expresses should serve as a challenge to those who strive for a better society—more attentive to the needs and welfare of its citizens. To accept such defeatism without a fight can only fan the discontent of the poor and the disillusionment of large segments of our population. Still another view is that new forms of medical services and new methods for organizing health personnel are needed to bring better health care to the ghettos and rural areas. Although there is much merit in some of these suggestions—it is indeed important to develop new training programs and to change some of our restrictive licensing practices—such proposals pose a danger of supplying two classes of medical services, which much

* I have studied this problem in some detail in the context of panel practice within the English National Health Service. See D. Mechanic, 1970, "Correlates of Frustration Among British General Practitioners." *Journal of Health and Social Behavior*, 11:87–104; also see Chapters 8 & 10 in the present volume.

of the population will find unacceptable and which may be highly divi-
sive. Such innovations may be useful in extending services to previously
disenfranchised populations and in increasing the effectiveness of physicians, but they must not have the effect of further stratifying our system
of medical care.*

The most frequently discussed solutions to the growing demands for
medical care are group practice, the development of health centers, and
prepaid health care. There is much to be said for each of these ideas, but
the contention that such changes in medical care will bring more and
better services to more people at lower cost is untenable. Well-organized
groups or health centers based on the prepayment insurance principle
—if they are to meet the various needs of good social, preventive, and
technical medical care—will not be inexpensive and will not constitute
a substantial remedy to the growing costs of medical care. Such plans,
however, do have strong potential for eliminating many of the abuses and
inefficiencies of the current organization of medical care, for moderating
patterns of excessive use of hospitals, for providing greater continuity
between preventive and other aspects of medical care, and for facilitating
a high level of technical health care making optimal use of ancillary
assistance and good technical facilities.[11-13]

A major function of group practice is to better meet demand through
specialization and more efficient use of facilities and ancillary personnel.
By pooling resources and providing supporting facilities, there is greater
potential for optimally using the doctor's efforts† and, from his personal
viewpoint, for alleviating some of his continuing responsibility for patients. But the advantages of organized practice are also its disadvantages.
Relieving the doctor's continuing responsibility means that the patient
cannot always obtain access to his doctor; growing specialization of function means that more individuals are involved in the patient's care, and
medical services are more segmented. Group organization itself means that
the doctor practices in a context with other doctors and is less dependent
on his individual patients; and, as Freidson has noted, this may mean
that he orients himself to a larger extent to the concerns and standards

---

* For an example of such efforts that have been successful, see S. Bellin, and H. J.
Geiger, 1970, "Actual Public Acceptance of the Neighborhood Health Center by the
Urban Poor." *Journal of the American Medical Association*, **214**:2147–2153; and S.
Bellin, *et al.*, 1969, "Impact of Ambulatory-Health-Care Services on the Demand for
Hospital Beds." *New England Journal of Medicine*, **280**:808–812.

† There are at least two separate issues involved here, the savings due to economy of
scale and the total efforts the doctor puts into his practice. For an interesting skeptical
perspective on group practice, see R. Bailey, 1970, "Philosophy, Faith, Fact, and Fiction in the Production of Medical Services." *Inquiry*, **7**:37–53.

of his colleagues and less to the demands and wishes of his patients.[14] The effect of all this may be a higher standard of technical care and greater efficiency, but it also may result in greater inflexibility and less sensitivity to the individual problems and concerns of patients. The issue to be solved, then, is how can medicine be organized so as to be technically excellent, sensitive to human problems and the personal needs of patients, and sufficiently responsive to the demand for care so that those who need health services can receive them at reasonable cost. There are no easy solutions to these requirements, but the importance of the issue has led to attempts to develop models that presumably meet the three basic requirements of technical quality, responsiveness to personal needs, and accessibility at reasonable cost. One such model which has received serious attention is that developed by Doctor Sidney Garfield,[15] who has been involved with Kaiser-Permanente for some thirty years. A careful examination of this model and its limitations will suggest the difficulties in organizing health care services so that they are responsive to personal and social need.

The Garfield Model

Doctor Garfield argues that since it is the patient who usually decides when he needs care, such decisions create a variety of types of patients seeking services: the "well," the "worried well," the "early sick," and the "sick." Garfield maintains that the fee for service has been a traditional regulator in who seeks care resulting in a limitation of "early sick" patients. He states therefore, that "elimination of the fee has always been a must . . . since it is a barrier to early entry into sick care." Garfield further argues, however, that the removal of the barrier results in an uncontrolled flow:

The result is an uncontrolled flood of well, worried-well, early-sick, and sick people into our point of entry—the doctor appointment—on a first-come, first-served basis that has little relation to priority of need. The impact of this demand overloads the system and, since the well and worried-well people are a considerable proportion of our entry mix, the usurping of available doctors' time by healthy people actually interferes with the care of the sick.

Garfield maintains that it is necessary to find a new regulator to substitute for fee-for-service, and suggests Multiphasic Health Testing as an adequate and appropriate regulator. Garfield presents his case as follows:

As a new entry regulator, health testing serves to separate the well from the sick and to establish entry priorities. In addition, it detects symptomless and early illness, provides a preliminary survey for the doctors, aids in the diagnostic process, provides a basic health profile for future reference, saves the doctor (and patient) time and visits, saves hospital days for diagnostic work and makes possible the maximal utilization of paramedical personnel. Most important of all, it falls into place as a heart of a new and rational medical-care delivery system.

Garfield proposes that patient flow should be directed to each of three distinct services. One group of patients, the healthy, would be sent to a new type of health facility, where they would have lectures, health exhibits, audiovisual tapes, counselling, and other services. Garfield notes that whether or not this will keep people healthy is not the point; he argues that it is essential for meeting increasing demand for information, and for taking the load off doctors. A second group of patients would be dealt with in a preventive-maintenance service dealing with high incidence chronic illness that requires routine treatment and followup. This service would prevent complications and the progression of illness, and would largely be run by paraprofessional personnel. Finally, a sick care service would allow doctors to use their time productively in caring for those who require diagnosis, treatment, intensive and extended therapy, and the like.

Although Garfield's model has a certain logic to it, it is based on a faulty set of assumptions as to reasons for people's use of health facilities, the basic problems underlying their complaints, and their relations to doctors and health services generally. Let us consider briefly each of these points.

Selection Into Medical Care

Garfield's notion that fee-for-service is the major regulator governing care, and that the elimination of the fee results in an uncontrolled flood that overloads the system and interferes with the care of the sick, is contrary to fact. Data are available, for example, from the Health Insurance Plan of New York, a large prepaid group in New York City where the fee-for-service has been eliminated. These data show the average number of physician services per person in 1968 was 4.3, no different from the national average for the same year, 4.2.[16,17] Data are also available for the Kaiser Foundation Health Plan, Oregon Region, where a nominal fee of a dollar or two has been charged for out-of-hospital physician visits. These data covering the years 1949 to 1966, show a high of 4461 outpatient doctor's office visits per 1000 members in 1949 to a low of 3332 visits per 1000 members in 1966, an average lower than the population as a whole which, in the period from July, 1966 to June, 1967, averaged 4.3 visits per person per year.[18,19] These figures are not exactly comparable and they refer to populations with varying characteristics, but the biases that exist in the character of the populations dealt with would probably favor a higher rate of utilization at Kaiser than in the population as the whole. The significantly lower rate clearly refutes Garfield's contention. It is difficult to account for these low levels of utilization at Kaiser, given the extremely low fees for service, and if there is a regulatory mechanism, it must exist elsewhere. Similarly, data from other situations where the fee barrier has been removed hardly support the contention of excessive or irresponsible use of health services.[20]

There is a variety of personal, social, and organizational features that affects the way health services are used. Considerable literature exists on the cultural, social, and social psychological variations in the use of medical services among different groups in the population.* Similarly, utilization of services depends not only on the inclinations of consumers but also on the availability of such services, the distance involved, transportation routes, waiting time, convenience, the manner in which patients are treated, and the like. Data are available, for example, from the Kaiser Plan which demonstrate the way in which distance from an outpatient facility affects the rate of utilization,[21] and such barriers as difficulty in getting an appointment are frequently noted among Kaiser enrollees. It is not at all clear that the medical care system requires a medical regulator, much less one formally constructed to keep people from seeing a doctor when they have decided to see one.

The Character of Patient Morbidity

Garfield proposes to use Multiphasic Health Testing for sorting patients into appropriate groups for the varying services. Such sorting, however, is not generally appropriate for most of the common illnesses for which patients typically seek routine primary care. A vast majority of such complaints are self-limited acute illnesses frequently compounded by worry and anxieties.[22-23] The patient's decision to seek care at a particular point in time results from some interaction between the occurrence of symptoms, their impact, and the situational and personal contingencies that affect his or her orientations.

Ignoring the question as to whether Multiphasic Health Testing is a useful, valid, or economic approach, which has been hotly debated,† it is

* For a review of these, see D. Mechanic, 1968, *Medical Sociology: A Selective View*. New York: Free Press; also see Chapter 12 in the present volume.
† For some critical reviews of health testing, see T. McKeown, *et al.*, 1968, *Screening*

perfectly clear that the kinds of illness which can be identified through this mechanism constitute only a small fraction of what is ordinarily conceived of as comprising usual primary medical care,* and Garfield never makes clear how he would sort such illnesses. Moreover, the approach suggested by Garfield regards with little seriousness the degree to which emotional factors affect the need to consult doctors, or the course of an illness. Although estimates of psychiatric morbidity are always tricky because of varying criteria, different studies suggest that anywhere from 5 to 10 per cent of patient populations have formal psychiatric disorders, with approximately one in twenty of such patients suffering from an acute psychosis. When one adds to this group, patients with significant psychological distress, those with psychophysiological problems, those with disorders like asthma and duodenal ulcer—which seem to be readily responsive to stress—and those whose symptoms have no apparent organic basis, then as much as a quarter to a half of all patients have difficulties complicated by emotional factors. Screening for such cases through psychological testing is notoriously poor;[24] but, even if adequate screening techniques were available, the issue is more difficult than such screening implies. There is evidence that even those patients with acute illnesses, such as respiratory conditions, or other common complaints are more likely to seek assistance from a doctor when their symptoms occur concomitantly with psychological distress, and such distress affects the course and outcome of a wide range of illnesses which are ordinarily not seen as psychosomatic in any sense.[25-28] To ignore such factors, or to attempt to deal with them as if they are of little significance, is to neglect essential components of good medical practice.

How Patients Relate to Medical Services

Just as it is difficult to separate the extent to which persons who seek medical care do so because of their physical symptoms, as opposed to other circumstances in their lives, so it is also difficult to separate these dimensions after patients seek help. Some patients have a receptivity to

in *Medical Care: Reviewing the Evidence*. Fair Lawn, N.J.: Oxford University Press. Also see R. Thorner, 1969, "Whither Multiphasic Screening." *New England Journal of Medicine*, **280**:1037–1042.

* In discussing Automated Multiphasic Health Testing in this context, I am not attempting to evaluate its overall utility or effectiveness in the provision of health services. There has been some attempt to develop provisional guidlines for such health testing and to define various aspects of the problem requiring research. See Center for Health Services Research and Development, *Provisional Guidelines for Automated Multiphasic Health Testing and Services, Volume 1*. Public Health Service, 1970. Washington, D. C.: U. S. Government Printing Office.

seeing their difficulties in social and psychological terms, while others come to present their distress in a physical language.[9] Such patients as the latter may not be amenable to a simple redefinition of their problem, as the Garfield model implies, and such attempts may only exacerbate distress and the patient's difficulties. The suggestive powers of a trusted physician are very substantial,[29]* and doctors and other health workers are in a position to greatly reduce the distress of their patients by small gestures and behavior that shows an awareness and concern for the patient and a willingness to provide needed instruction.[30,31] To be effective, such gestures may require the doctor to accept the patient's general presentation of his symptoms but to work subtly and indirectly in addressing himself to what he really feels is the patient's underlying difficulty. A labeling and sorting process may make sense logically, but it might readily violate the psychological logic of effective doctor-patient understanding and communication. We should be careful in discarding the subtle skills of the sensitive physician who recognizes that there is more to the problem than the patient will say and who takes such factors into account in the management of his patient. Developments in technical medical care have been quite dramatic, but a large percentage of medical care is still more of an art than a science.†

Toward Models of Humane and Socially Responsive Care

Despite its capacity for personalized relationships with patients, individual medical practice is increasingly outmoded. Not only is such practice inefficient and technically limited but it is also not easily adaptable to growing technology and the complexity of medical knowledge. In adapting to these conditions through more organized forms of practice, it is inevitable that more personalized elements of medical care will be threatened. Models for the future must not only develop the physician's role so that he is responsive to the kinds of issues discussed above; they must develop, as well, entirely new types of workers, whose prime concerns will be the continuity of health care, the health education of the

* For a general review of the placebo effect area, see D. Mechanic, 1968, *Medical Sociology: A Selective View.* New York: Free Press.
† A very significant but neglected issue in medical care is the large proportion of patients who fail to conform to medical regimens. See, for example, M. Davis, 1966, "Variations in Patients' Compliance With Doctors' Orders: Analysis of Congruence Between Survey Responses and Results of Empirical Investigations." *Journal of Medical Education,* 41:1037–1048. Also see V. Francis, B. Korsch, and M. Morris, 1969, "Gaps in Doctor-Patient Communication." *New England Journal of Medicine,* 280:535–540.

patient, and the coordination of the technical and social aspects of health care service. Such new elements must not be mechanisms to draw off patients who "waste" the physician's time; they must be, rather, an integral part of the entire health service, bringing together that which technical developments and increasing organization have segmented. The particular forms that such new specialties will take and what the receptivity of patients and doctors toward them will be are still unclear; but a variety of new workers is now being introduced on a trial basis, and something valuable and lasting is likely to result from these new experiments.*

One possibility for the future development of such personnel would be someone who functioned as a medical ombudsman. Such a person would have sufficient technical training to know his way around medical settings and the variety of medical specialties, but also would be sufficiently trained to be sensitive to the social and behavioral aspects of care, the coordination of services, and the need for and availability of social services in general. Such a person might serve to improve communication and coordination among the various persons involved in providing health care, contribute to educating the patient about the nature of his care and health status generally, and serve as the point of unification of all medical, rehabilitative, and social services provided for the patient within the context. He can also serve as a link for the patient between a particular medical service and other health services to which the patient requires referral. In more "elite" systems of medical care services, especially trained physicians will play such a role. At the present time, physicians neither appear inclined toward nor are they, in fact, effectively performing such a role. It is essential that trained workers undertake this responsibility, and if physicians are unwilling to do so, then we had better begin to develop new types of professionals who will. This suggestion is not provided with the assurance that it is necessarily the most appropriate way of dealing with the coordination of a highly complex set of services, but rather with the understanding that events will require us to develop new solutions to old problems.

In the final analysis, we must be sensitive to the fact that health institutions are responding to the same forces in society as other social institutions. Social life generally is becoming more technically complicated, more differentiated, and more bureaucratized. There is a growing sense

---

* Some results are more promising than others. See, for example, C. E. Lewis and B. A. Resnik, 1967, "Nurse Clinics and Progressive Ambulatory Patient Care." *New England Journal of Medicine*, **277**:1236–1241. Also see G. Silver, 1963, *Family Medical Care*. Cambridge: Harvard University Press; and E. Freidson, 1959, "Specialties Without Roots: The Utilization of New Services." *Human Organization*, **18**:112–116.

of loss of community, and social relationships are more segmented and less personalized. As the opportunities for catharsis become less prevalent in the community at large, there is a special responsibility on the part of the health sector and other helping institutions to develop mechanisms that support and sustain persons who seek and need help. Yet the helping institutions themselves are responding to these very same social forces and are increasingly less capable of providing these needed services. As we begin to restructure health care services in America, we must be constantly aware that the need for and provision of medical care existed before there was any significant health technology. The forces that brought the sick to the early practitioner and the nonliterate to the shaman are no less existent today than in prior times, and the recognition of and response to these forces define the nature of a civilized society.

Notes

1. McNamara, M. E., and C. Todd (1970). "A Survey of Group Practice in the United States, 1969." *American Journal of Public Health,* **60:**1303–1313.
2. Ginzberg, E., and M. Ostow (1969). *Men, Money, and Medicine.* New York: Columbia University Press.
3. Mechanic, D. (1967). "The Changing Structure of Medical Practice." *Law and Contemporary Problems,* **32:**707–730.
4. Ginzberg, E. (1966). "Physician Shortage Reconsidered." *New England Journal of Medicine,* **275:**85–87.
5. McNerney, W. J. (1970). "Why Does Medical Care Cost So Much?" *New England Journal of Medicine,* **282:**1458–1466.
6. Mechanic, D. (1970). "Problems in the Future Organization of Medical Practice." *Law and Contemporary Problems,* **36:**233–251.
7. Mechanic, D. (1968). *Medical Sociology: A Selective View.* New York: Free Press.
8. Duff, R., and A. Hollingshead (1968). *Sickness and Society.* New York: Harper.
9. Mechanic, D. (1969). "Hypochondriasis: A Sociological Perspective." *Psychiatric Opinion,* **6:**12–24.
10. Fein, R. (1967). *The Doctor Shortage: An Economic Diagnosis.* Washington, D. C.: The Brookings Institution.
11. Donabedian, A. (1965). *A Review of Some Experiences With Prepaid Group Practice.* Bureau of Public Health Economics. Research Series No. 12. Ann Arbor: University of Michigan, School of Public Health.
12. Shapiro, S. (1967). "End Result Measurements of Quality Medical Care." *Milbank Memorial Fund Quarterly,* **45:**7–30.
13. Saward, E. (1969). "The Relevance of Prepaid Group Practice to the Effective Delivery of Health Services." Washington: U. S. Department of Health, Education, and Welfare, Office of Group Practice Development.

14. Freidson, E. (1961). *Patients' Views of Medical Practice.* New York: Russell Sage Foundation; (1970), *Profession of Medicine,* New York: Dodd-Mead.

15. Garfield, S. R. (1970). "The Delivery of Medical Care." *Scientific American,* **222:** 15–23.

16. Health Insurance Plan of New York (1970). *H.I.P. Statistical Report: 1968–1969.* New York: Division of Research and Statistics.

17. National Center for Health Statistics (1970). *Current Estimates from the Health Interview Survey.* PHS Series 10, No. 60. Washington: U. S. Government Printing Office.

18. Saward, E., J. Blank, and M. Greenlick (1968). "Documentation of Twenty Years of Operation and Growth of a Prepaid Group Practice Plan." *Medical Care,* **6:**239–244.

19. National Center for Health Statistics (1968). *Volume of Physician Visits: U. S., July 1966–June 1967.* PHS Series 10, No. 49. Washington: U. S. Government Printing Office.

20. Mechanic, D. (1971). "Experience of the English National Health Service: Some Comparisons with the United States." *Journal of Health and Social Behavior,* **12:** 18–29.

21. Weiss, J., and M. Greenlick (1970). "Determinants of Medical Care Utilization: The Effect of Social Class and Distance on Contacts with the Medical Care System." *Medical Care,* **9:**296–315.

22. Huntley, R. (1963). "Epidemiology of Family Practice." *Journal of the American Medical Association,* **185:**175–178.

23. Shepherd, M., *et al.* (1966). *Psychiatric Illness in General Practice.* London: Oxford University Press.

24. Dohrenwend, Bruce, and Barbara Dohrenwend (1969). *Social Status and Psychological Disorder.* New York: Wiley.

25. Gardner, E. (1970). "Emotional Disorders in Medical Practice." *Annals of Internal Medicine,* **73:**651–652.

26. Mechanic, D., and E. H. Volkart (1961). "Stress, Illness Behavior, and the Sick Role." *American Sociological Review,* **26:**51–58.

27. Mechanic, D. (1963). "Some Implications of Illness Behavior for Medical Sampling." *New England Journal of Medicine,* **269:**244–247.

28. Balint, M. (1957). *The Doctor, The Patient, and His Illness.* New York: International Universities Press.

29. Frank, J. (1961). *Persuasion and Healing.* Baltimore: Johns Hopkins Press.

30. Egbert, L. D., *et al.* (1964). "Reduction of Post-Operative Pain by Encouragement and Instruction of Patients." *New England Journal of Medicine,* **270:**825–827.

31. Skipper, J. K., Jr., and R. C. Leonard (1968). "Children, Stress, and Hospitalization: A Field Experiment." *Journal of Health and Social Behavior,* **9:**275–287.

CHAPTER V

Inequality, Health Status, and the Delivery of Health Services in the United States*

Innumerable studies have demonstrated that the poor have a greater prevalence of illness, disability, chronicity, and restriction of activity because of health problems than those of higher status, and that they have less accessibility to many types of health services and receive lower quality care.[1-7] There are, of course, distinctions to be made, since the "poor" include a variety of persons and groups, different health and disease conditions are associated with varying causal factors, and failures in maintaining a good level of health and having access to necessary services are the product of a variety of sociocultural and environmental circumstances. Yet, it is a widely known fact that the environmental resources that influence the maintenance of health, the prevention of illness, and the amelioration of disease and disability are distributed in society in relation to the abilities of various groups to economically command them.

In this essay I shall focus on the poor as a special group, since it is clear that the prevalence of disease and levels of health are not related to socioeconomic status in a simple linear fashion. Most existing data suggest, in contrast, that particularly poor health levels and a high vulnerability to disease and disability predominate in the poverty group, and that after a minimum income level is reached such differences tend to be more modest relative to differences in economic status. There are several factors that contribute toward this trend. Old people make up a disproportionate number of low income persons, and they also suffer

* Paper presented at the Annual Meeting of the American Sociological Association, Denver, Colorado, August, 1971.

from greater illness and disability. Furthermore, persons with physical difficulties and disabilities are frequently limited in employment possibilities which result in low socioeconomic status. Moreover, given the existing health insurance situation, once a person reaches a certain income level the probability is high that he will have some minimum insurance coverage to deal with serious episodes of illness requiring hospitalization. Although such insurance may be less than optimal, it will usually provide services in cases that involve emergencies or serious illness. Although level of income may determine the amount and quality of services that persons can afford beyond the minimum that typical insurance policies provide, these probably have only limited effect on health status and resulting disability. I do not mean to suggest that middle income persons do not face difficulties in finding adequate medical services at a price they regard as reasonable, and certainly most of the population would face profound difficulties in the face of such catastrophic conditions as chronic uremia. I focus on the poor, however, because I believe that it is particularly this group that faces the most serious consequences relative to illness and inadequate health care and that their problems are most difficult to resolve from the standpoint of public policy.

Social programs to ameliorate the consequences of illness, disability, and poverty have evolved slowly in the United States, and they have been typified by strong moral overtones and a tight hold on the purse strings.[8] Throughout most of our early history, a strong sense of social darwinism prevailed, and poverty was viewed as the outcome of natural selection which brought to the bottom those who were defective, lazy, or otherwise held in contempt. With time, there was a growing appreciation that chronic illness and disability were unpredictable, and public subsidy for the poor developed to supplement charity made available by religious and philanthropic groups. Public aid was always provided penuriously and frequently with the implication that those who required help did so because of their own personal failures or their unwillingness to make the necessary effort to look after their own needs. As social programs developed, they increasingly made distinctions between the deserving poor, those whose poverty was the consequence of unpredictable life events— such as the blind, the aged, the permanently disabled, and children—and the undeserving poor who were frequently seen as unwilling to work. With the depression and the unemployment of vast numbers of "respectable" able-bodied workers, the view of the deserving needy was extended to the temporarily unemployed, and social programs were developed to aid them. But general assistance in this country, and in the tradition of the English poor laws, has always been grudgingly provided with a conviction on the part of many that those on welfare or receiving other social benefits are undeserving and must be policed, supervised, or otherwise discouraged from becoming too dependent on the taxpayer.

In the area of health services, similar attitudes have prevailed. Although there have been many areas of the country, particularly in large cities, where the poor have been able to obtain health services from municipal or university hospitals, such services have often been characterized by fragmentation and impersonality and have frequently affronted patients' human dignity. Moreover, the *quid pro quo* was that since the patient was receiving free care, hospital personnel could use him as they wished to promote their teaching and research efforts, and a very different style of medical care prevailed on the public as compared with the private services.[9] By whatever criterion one wishes to adopt, whether it be the availability of services, the accessibility of most specialized personnel, or the courtesy and thoughtfulness with which services are rendered, it is clear and unequivocal that these aspects of care have been and continue to be directly related to the socioeconomic status of the patient.

Implicit in the criticism of the current state of affairs is a value judgment that health care services are more important than other consumer goods, and that their availability should be determined on a basis other than the ability to economically command them. Some dispute such "importance," but the fact that health services may not be as crucial to life as many believe is less important than the fact that people regard them so.[1] Given the nature of our social and economic system, there is little reason to believe that if health resources are scarce the poor can substantially improve their access. Indeed, if we are to make a commitment in this country to provide a reasonable level of care to all Americans irrespective of their socioeconomic circumstances, a general expansion of the health sector must continue to take place, and there must be further development of health personnel, facilities, and services.

It is ironic that some economists and manpower experts, such as Eli Ginzberg of Columbia University, who recognize the role of the market in distributing health services, and who defend market mechanisms, are precisely those same economists who have opposed substantial increases in the provision of physicians and other services.[10,11] It seems fairly evident that even if financing is made available for the poor to compete in the purchase of care, the more aggressive, demanding, and knowledgeable affluent will have major advantages in a marketplace of scarce personnel and resources. As Ginzberg argues:[12]

Large-scale governmental financing can shift the relative position of various groups in their access to medical services, but there is little or no prospect—no matter how much money government invests—of equalizing the claims of all citizens so that need, rather than income determines the services rendered to each individual . . . any serious proposal to establish a more equitable system of medical care within our present society has no prospect of success unless profound structural alterations occur in our free-market economy. . . . With none of these changes even remotely possible, augmented purchasing power in the hands of the poor cannot effect any significant redistribution of medical services.

Following Ginzberg's reasoning, a condition for providing better care, barring profound structural changes, would involve some relief in the competition for scarce supply. At this point, Ginzberg shifts his argument and maintains that we already have enough doctors; what we need is greater doctor productivity and a more efficient health services system. But Ginzberg, in another context, has already recognized that profound structural changes are unlikely, and the kind of efficiency he is talking about is no more realistic. It is obvious that the efficiency of the health services system must be improved, but it is also reasonably certain that health progress for the poor will not be a product of improved efficiency in health organization alone.

In discussing social inequality and health, we cannot neglect the fact that stratification in health care is based not only on income, ethnicity, and race, but also on a variety of other implicit value systems that order the availability of care in terms of the character of the disorder, the age of those affected, the degree of chronicity and disability, and the like.* Differential attitudes in the delivery of health services persist in relation to patients with irreversible chronic diseases, geriatric patients, alcoholics, drug addicts and psychotics, and other patients who require intensive rehabilitation services.[13] Many of these categories of need tend to be associated as well with low income and minority status, but they pose more general problems.

Also, medical and other health priorities reflect the ethos of the society. A recent analysis, for example, illustrated that research in sickle-cell anemia, a problem concentrated among black Americans, received only a small fraction of the support and interest given to many other diseases causing less overall morbidity but which affect the more affluent.† Since

---

* The impact of such influences on the care of the dying patient is described by L. Lasagna, 1970, "Physicians' Behavior Toward the Dying Patient." In O. Brim, Jr., H. Freeman, S. Levine, and N. Scotch (eds.), *The Dying Patient*. New York: Russell Sage Foundation. Similar observations were made by D. Sudnow, 1967, *Passing On: The Social Organization of Dying*, Englewood Cliffs, N. J.: Prentice Hall.

† "Sickle cell anemia occurs about one in 500 Negro births and median survival is still only 20 years of age. In 1967, there were an estimated 1155 new cases of SCA, 1206 of cystic fibrosis, 813 of muscular dystrophy, and 350 of phenylketonuria. Yet, volunteer organizations raised $1.9 million for cystic fibrosis, $7.9 million for muscular dystrophy, but less than $100,000 for SCA." (R. B. Scott, 1970, "Health Care Priority and Sickle Cell Anemia." *Journal of the American Medical Association*, 214:731–734.)

then, the federal government has initiated a more significant program. The previous failure to develop a reasonable program in this area had little to do with the potential researchability of the field or the promise of new developments. In the past decade, the concentrated efforts and attention devoted to attacking paralytic polio, in contrast to feeble efforts in closing gaps in infant mortality, must be understood within the context that the incidence of polio was higher in the middle classes than in the lower classes.[14] The areas receiving official recognition and attention depend, in large part, on the ability of affected groups to make their needs known and to organize in order to stimulate official response. In this context, the problems that most affect the poor have less public visibility and less impact on political and administrative processes. Clearly, we must give more attention to considering how social priorities are determined and how the needs of those less vocal or sophisticated can be properly weighed against the claims of other groups.

Some Aspects of the Relationship Between Social Inequality and Health

Inequalities in health and health care develop in a variety of ways. I can appreciate that when the needs are so pressing, one becomes impatient with subtle distinctions in theory and concept. Such distinctions, however, are helpful and it is necessary to understand them in effectively closing the gaps in accessibility to health care and differential health status. Whatever our aspirations might be, there are no indications that in the near future we will experience a radical transformation in our values, our economic system, or in the distribution of wealth; and thus we must anticipate attacking the problems of health in an arena of scarce resources. The resources that become available must be used effectively in closing the gaps that we know exist and in preventing the further occurrence of differentials in areas where preventive intervention has some possibilities for success.

It is widely appreciated that the relationship between poverty and health status is part of a vicious cycle. Illness and disability are major causes of dependency and low socioeconomic status,[15] and traditionally the lower income of the poor has limited their opportunities to receive services to increase their functional capacities and, indirectly, their income potential. Although in recent years the Medicaid program has improved the medical care situation of many poor persons, it is generally true that rehabilitation of the functional capacity of the ill and disabled is an underdeveloped aspect of our entire health care system, and frequently adequate services are just not available. In addition, persons who are seriously disabled and visibly handicapped are exposed to various forms of discrimination in employment as well as in other life areas, and often cannot use the skills and education they have because of arbitrary exclusion from the work force. Much social legislation for health services in the United States is oriented toward the irreversibly disabled (the deserving unfortunate), and frequently persons who are rehabilitable cannot receive public support for rehabilitation without first becoming indigent. Thus, social legislation often produces incentives against rehabilitation and gainful employment, and our social ethos defines the ill and disabled as lesser citizens.

Although the literature is uncertain concerning the relationships between the occurrence of disease and socioeconomic status—and, of course, this varies from disease to disease—it is clear and unequivocal that when the poor become ill, they suffer consequences more serious than those experienced by more affluent classes. The poor are less likely to receive adequate treatment, are more likely to come into treatment during more advanced stages of their illness, and are more likely to experience persistent morbidity and disability.[16–18*] Moreover, the social position of the poor exposes them to lesser social protection for themselves and their families in that their jobs are generally less secure, they have less income to tide them through a serious illness, they are less protected by sick leave and other social arrangements, their illness is more likely to impinge on the performance of their work, and their living environment is less conducive to recovery and freedom from worry. The consequences of illness for the poor make illness a more frightening and disruptive experience, and probably encourage denial of illness and reluctance to enter treatment during its less evident stages of development.[19]

I raise these issues, in part, because the problems characteristic of the cultural orientations and inclinations of the poor-sick for receiving medi-

* This conclusion has as its basis a wide variety of studies which demonstrate greater chronicity and disability among the poor. Although it is difficult to find studies that compare the poor and more affluent on chronicity who have suffered from similar morbidity incidents, the general consistency in the literature supports the overall conclusion. There is evidence, however, that government programs in recent years have significantly increased the access of the physician for the poor, and as access to health services improves among the poor, we might anticipate some reduction in disability days. Bice and Eichhorn, in reviewing utilization trends, have found that average use of physician services among those with lowest incomes has increased in recent years. (T. W. Bice and R. L. Eichhorn, 1971, "Socioeconomic Status and the Use of Physicians' Services." Paper presented to the American Public Health Association, Minneapolis, Minnesota.) Recent data on access to more specialized services or the quality of care are not available.

cal care must be understood within the existential situation they face. When some segments of the poor come into contact with large medical bureaucracies, professionals often define their behavior as ill-adapted, and complain of the difficulties of delivering necessary health services to the poor. The poor, of course, are in no sense monolithic, and it is dangerous and misleading to offer generalizations about them as a special class. Yet a variety of studies have shown that one more frequently finds among the poor tendencies which make them less receptive to preventive care, less likely to conform to medical regimen, less oriented toward taking precautions necessary to maintain their health, less informed about health matters, and the like.[20-22] To some extent, such responses reflect limited education, cultural and social deprivation, apathy and neglect, and fear. The responses also indicate the experience of the poor with impersonal medical institutions, inconsiderate personnel, and resulting humiliation. But such tendencies also reflect a problem of fit between social institutions developed by middle class Americans with middle class concepts that are not adaptive or sensitive to the special difficulties the poor may have in accommodating to such forms of delivery of health care.[23] In agreeing that there is a great deal more that can be done in structuring preventive and other services so that those in need of them find them more compatible with their orientations and understandings, we must also recognize that there are significant differences in the manner in which populations orient themselves to health and health institutions, and that such differences cannot all be explained by the lack of commitment, interest, or other limitations of health personnel.* The poor have special needs and problems that must be taken into account, but in any situation of scarcity of personnel and other resources, health facilities similarly face serious operational difficulties. We know that many medical and social programs oriented toward the poor and disabled frequently end up servicing those with lesser need. Such programs can be structured so that they are more responsive to the hard-core poor and disabled, but it is unlikely that the problems of providing access and service can be remedied if we underestimate the degree to which the client's orientations and reactions may be an important barrier to bringing about some reasonable fit. It is only when we recognize such facts that we begin to develop programs and procedures that overcome them.

* There is a rather vigorous dispute in the behavioral sciences as to the existence of a "culture of poverty." Existing evidence would suggest that although some poor tend to have orientations that exacerbate their condition and interfere with successful coping, the argument is frequently overstated. For a middle position, see S. Parker, and R. J. Kleiner, 1970, "The Culture of Poverty: An Adjustive Dimension." *American Anthropologist,* 72:516–527.

Inequality and Mortality

The reduction of mortality, improvement of longevity, and the maintenance of a high level of health status is largely the result of improvements in nutrition, housing, sanitation, and the quality of life.[1,24] At the present time, the major causes of mortality and morbidity in the population—such problems as heart disease, cancer, stroke, accidents, mental disorders, and the like—are not impressively affected by medicine as it is practiced, and much of the medical care provided is ameliorative and supportive. Such care is important and should not be disparaged, but a realistic attack on the problem of health must recognize the true potentialities and limitations of medical practice. Similarly, major problems of health among the disadvantaged young—such as drug addiction—have not been easily amenable to medical control, and much of the solution to these problems may lie outside the traditional practice of medicine. Moreover, the unhappiness and the despair of the old, abandoned in their later years without function or status, or the alienation of the young depend more on social values and conditions generally than on the activities of health workers. I raise these issues because many of the problems of health related to inequality will not be simply responsive to the expansion of services, but require a more profound recasting of social values, practices, and priorities. This will demand efforts more pervasive than those that can be mustered by the health sector alone.

In this essay, I shall restrict my attention to efforts possible through the health sector as it is traditionally seen with the understanding that health does not operate in a vacuum, but is responsive to the larger forces that shape society and people's lives.

The most persistent and impressive inequality in the health care area is the disparity between white and nonwhite infant mortality in the United States. Such differences are extremely large; the nonwhite rate has been almost double the white rate for some years, and although both whites and nonwhites have made progress in recent decades, the gap itself has persisted and has even given evidence of increasing. In 1968 the nonwhite rate was 34.5 deaths per 1000 live births in contrast to a rate of 19.2 among whites.* Even the white rate is considerably higher than the prevailing rate in several other highly developed industrialized coun-

---

* Estimates by the National Center for Health Statistics for 1969 and 1970 indicate white rates of 18.4 and 17.4 and nonwhite rates of 31.6 and 31.4. See *Monthly Vital Statistics Report,* Provisional Statistics, September, 1971, Annual Summary for the United States, 1970. Public Health Service. Washington: U. S. Government Printing Office.

tries, and excluding nonwhites from the total would not change our position substantially. Thus, although the factors leading to infant death in America are exaggerated among nonwhites, they exist generally and contribute to what might be regarded as an excessive rate of infant death.

The factors affecting infant mortality are intertwined in a complex web, and it is not easy to isolate one or another factor as a major determinant. The opportunity of a new infant to survive is affected by the stature and health of the mother, which is in turn affected by her early nutrition and development, which may be a product of her social background, the economic status of her family, and so on.[25] Similarly, socioeconomic status is associated with the rate of illegitimate births, parity of the mother, age at the time of childbearing, quality of medical care received, and the like. Much of the data on which national trends are ascertained are collected in a fashion that does not allow for a detailed description of the manner in which these variables relate to one another, but further information is obtained from studies restricted to more limited populations.

The best predictor of infant survival is the birth weight of the infant which is correlated with the period of gestation, but there are significant variations in average weight at any gestation stage. The rate of infant mortality among infants weighing five and a half pounds or less at birth is seventeen times the rate among infants with higher weights at birth. In the first four weeks, the ratio is thirty to one. The experience of low-weight infants who survive the early period following birth continues to involve high risk. Low-weight infants who survive also have a high risk of such disorders as mental retardation, cerebral palsy, and epilepsy.[26, 27]*

Low-weight infants are more likely to be born to mothers who are under 15 years of age, nonwhite, of lower socioeconomic status, of less education, and among those who smoke. Current statistics suggest that low-weight nonwhite infants have a slightly better chance of survival than white infants of comparable weight,[28] but it is not clear whether this is a true advantage or whether it is a product of classification variations or differences in gestation of infants at comparable weight. In any case, it is reasonably clear that low-weight infants who constitute less than 10 per cent of all births are a group at special risk, and it is imperative that this population receive effective prenatal and postnatal care and other types of health services. It is not clear, however, how this group can be most effectively identified.

---

* I have depended heavily in this section on H. Chase's very excellent review of the demographic evidence.

There are a variety of other factors correlated with the occurrence of infant mortality, but none of these has an effect as large as birth weight. These factors include race, parity, maternal age, socioeconomic status, and illegitimacy. Although maternal age and parity are important, the combination of the limited influence of such variables, and the limited extent to which extreme values on these variables are characteristic of birth, results in a very small total impact on the overall rate of infant mortality.[27] It seems unlikely that a coherent public policy can be built around such risks.

The situation is somewhat different among nonwhites, the poor, and illegitimate births and, of course, these three categories are associated with one another. Among both whites and nonwhites, the absence of a father recorded on the birth certificate is associated with a marked increase in rates of infant mortality and, similarly, one finds among both whites and nonwhites highest infant mortality in the lowest occupational groups. This social status effect is not uniform or clearcut, and it is apparent that certain cultural patterns and behavior can support a low infant mortality rate even in relatively impoverished circumstances.[29] The crucial point, however, is that extreme poverty is often associated with a pattern of living and orientations that involve extremely high risks of infant mortality, and this argues very strongly for particular attention to such high risk areas which insure the development of adequate patterns of prenatal, maternal, and child care.

It is reasonably clear that well-organized public health efforts, associated with improvement in the overall life conditions of the poorest segments of our population, can result in a substantial decrease in the magnitude of infant mortality in the United States. It is extremely difficult to estimate specifically what constitutes a reasonable reduction in infant mortality given the tremendous variations characteristic of the living environments and cultures of the United States. Speaking relatively conservatively, I see no good reason why the national rate cannot in the coming years be reduced to a level of 15 or 16 deaths per 1000 live births, which is higher than the present rate in Sweden.*

The low rate of infant mortality, characteristic of the Scandinavian countries, is probably attributable to a variety of factors: the relatively limited variations in the social status of the population, biological char-

---

* In 1967, the United States ranked fourteenth in the world in favorable infant mortality experience with an overall rate of 22.4. The rate in Sweden was 12.9. There are many who are skeptical about statistics from other countries. One, however, need look no further than variations within the United States. Communities vary widely, some as low as Sweden; other communities in the same states have rates three or four times as high.

acteristics of the population, the cultural homogeneity and development of the countries involved, the well-organized social services, and particularly those in relation to child and maternal care. These countries place a high value on child and maternal health, and have well-developed public programs to insure a satisfactory outcome of pregnancy.

Although the experience of other countries is instructive and useful, there are usually wide gaps in culture and traditions from one society to the next, and it is particularly instructive to seek evidence from situations that are as comparable as possible to the circumstances for which one wishes to design programs. Although there is not a great deal of carefully collected data relevant to the issue at hand, we have some evidence from the United States relevant to the relationship between infant mortality and the delivery of health services.

Some valuable data result from a study comparing rates of mortality among subscribers to the Health Insurance Plan of New York (HIP), a large prepaid group practice program in New York City, in comparison to women in the general population of New York City.[30,31]* This study involving live births, fetal deaths, and infant deaths from 1955 to 1957 was executed carefully and with considerable attention to possible intervening factors that could affect the results. The investigators found that a higher proportion of the women in HIP initiated their prenatal care in the first trimester of pregnancy and that prematurity and perinatal mortality rates were lower than in New York City as a whole. When the New York City comparison sample was restricted to women delivered in a hospital by a private doctor, the difference in proportions of women seeking prenatal care was eliminated. HIP still retained a small advantage in respect to prematurity and perinatal mortality rates. This analysis took account of differences in demographic characteristics between HIP women and women in the city as a whole and other possible biasing factors.

The HIP study is suggestive, but one might reasonably suspect that persons choosing to obtain their care from a prepaid group, regardless of economic status, are somewhat more interested in their health, more knowledgeable about health matters, and the like, and thus it is difficult to generalize from this study to particularly high risk subgroups of the population. The HIP study did show clearly that among both whites and nonwhites, women using general ward services did considerably worse than women using either HIP or private physicians in New York City.

---

* Similar findings on improved outcomes for the indigent aged are reported by S. Shapiro, *et al.*, 1967, "Patterns of Medical Use by the Indigent Aged Under Two Systems of Medical Care." *American Journal of Public Health*, **57**:784–790. For a general review of such end result measurement studies, see S. Shapiro, 1967, "End Result Measurements of Quality Medical Care." *Milbank Memorial Fund Quarterly*, **45**:7–30.

These results are attributable probably to a variety of factors: selective factors both in terms of socioeconomic status and health risk among those using ward services, differing degrees of health consciousness in this group, and the fragmented and ineffective character of the New York City ward services relative to the problem. In New York City as a whole, at the time, 61 per cent of white women were found to obtain prenatal care, primarily from private physicians. Among nonwhites and Puerto Ricans, the comparable statistics were 16 per cent and 13 per cent. Although the use of such services among white women increased only slightly within HIP, very large improvements took place among nonwhite and Puerto Rican women in HIP. The nonwhite percentage went from 16 per cent to 55 per cent, and the Puerto Rican percentage increased from 13 per cent to 48 per cent. Although these data are suggestive, we have no way of ascertaining how representative nonwhite and Puerto Rican women in HIP were of all nonwhite and Puerto Rican women.

Some very suggestive data are available from the City of Denver, Colorado, where in the period from 1964 to 1969 the Department of Health and Hospitals has developed a coordinated system of health services for the poorest areas of the city to attempt to meet the health needs of this population. Among the services provided were a neighborhood health center, conveniently located health stations, and more specialized clinic and hospital facilities. The program utilized specially trained nurses to assist physicians as well as a variety of workers from the areas serviced who received special training. Data are available comparing Denver's twenty-five lower socioeconomic ranked census tracts served by these new programs with the remaining census tracts in the city. In 1964 the twenty-five lowest tracts had an infant mortality rate of 34.2 as compared with a rate of 23.5 in the remaining tracts. In the twenty-five lowest tracts, the infant mortality rate decreased from 34.2 in 1964 to 21.5 in 1969. Rates of postneonatal mortality decreased from 11.3 in 1964 to 7.3 in 1969. Among the remaining tracts, infant deaths declined from 23.5 in 1964 to 19.7 in 1969. By 1969 infant mortality differences between the least favored socioeconomic tracts and other tracts had been largely eliminated (information received from the Denver Department of Health and Hospitals). Although we would want to know a great deal more about other changes that took place in these census tracts and the specific relationships between changes in services and reductions in infant mortality, these gross data suggest that it is possible to significantly reduce infant mortality. Similar findings have been reported by O.E.O. neighborhood health centers established in poor underserviced areas.

Mortality among adults also varies significantly by race and socioeconomic status. At almost every age, nonwhites and the poor suffer a higher risk of mortality; and, overall, adult rates of mortality in the

United States lag behind other nations as well.[32] Although the trends are approximately similar to the situation described relevant to infant mortality, it is more difficult to provide evidence that these differentials can be markedly influenced by changes in the organization of medical care rather than more basic changes in the life circumstances of the poor.

There are no doubt circumstances where, for example, the lack of availability of medical facilities decreases the longevity of nonwhites and the poor relative to whites and those better off—for example, such as access to good medical care following a heart attack—but much of the differential is a product of more embracing life disadvantages that the poor must face. Just as it is difficult to specify precisely the effects of medical care in general relative to other life forces, so it is difficult to specify how much specific gain can be achieved through better medical services as compared with a decent job, adequate housing, and a neighborhood free of the pathologies of drug addiction, alcoholism, and alienation. Improved access to medical care for all does not necessarily depend on any particular assessment of impact but can be based on a concept of social justice. Medical care is an important right as much because people see it as such as it is because of its specific impacts on the health of the population.

Some Notes on Forms of Health Care Delivery and the Poor

Much of the problem of bringing health care services to the poor involves eliminating economic barriers to care and providing the required manpower and facilities for providing adequate care. There is evidence that suggests that major gaps in care can be closed if such conditions are fulfilled in a reasonable way.* The utilization of health services, of

---

* In general, there is evidence that systems that eliminate economic barriers to care are able to close the gap in medical utilization between the poor and the more affluent (A. Cartwright, 1967, *Patients and Their Doctors: A Study of General Practice*. London: Routledge and Kegan Paul). Making available comprehensive services apparently leads to a higher level of utilization which cannot be accounted for by trivial and unnecessary uses of services (B. Darsky, N. Sinai, and S. Axelrod, 1958, "Problem in Voluntary Insurance: Some Answers from the Windsor Experience." *American Journal of Public Health*, **48**:971–978). A recent study of the Tufts-Columbia Point Health Center in Boston found that when economic barriers were removed, and attractive and convenient services were provided, the average rate of utilization of low income persons was considerably higher than for the population as a whole (S. Bellin and H. J. Geiger, 1970, "Actual Public Acceptance of the Neighborhood Health Center by the Urban Poor." *Journal of the A.M.A.*, **214**:2147–2153). For a general comparison of health care in the United States with health care in England, where economic barriers have been largely eliminated, see Chapter XI.

course, will also depend on social and cultural orientations toward the types of care provided, the manner in which care is organized, and the responsiveness of health personnel to medical consumers. Access to medical care decreases as costs increase, and costs must be measured not only in money terms, but also in terms of time, inconvenience, distance, embarrassment, or whatever.

Traditionally the poor, particularly in large cities, have depended very heavily on public clinics and outpatient departments for their care. Data collected during the interval of July 1965 to June 1967 indicate that physician visits in the United States no longer show any large variation by socioeconomic status, although nonwhites continue to have a lower level of utilization than whites among both men and women (age-adjusted data).[33] Also, the children of the more affluent receive more physician services than those in families with more modest incomes.[34]* Overall, the change in the trend suggests that new programs for the medically indigent have had some impact on their rate of utilization of services which in the period from July 1965 to June 1967 resembled the level characteristic of the nation as a whole, but major gaps in access to medical care appear in many places, as the data on white-nonwhite differences suggest. There is also evidence that differences in the basic pattern of use of services continue to persist. While approximately 8 per cent of whites received their medical care at emergency rooms or hospital clinics, more than one-quarter of nonwhites received their care in such locations. Nonwhites with incomes of $7000 or more, however, were more likely than other nonwhites to see the physician in his office.[33] The medical significance of this varying pattern of care is in dispute, with some experts suggesting that the pattern of care available in large outpatient departments of teaching hospitals is superior to that available from private physicians in their offices. There may be some merit to this view but, as Duff and Hollingshead have so dramatically indicated, the potentialities for good technical medical care are not the same as high quality health care.[9]†

---

* In the period from July 1966 to June 1967, among children under age 17, whites averaged 3.9 physician visits a year and nonwhites averaged 2.0 visits a year. Among children with family incomes of less than $3000 the average was 2.5 visits, while among those with $7000 or more the average was 4.1 visits. Data collected for the period from July 1963 to June 1964, indicate that 66 per cent of nonwhite children under 17 had never seen a dentist, and 62 per cent of those with family incomes of less than $3000 were in a similar situation. The comparable figure among white children was 39 per cent.

† This pattern is not unique to the United States (Ann Cartwright, 1964, *Human Relations and Hospital Care*. London: Routledge and Kegan Paul; and G. Forsyth and F. L. Logan, 1968, *Gateway or Dividing Line: A Study of Hospital Out-Patients in the 1960's*. New York: Oxford University Press).

Those with less knowledge and sophistication in particular, but probably all of us as well, require more than the episodic and fragmented care characteristic of the large hospital outpatient clinics. Although the well-educated and sophisticated consumers of medical care complain about the growing impersonality of care and the lack of responsiveness of medical personnel, such persons are often able to exploit existing resources through their aggressiveness, their ability to obtain information, and their demands for respect and courtesy. Those who are less sophisticated and assertive, because of lack of education or cultural orientations, are frequently confused and intimidated by the vastness and complexity of the large medical bureaucracy, and by the interchangeability of people and roles. The poor family with multiple difficulties, in particular, must deal with a variety of agencies and personnel to obtain needed care involving great time, patience, and initiative. Not only is the location of such care fragmented and confused but, frequently, no serious attempt is made to coordinate services or to deal with the array of health problems in its family context or in any relationship to one another. No matter how good any particular service may appear, when poorly coordinated, the overall pattern of care may be inferior and poorly fitted to the needs or social conditions of the persons involved.

The Crisis in Health Care and Its Relationship to the Problems of the Poor

The present crisis in health care stems from the inability of the health sector to accommodate effectively to the developments in medical knowledge and technology, the growth of more specialized activity, resulting failures in providing comprehensive and coordinated care, and rising aspirations for more and better health care. As the medical product becomes more valuable, and as the population becomes more sophisticated, more people seek services; and those who have been traditionally without equal access feel the lack of availability of services more acutely. Thus the crisis results from internal changes in the health sector, changing demographic and social aspects of the population, a redefinition of the role of medical care and its relevance on the part of the population, and the resulting increased demand, problems of cost and financing, and inflation in the medical care sector.

The growing sense of crisis is the product of various forces that have differentially affected varying interest groups in the population. Those in the urban ghettos and rural areas acutely feel their lack of access to physicians and other health services and demand change so that their needs can be met. Government officials, representatives of insurance companies, labor, and management are all alarmed at the growing escalation of medical care costs and the difficulties in stemming the inflationary tide that affect their programs and have financial implications for them. The providers—the hospitals, medical schools, clinics, and the like—are similarly concerned with growing costs, and particularly seek greater reimbursement or other more attractive financial arrangements. The average person is increasingly concerned about changing patterns of practice characterized by impersonality and bureaucracy, the difficulty of finding a personal physician who is responsive to his concerns, and alarm at the growing difficulty of obtaining a reasonable level of service at a price he can afford.

Although one might wish that the movement toward reorganization of medical services and National Health Insurance were based on a growing consciousness of social justice and an increased compassion for the plight of the poor, the fact is that this is only a subsidiary theme in what most centrally is a concern with costs and efficiency. As health care prices have risen, and as demands for care on the manpower pool have become more intense, federal and state officials have been concerned with establishing a ceiling on the uncontrollable costs of medical care within the programs they finance. Similarly, various third parties find that they must persistently increase their premiums to meet expenses resulting in continuing criticism from the public. It is this type of generalized concern that has stimulated much of the apparent activity, and if one considers the types of solutions being seriously entertained it is fairly apparent that they apply to the needs of traditional interest groups as much, if not more, than the special health needs of the poor.

Problems of Financing Health Care

Although existing problems have been recognized for some time, they have been highlighted in the past few years. Few public commentators anticipated the inflationary impact of Medicare and Medicaid on the health services sector, nor was it appreciated to what extent rising costs under these programs in the context of other public expenditures would strain federal and state budgets encouraging re-examination of the entire issue of medical care. To some extent the growing costs reflected the buildup of need among the aged and the poor for medical services but, more acutely, it demonstrated that to invest in medical care without attempting to rationalize and organize health services delivery would be costly and only marginally successful. Attention has now moved from the earlier focus on providing assistance to special needy groups to means of providing health care in a more efficient and structured way.

The Physician Shortage and the Crisis of Manpower

A prerequisite for effective health care is a reasonable quantity and distribution of facilities and manpower. The need for facilities and manpower is dependent, of course, on a variety of factors: how well they are distributed in the population, the patterns of need existing, the patterns of health service utilization in the population, and the like. Although the usual indicator of availability of manpower is the number available relative to some unit in the population, such figures can be highly deceptive since they often mask the factors described above. Moreover, such figures do not take into account such crucial matters as the types of tasks performed, relative efficiency in performing them, and the distribution of activities generally. Manpower shortages may result from too few professionals, from uneven distribution of professionals from one area to another, from uneven task allocation among professionals, and between professionals and ancillary workers, or from any combination of these factors.

In recent years there has been a slight increase in the number of physicians available relative to the size of the American population. For example, from 1950 to 1960 there were approximately 150 doctors per 100,000 population including doctors in nonpatient care activities. By 1967 this figure had risen to 158.[35] The increase has been sustained by some growth in the number of medical school graduates, but it is also the product of significantly relying on manpower trained by foreign medical schools who may often have significant handicaps in their medical training, the understanding of English, and appreciation of the patient's cultural patterns. If physicians not delivering patient care are excluded from these totals, then there were 132 physicians per 100,000 population in the United States in 1967. Even using such large aggregates as states, one finds enormous variation from one unit to another, ranging from 320 nonfederal physicians providing patient care per 100,000 population in Washington, D. C., and 203 in New York state to 69 in Mississippi and 75 in Alabama.[35]

Such aggregates, however, are highly misleading since doctors tend to concentrate in metropolitan areas and in suburbs. There are, for example, almost four times as many doctors in metropolitan areas per unit population as there are in isolated rural areas. If one considers more meaningful units, more closely fitted to the distances within which people can reasonably seek medical care, such discrepancies become enormous. For example, in urban ghettos such as East Garfield, Chicago, there are 13 physicians for 63,000 residents while in Kenwood-Oakland, Chicago, 5 physicians serve 45,400 blacks.[36] A similar situation exists relative to many rural communities. Even these data do not reflect the magnitude of the problem in that doctors in ghettos and rural areas tend to be older than the average, and it is clear that even the few that exist are not being replaced when they die or retire.

Similar problems exist relative to most other health personnel, although the rates of such personnel are more easily enlarged. A notable exception is dentistry, where the dentist-patient ratio has not changed in the past two decades, being 57 in 1950, and 56 in 1967. In considering these ratios, it is important to recognize that dentistry is usually given relatively low priority compared to other health services, and that it is only recently that we have begun to be concerned with inadequacies in the distribution of dental care. As people become more affluent, they are more able to afford dental care and more likely to seek it, yet it is ironic that a commensurate increase in the number of dentists has not accompanied growing demand for dental care. Dentists have learned to practice with greater efficiency in recent years, many making use of dental assistants, and thus the situation may not be quite as bleak as it appears—but it is bleak nevertheless. National data show that many Americans receive very poor dental care, and the pattern of dental care is clearly and substantially related to race and socioeconomic status.[37]

The basic problems of distribution of health manpower in general are similar to those involving doctors. Although there were 313 employed registered nurses in the United States per 100,000 population in 1967, these rates varied from 157 in Mississippi to 536 in Connecticut.[35] Many types of health personnel are largely hospital-based in their activities, and their pattern of distribution follows the pattern of location of hospitals. But even when hospitals exist, they often face problems in recruiting doctors, nurses, and other highly skilled manpower when they are in urban ghettos and more isolated areas.

The physical location of doctors and other personnel is only part of the distribution difficulties. A major aspect of the problem, which has been creating increasing dissatisfaction in recent years, has been the manner in which health tasks have been distributed between doctors and among the health professions in general. Although the total pool of doctors relative to the population has been increasing, the number and proportion of doctors delivering primary medical care have been steadily decreasing. General practitioners are increasingly becoming defunct, and now constitute less than one-quarter of all doctors. A more realistic estimate of the availability of primary care physicians is to consider not only general practitioners but also internists and pediatricians, the latter taking considerable responsibility for primary health services. But even these figures are discouraging. In 1931 there were 94 primary care physicians per 100,000 population. This rate has shown a continuing trend downward to 89 in 1940, 75 in 1949, 60 in 1957, and 50 in 1965.[38] The downward trend is probably continuing.

It is somewhat surprising to find that the largest component of the medical profession is in the surgical specialties, and their size relative to the rest has been increasing, now accounting for approximately one-third of all specialists.[39, 40] The largest group among the surgeons is the general surgeons, and they are in competition as well with general practitioners and others who also perform some surgery. One overall effect of this concentration of surgically inclined doctors is the completion of a high rate of surgical activity relative to other health care activities.[41, 42]

Providing Health Services for the Poor

More recently, there has been an outpouring of analyses on the health care crisis. The typical discussion concludes with the recommendation that the solution to these problems lies in the development of widespread prepaid group practice, preventive care and health maintenance, and the use of a variety of new paramedical personnel as well as more effective use of those already in evidence. I do not wish to belittle these recommendations for there is much in their favor. But we should be aware that the central feature in current discussions of health care has continued to be the growing cost of services. As such costs have risen, they have put pressure on many different interest groups who together make up a powerful force in political affairs. As government through an incremental process has assumed payment for a greater proportion of the costs of medical care for the old and the poor, resulting inflation in the health care area and higher taxes has aroused many middle class consumers and has put considerable financial pressures on state finances as well as on the federal treasury.

Although the health problems of the poor are of concern to governmental and other groups, these interests are only part of the larger set of interests which are coalescing and forming a countervailing force against more traditional interests in the health field. It is not at all clear from current discussions how well the poor will do within the context of the types of reforms generally being advocated, but it is reasonably clear that in the absence of general reforms of our health care system, which bring benefits to many segments of the American population, the benefits provided to the poor will be unequal to the scope of the problems they face. It is already clear from the Medicaid program that coverage for the poor or near-poor will be fragmentary and uneven from area to area if the approach is a categorical one and if it is heavily dependent on tax support from the states and localities.

In the last analysis, we must recognize that the health care problems of the poor are a product of the larger sociopolitical system and of the more general organization of health care services in America. As long as these problems are seen as nothing more than slight maladjustments of what is basically a constructive approach to meeting the health needs of the country, it is unlikely that an adequate solution will be found. The poor are not a sufficiently powerful interest group to effectively compete in the establishment of priorities or in the distribution of available facilities, manpower, and services. Moreover, the problems of health care are only one part of a more complex pattern of social, economic, and environmental difficulties. It appears then that the health care needs of the poor can most constructively be met within a larger and more basic reconstruction of health care institutions in America, which insure access to medical care for all and which establish a minimal level of health service available irrespective of social status or geographic area. It is doubtful that this can be achieved without greater direction over professional behavior. Access to care for all is available elsewhere in the world and under social and economic circumstances that pose greater pressure on national resources. The fact that the United States has still failed to achieve such modest goals is shameful. But even when we do, we will have hardly begun to face the underlying conditions that make the plight of the poor so difficult and their pathologies so prevalent. These problems will require a more frontal attack on our national values, our priorities, and our system of social stratification itself.

Notes

1. Mechanic, D. (1968). *Medical Sociology: A Selective View*. New York: Free Press.
2. Kosa, J., A. Antonovsky, and I. Zola (eds.) (1969). *Poverty and Health: A Sociological Analysis*. Cambridge: Harvard University Press.
3. Norman, J. C. (ed.) (1969). *Medicine in the Ghetto*. New York: Appleton, Century, Crofts.
4. Medical and Health Research Association of New York (1967). *Poverty and Health in the United States: A Bibliography with Abstracts*. New York: Medical and Health Research Association.
5. Dohrenwend, Bruce, and Barbara Dohrenwend (1969). *Social Status and Psychological Disorder*. New York: Wiley.

6. National Center for Health Statistics (1970a). *Annotated Bibliography on Vital and Health Statistics*. PHS Publication No. 2094. Washington: U. S. Government Printing Office; (1970b) *The Health of Children*—1970. PHS Publication No. 2121. Washington: U. S. Government Printing Office.

7. Ferman, L., J. Kornbluh, and A. Haber (eds.) (1968). *Poverty in America*. Revised Edition. Ann Arbor: University of Michigan Press.

8. Handler, J. (1972). *Reforming the Poor: Welfare Policy, Federalism, and Morality*. New York: Basic Books.

9. Duff, R., and A. Hollingshead (1968). *Sickness and Society*. New York: Harper.

10. McNerney, W. (1970). "Why Does Medical Care Cost So Much?" *New England Journal of Medicine*, **282**:1458–1466.

11. Ginzberg, E. (1966). "Physician Shortage Reconsidered." *New England Journal of Medicine*, **275**:85–87.

12. Ginzberg, E. (1969). *Men, Money, and Medicine*. New York: Columbia University Press.

13. Mechanic, D. (1969). *Mental Health and Social Policy*. Englewood Cliffs, N. J.: Prentice Hall.

14. Simmons, O. G. (1958). "Social Status and Public Health." Social Science Research Council Pamphlet No. 13.

15. Lawrence, P. S. (1958). "Chronic Illness and Socio-Economic Status." In E. G. Jaco (ed.), *Patients, Physicians, and Illness*. New York: Free Press.

16. Hollingshead, A., and F. Redlich (1958). *Social Class and Mental Illness*. New York: Wiley.

17. National Center for Health Statistics. See various publications from Public Health Service, Series No. 10. Washington: U. S. Government Printing Office.

18. Howard, J. (1965). "Race Differences in Hypertension Mortality Trends: Differential Drug Exposure as a Theory." *Milbank Memorial Fund Quarterly*, **43**:202–218.

19. Koos, E. (1954). *The Health of Regionsville: What the People Thought and Did About It*. New York: Columbia University Press.

20. Rosenstock, I. (1969). "Prevention of Illness and Maintenance of Health." In J. Kosa, A. Antonovsky, and I. Zola (eds.), *Poverty and Health: A Sociological Analysis*. Cambridge: Harvard University Press.

21. Mechanic, D. (1969). "Illness and Cure." In J. Kosa, A. Antonovsky and I. Zola (eds.), Poverty and Health: A Sociological Analysis. Cambridge: Harvard University Press.

22. Green, L. (1970). *Status Identity and Preventive Health Behavior*. Public Health Education Reports, **1**:13–53. Schools of Public Health: University of California-Berkeley; University of Hawaii-Honolulu.

23. Strauss, Anselm (1969). "Medical Organization, Medical Care, and Lower Income Groups." *Social Science and Medicine*, **3**:143–177.

24. McKeown, T. (1965). *Medicine in Modern Society*. London: Allen and Unwin.

25. Illsley, R. (1967). "The Sociological Study of Reproduction and Its Outcome." In Stephen Richardson and A. Guttmacher (eds.), *Childbearing: Social and Psychological Aspects*. Baltimore: Williams and Wilkins.

26. Birch, H., and J. Gussow (1970). *Disadvantaged Children: Health, Nutrition and School Failure*. New York: Harcourt, Brace and World.

27. Chase, H. (1970). "Influence of Selected Demographic, Sociologic, and Biologic Factors on Infant Mortality." Unpublished report prepared for the Board on Medicine, National Academy of Science.

28. Shapiro, S., E. Schlesinger, and R. L. Nesbitt, Jr. (1968). *Infant, Perinatal, and Childhood Mortality in the United States.* Cambridge: Harvard University Press.

29. Anderson, O. (1958). "Infant Mortality and Social and Cultural Factors: Historical Trends and Current Patterns." In E. G. Jaco (ed.), *Patients, Physicians, and Illness.* New York: Free Press.

30. Shapiro, S., L. Weiner, and P. M. Densen (1958). "Comparison of Prematurity and Perinatal Mortality in a General Population and in the Population of a Prepaid Group Practice Medical Care Plan." *American Journal of Public Health,* **48:**170–187.

31. Shapiro, S., H. Jacobziner, P. M. Densen, and L. Weiner (1960). "Further Observations on Prematurity and Perinatal Mortality in a General Population and in the Population of a Prepaid Group Practice Medical Care Plan." *American Journal of Public Health,* **50:**1304–1317.

32. Anderson, O. (1972). *Health Care: Can There Be Equity: The United States, Sweden and England.* New York: Wiley-Interscience.

33. National Center for Health Statistics (1969). *Differentials in Health Characteristics by Color—U. S., July 1965–June 1967.* PHS Series 10, No. 56. Washington: U. S. Government Printing Office.

34. National Center for Health Statistics (1968). *Volume of Physicians—U. S., July 1966–June 1967.* PHS Series 10, No. 49. Washington: U. S. Government Printing Office; (1970) *The Health of Children—1970.* PHS Publication No. 2121. Washington: U. S. Government Printing Office.

35. National Center for Health Statistics (1970). *Health Resource Statistics: Health Manpower and Health Facilities.* PHS Publication No. 1509. Washington: U. S. Government Printing Office.

36. Ferguson, L. A. (1970). "What Has Been Accomplished in Chicago?" In J. C. Norman (ed.), *Medicine in the Ghetto.* New York: Appleton, Century, Crofts.

37. National Center for Health Statistics (1965). *Volume of Dental Visits: U. S.— July 1963–June 1964.* PHS Series 10, Washington: U. S. Government Printing Office; (1966) *Dental Visits: Time Interval Since Last Visit, U. S.—July 1964–June 1965.* PHS Series 10. Washington: U. S. Government Printing Office.

38. Fein, R. (1967). *The Doctor Shortage: An Economic Analysis.* Washington, D. C.: The Brookings Institution.

39. Stevens, R. (1971). "Trends in Medical Specialization in the United States." *Inquiry,* **8:**9–19.

40. American Medical Association (1970). *Distribution of Physicians, Hospitals, and Hospital Beds in the United States, Vol. 1.* Chicago: Department of Survey Research.

41. Bunker, J. P. (1970). "Surgical Manpower: A Comparison of Operations of Surgeons in the United States and England and Wales." *New England Journal of Medicine,* **282:**135–144.

42. Lewis, C. (1969). "Variations in the Incidence of Surgery." *New England Journal of Medicine,* **281:**880–884.

CHAPTER VI

A Note on the Concept of "Health Maintenance Organizations"

The largest proportion of ordinary medical practice takes place outside the hospital, and there are strong economic reasons to minimize the unnecessary use of inpatient hospital care. Screening and allocating patients to various facilities and caring for the more common and less complicated conditions constitute the major functions of the general practice of medicine. However, as medicine has advanced on a scientific and technological level, it has become less clear how to properly organize these functions and to fit them appropriately within the larger context of care and make them consistent with the scientific stance encouraged by modern medical developments.

As noted earlier in this book, the typical adaptation to the growing complexity of scientific medicine has been increased specialization, but its overelaboration has produced new strains and difficulties which may outweigh its advantages. Most clearly, there has been a significant failure with increasing specialization to coordinate the various aspects of medical care and to provide necessary services within reasonable economic limits. Wherever one travels in the Western world these problems are of concern, and countries varying widely in their ideologies are considering similar alternatives for a more organized, effective, and economical structure for providing as much of medical care as possible in ambulatory settings. The most frequently discussed alternatives tend to be health centers and prepaid group practice or, using more recent terminology, health maintenance organizations.

The Organization of Community Medical Practice in the United States

The solo practitioner and small partnership continue to constitute the basic framework of community medical practice, although in recent years a greater diversity of practice forms has appeared. Since 1950 the proportion of physicians in private practice has shifted from approximately three-fourths to three-fifths, and there has been extensive growth in the very small group practice base in recent years.[1] In 1959 there were only about 13,000 group practices, but by 1969 there were more than 40,000 such practices. The vast majority of these are very small and continue to constitute a relatively small proportion of the 340,000 medical practitioners in the United States. However, the annual increase has been substantial, averaging 18 per cent from 1959 to 1965, and 10 per cent from 1965 to 1969. It is also apparent that younger medical graduates are more oriented toward groups than in the past, and we can anticipate a steady development of the group practice trend.

Group practice as an innovation in medical care can be organized mainly for the convenience of the physician, for the purpose of providing a higher level of services for the patient, or both. For the most part, existing data suggest that such groups are presently organized more to serve physician advantage, and most such groups do not appear to offer services that are vastly different from those provided by solo practitioners or partnerships. Three-quarters of the groups in the United States have five or less doctors, and more than 90 per cent of the general practitioner groups have four or less doctors. The largest units tend to be multispecialty groups, but even here more than half include five or less physicians. A better indication of the capabilities of presently existing groups is suggested by their ratio of allied help to physicians. A well-organized health center might include as many as 6 to 10 other health workers for each physician, but the typical pattern in existing group practice is for a very low ratio of such workers per physician. On the average, groups in 1969 had 2.5 workers, and more than half of the total is accounted for by clerical, laboratory, and x-ray assistance. Only a very small proportion of the ancillary work force provides direct patient services of any kind. In short, most of the existing groups are variants on traditional patterns of providing health care.

The prepaid groups, which presently provide services to less than one-tenth of the population, appear to offer a greater variety of services to the consumer, but even here the picture seems to be dominated by the presence of a few very large practices, such as the Kaiser Plan on the West

Coast and the Health Insurance Plan of New York. Although the average size of prepaid groups is 16.5 physicians, the elimination of the giant prepaid practices brings the average to less than five physicians per group. It is significant to note that approximately three-quarters of the prepaid groups have eight or fewer physicians. Most of the research on prepaid group practice comes from the study of a few giants, which are in no sense representative of all such groups.

The Rationale for "Health Maintenance Organizations"

One of the major goals of several alternative proposals for National Health Insurance, and recent proposals for a Health Maintenance Organization alternative for Medicare recipients, is to increase the group organization of physicians and the extent of prepaid group practice. The basic justifications for such goals are based on the belief that group organization and prepayment improve the potentialities for the practice of scientific medicine, provide economies of scale in the use of medical technology and ancillary personnel, and, most important, result in a reduction in hospitalization and surgical rates and other expensive services. Group practice, it is argued, not only offers better technical facilities, easy availability of peer consultation, more efficient use of paraprofessionals and ancillary services, and the like, but also provides physicians additional benefits through regularized schedules, leisure time, and opportunities for continuing professional development.

The federal government, in putting emphasis on the HMO concept, cites the following arguments as its basic justification.

Because HMO revenues are fixed, their incentives are to keep patients well, for they benefit from patient well-days, not sickness. The entire cost structure is geared to preventing illness and, failing that, to promoting prompt recovery through the least costly services consistent with maintaining quality. In contrast with prevailing cost-plus insurance plans, the HMO's financial incentives encourage the least utilization of high cost forms of care, and also tend to limit unnecessary procedures.

HMO's provide settings for innovative teaching programs (using the entire team of health professionals and supporting personnel), as well as for continuing education programs for practitioners. They also provide a setting in which new technologies and management tools can be most effectively employed, in which the delegation of tasks from physicians to supporting personnel is encouraged, and in which close and constant professional review of performance will provide quality controls among colleagues.[2]

Although the advocates of HMO's cite Kaiser Permanente as the prototype of the kind of organization they have in mind, it is clear that the concept also contains some diversity of models varying significantly on several dimensions. The effectiveness of prepaid group practice may vary by size, the nature of group organization, the types of controls developed, the characteristics of doctors and patients who make up the organization, the proportion and use of ancillary health personnel, the level of technology, the comprehensiveness and innovativeness of its special programs, the priorities it gives to varying health programs, and many others. In considering the likely effects of HMO's there is a tendency to talk as if one would not anticipate considerable variations in their levels of performance. Although the concept, in my estimation, has considerable merit, it is ill-advised not to consider very carefully the diversity of variables that affect the performance of HMO's and the integrity of the data that are cited in their support.

Some Consideration of the Prototypes: Kaiser Permanente and the Health Insurance Plan of New York

Most of the organizational research and outcome studies that pertain to HMO's refer to the two major prototypes: Kaiser Permanente and the Health Insurance Plan of New York. Even these two models are somewhat different; most pertinent is the fact that Kaiser Permanente maintains its own hospital system while HIP does not. The Kaiser Permanente Plan is a voluntary plan of about 30 years duration encompassing approximately 2 million subscribers mostly on the West Coast. In planning for its facilities, Kaiser estimates that for every 100,000 subscribers it requires 180 hospital beds, 90 physicians organized in groups, 800 ancillary personnel, and approximately $12 million in capital investment. Ernest Saward,[3] former Medical Director of the Kaiser-Portland medical group, has noted the following important components of the Kaiser prepayment plan: (1) its nonprofit and self-sustaining status; (2) prepayment mechanisms based on community cost rating; (3) self-governing and autonomous group medical practices which contract with the prepayment organization on a capitation basis; (4) hospital-based group practice in institutions controlled by the Plan; (5) voluntary enrollment involving a choice between Kaiser and some alternative plan; (6) the concept of payment through capitation; (7) comprehensive services; and (8) the development of special programs.

The HIP of New York involves greater diversity, since it involves contracts with some thirty medical groups, some of which are hospital based. Enrollees in the prepayment plan are provided preventive, diagnostic, and treatment services, and hospital care is financed through a Blue Cross type policy. The medical groups tend to vary in size, but each includes physicians in twelve basic specialties, and approximately half of all physician services are provided by specialists. More specialized facilities are supported by HIP on a citywide basis. HIP is a less attractive national prototype than Kaiser because it does not control the hospitals it depends on, and it is believed that the incentives for economy that can be developed under such circumstances are considerably weaker than those at Kaiser where doctors can allegedly be penalized for excessive use of hospital facilities.

Despite the fact that these two models exaggerate desirable qualities characteristic of prepaid group practice, such as the range of specialty care available, a higher ratio of ancillary help per physician, and more specialized and innovative programs, the form of medical practice carried out in these groups does not appear to differ dramatically from more traditional forms of medical care in the community.[4] For the most part, these groups have not made major modification in the use of manpower, developed a more efficient utilization of physicians, nor emphasized a practice that is preventive and health maintaining as opposed to the typical pattern of caring for the sick. Although there have been experiments within these groups that encompassed innovative features relative to such goals,[5-8] generally the lofty object of medical groups organized around the goal of maintaining health is more honored in theory than in fact. Moreover, we cannot assume that those qualities that the prototypes have developed will inevitably develop in newly formed prepaid group practices. Not only are they larger than those most likely to develop but, as experiments, they may have attracted physicians and patients who shared a philosophical propensity toward group practice and a desire to make it work. As such practice encompasses a larger proportion of doctors, other health workers, and patients, we cannot assume that they will share such propensities. As prepaid practice comes to involve a larger pool of doctors, it may not be able to attract physicians with the same levels of competence and commitment that Kaiser and HIP have, thus far, been able to maintain.

In considering what can reasonably be expected from HMO's, we begin by assessing the implication suggested by its name that it has special capacity to maintain health and prevent illness. The basis of this alleged capacity comes from the assumed economic incentives that doctors have to keep people healthy, greater access among consumers to preventive services and early treatment, and new possibilities for innovative preventive health programs. It is maintained that because doctors wish to avoid the need for expensive treatments under capitation plans, they provide a range of preventive services that serve to keep people healthy, and that because of the prepaid aspect of the plan, patients seek preventive services and get treatment before their illnesses become advanced or chronic. The data to support these contentions are fragmentary, indeed, although there is some suggestion that the HIP has had advantages over other forms of practice.

The small differences found favoring HIP relative to more traditional practices must be taken seriously, but they may be a product of the special virtues of HIP in contrast to prepaid group practice in general. Moreover, these studies compared groups that elected to receive their care from HIP in contrast to alternative forms of care, and it is certainly conceivable that persons who elected to receive their care from HIP were more health conscious, were more attuned to preventive care, and the like. Thus it is not apparent whether prepaid care or the types of people attracted to such care is the more important factor in accounting for the differences found. But even more basic, if we are to assume that prepaid care maintains health by providing ready access to a variety of outpatient health services—thus negating the need for more expensive treatments— then we would expect prepaid medical groups to have a much higher outpatient utilization rate than is typical among more traditional alternatives. Although there are no data that allow precise comparisons, data available concerning outpatient utilization in both HIP and Kaiser suggest that rates of utilization are certainly no higher and perhaps lower than in more traditional types of medical practice.[6,9] It is not correct to assume that the elimination of economic barriers, in itself, provides greater access. There are many mechanisms through which a clinic may regulate utilization by increasing the difficulty and inconvenience required to obtain treatment. Busy medical practices, such as HIP and Kaiser, regulate utilization by making it difficult to schedule an appointment, by requiring patients to wait, and the like. Demand tends to adjust itself to the manpower available as a consultation becomes more inconvenient for the patient. Finally, it is not at all clear that many of the preventive features of medical practice—such as the annual checkup or multiphasic health screening—really have a major impact on the health of populations.[10] Although there is reason to believe that well-organized prepaid group practice can serve to enhance health and prevent illness, it is not apparent that this is actually the case; but if it is, it is unclear what special features of prepaid group practice make the difference.

A second argument in favor of HMO's is that they provide potentialities for taking advantage of economies of scale, although it is not abundantly clear that smaller HMO's could successfully do so. This argument has been seriously questioned by Bailey[11] who differentiates between economies of scale in medical practice and in group practice. He notes that many of the economies of scale that make group practice attractive can be achieved independently of group organization of the physicians themselves by pooling facilities and sharing expensive technology. Bailey fears that salaries and other forms of reimbursement that remove incentives for long work weeks on the part of physicians may have an overall effect of decreasing physician supply. To the extent that doctors in group practice work fewer hours, the total physician manpower pool is reduced, and compensating the loss may be very costly. Bailey's argument has some bearing on modes of reimbursement, but there is no obvious reason why group practice cannot incorporate incentives that promote maximal work efforts on the part of physicians to the extent that this is deemed desirable.

The crucial fact that makes HMO's so attractive to many is that it appears to be less costly than other alternative forms without evidence of significantly diminished quality. The estimates of the degree of savings vary, and they are complicated by considerations of the relative characteristics of the populations being compared in terms of demographic and selective characteristics and the extent to which use of services outside prepaid plans is taken into consideration. However, even when reasonably comparable data are obtained, there seems to be evidence that the prepaid plans use relatively less hospital days, less hospital admissions, and perform less surgery particularly in areas where surgery is highly discretionary. It appears that prepaid group practice may involve costs for comparable populations that are 15 to 20 per cent lower than in more traditional medical practices.

It seems clear that the major saving in prepaid group practice is achieved through preventing hospitalization. It is not clear what mechanisms contribute most strongly toward this trend. It is generally believed that savings result from the removal of an incentive for unnecessary work, peer influence, and group controls. If group controls and peer influence are influential, the processes through which such influence works are not well understood, and a study of peer influence in HIP suggests many reasons to doubt their efficacy.[12] Similarly, the argument that savings are achieved through good preventive care is not very persuasive for the reasons given earlier. Thus it appears most likely that the operating incentive against unnecessary work may be the key variable. However, we must not neglect the possibility that the availability of beds is the determining factor. Kaiser, for example, operates at a lower bed ratio than more traditional facilities, and it is well known that the availability of hospital beds creates its own demand. The extent to which doctors will use beds will depend on the difficulty of access to them, and it appears that doctors in Kaiser and other prepaid groups that demonstrate lower hospitalization rates have had less access than doctors at large.

The foregoing has implications for the diffusion of prepaid group practice. Although incentives that operate against the use of hospitals can theoretically have dangerous and undesirable effects, observers generally agree that the overall quality of the care provided by the large prepaid practices is reasonably good. It is not misleading, however, to suggest the possibility that, as prepaid practice develops in response to new economic incentives, some of these practices may not have the internal integrity and medical leadership characteristic among the existing prepaid giants. Thus there is more than a theoretical danger that incentives to avoid expensive care can lead to dangerous practices. The federal government has suggested various mechanisms to control against such abuses, involving audits and controls, on the one hand, and the test of the market place, on the other. By requiring HMO's to compete with other forms of practice for a mix of patients, it is assumed that incentives against such abuses will exist. This, of course, implies that medical consumers will have sufficient information to make informed choices and that they can judge competing forms of care on more than superficialities. There is also no particular reason to feel confident that the control features that the federal government has in mind will be sufficiently effective to prevent significant abuses. Although this is certainly possible, the case at this point is less than compelling.

It is clear that we need overall comparative studies of HMO's with other forms of medical practice. Such studies must be directed to more than one or another aspect of services, since different types of practice may invest differently in various aspects of their program. Even within Kaiser, for example, there has been no uniformity in special programs and priorities, and while some groups have emphasized health screening, others have chosen other areas of emphasis. We therefore need relatively comprehensive studies of the overall workings of alternative health services and their differential impacts on the populations they serve. Such studies are enormously difficult to execute and involve innumerable problems, but they must be undertaken, nevertheless.

Although one of the assumed advantages of HMO's is the possibility for imposing controls on the doctor's work, the stronger such controls, the less likely it is that doctors will be attracted to such groups. HMO's have always had some difficulty in recruiting doctors and, as such organizations tighten internal controls, they may become even more unattractive to physicians. Under external pressures doctors will be more receptive to peer review by immediate associates, but such controls can readily break down. Generally, men who associate daily as peers and friends tend to be reluctant to exercise discipline relative to one another. It may be that only the very grossest abuses can be checked by peer review. To the best of my knowledge, Freidson,[12] in his study of HIP, is the only one who has examined carefully the dynamics of peer controls, and his conclusions are not very comforting. For the most part, doctors were not visible to one another within a large group practicing in close proximity. Freidson believes that doctors tend to sort themselves into subgroups of similar abilities and orientations, and that such groups have low visibility relative to one another.

In short, there may be dangers in providing incentives for lower rates of hospitalization within HMO's without also providing effective checks and balances. To impose the types of checks that physicians find repugnant or which they see as interfering with their professional autonomy can create a serious problem in maintaining the viability of the group itself. The development of effective controls without arousing the opposition of physicians is an important goal, but there is not much evidence that we have developed an adequate solution to this problem. It is, perhaps, the character of medical care politics that encouraged proponents of HMO's to advocate this form of practice as a national goal with so few qualifications and so little good data. It would be more productive, in the long run, to view HMO's as mechanisms offering both the potentialities and disadvantages of group organization in general. How to maximize the expected advantages but control such consequences as impersonality, superficial treatment, and unresponsiveness to patient need is one of the most important issues our health care system will face in the coming years.

Notes

1. McNamara, M. E., and C. Todd (1970). "A Survey of Group Practice in the United States." *American Journal of Public Health,* **60:**1303–1313.
2. U.S. Department of Health, Education, and Welfare (1971). *Toward a Comprehensive Health Policy for the 1970's: A White Paper.* Washington: U. S. Government Printing Office.
3. Saward, E. (1969). "The Relevance of Prepaid Group Practice to the Effective Delivery of Health Services." Washington: Office of Group Practice Development, U.S. Department H.E.W.
4. U.S. Department of Health, Education, and Welfare (1967). *Report of the National Advisory Commission on Health Manpower, Vol. II.* Washington: U. S. Government Printing Office.
5. Silver, G. (1963). *Family Medical Practice.* Cambridge: Harvard University Press.
6. Health Insurance Plan of Greater New York (1970). *H.I.P. Statistical Report, 1968–1969.* New York: Division of Research and Statistics.

7. Greenlick, M. R., D. W. Burke, and A. V. Hurtado (1967). "The Development of a Home Health Program Within a Comprehensive Prepaid Group Practice Plan." *Inquiry*, 4:31–39.

8. Somers, A. R. (ed.) (1971). *The Kaiser-Permanente Medical Care Program.* New York: Commonwealth.

9. Saward, E., J. Blank, and M. Greenlick (1968). "Documentation of Twenty Years of Operation and Growth of a Prepaid Group Practice Plan." *Medical Care,* 6:231–244.

10. McKeown, T., *et al.* (1968). *Screening in Medical Care: Reviewing the Evidence.* London: Oxford University Press.

11. Bailey, R. (1970). "Philosophy, Faith, Fact and Fiction in the Production of Medical Services." *Inquiry,* 7:37–53.

12. Freidson, E. (1970). *Profession of Medicine.* New York: Dodd-Mead.

PART THREE

THE UNITED STATES AND ENGLAND: SOME COMPARISONS

CHAPTER VII

Medical Practice in the United States and England: Background Notes

The goal of any medical system is to organize for the provision and distribution of health services to those who need them, and to use the facilities, manpower, and technologies available to prevent and alleviate disease, disability, and suffering to the extent possible under prevailing conditions. There are alternative ways by which these goals may be pursued, and the form that health institutions take is related to the form of other social institutions, and to the economic, organizational, and value context of the society of which they are a part. Thus, it becomes necessary to consider not only "ideal patterns" of health organization but also those most desirable, given the economic limitations and value context within which medical decisions must be framed.

In comparing various aspects of British and American medicine, we must be aware of the difficulties inherent in such comparisons. Patterns of organizing and providing medical services have become increasingly complex and varied. In the United States alone, medical care will soon be a $100 billion business, and the variety and complexity of arrangements for financing and distributing medical care services are staggering. There is no study of the American system of medical care that even begins to describe, in any comprehensive way, existing medical arrangements, and we often lack even the most superficial information concerning the provision, distribution, and quality of care obtained for our vast investments. Comparative data are even more difficult to obtain, and it is prudent to begin our comparative discussion of the changing character of British and American medicine by becoming aware of the difficulties of such studies and by defining some of the possible dimensions of medical care systems that are comparable across nations.

115

Some Problems and Concepts in Studies of Comparative
Medical Organizations

One need not study other countries to meaningfully engage in comparative studies of medical organization. A medical care system as large and as varied as ours offers abundant opportunities for good comparative studies as is possible in comparing prepaid and fee-for-service plans, group and solo practice, new community health centers with more traditional forms of service, and the like. There are substantial advantages in staying within the same medical care system, since one is not faced with the difficult problems of assessing the consequences of comparing care programs which operate within varying cultural contexts having different histories, medical traditions, and forms of professional organization, and which are affected in very different ways by government regulations, planning, and economic circumstances in general. Modern medical systems have not evolved in accordance with any truly rational plan; the evolution of medical services has been greatly affected by necessary compromises with traditional practices and vested interests. These influences are very difficult to weigh when one undertakes comparative studies across nations.

Despite the real difficulties in carrying out studies across nations, there are at least two important justifications for giving more attention to such concerns. First, we need greater assurance that the hypotheses we develop and test within our own medical care system are not tied to the peculiarities of the system, and that our findings have applicability beyond the contexts studied. Ideally, we wish to test our hypotheses under widely varying conditions so as to ascertain their general applicability. Such comparative studies are made for the purposes of replication on the assumption that a hypothesis is more powerful if it holds true under widely varying circumstances than if it does not. In the United States, for example, it has been consistently found that the use of outpatient medical services is greater among persons of higher than persons of lower socioeconomic status. The assumption that this is purely a product of cost barriers has been questioned by those who have pointed out that even when medical care facilities are provided without cost, the differential pattern remains. Thus it is not clear to what extent such differences are a product of the medical care system itself and the manner in which it is organized and operated, or whether it reflects in some fashion the culture and perspectives of lower-class persons. The failure to find similar correlations between use of medical services and socioeconomic status within the National Health Service suggests that the differential in use of services in the United States is probably a result of factors inherent in the manner in which health services are organized and the viewpoints of professionals providing such services, although it is, of course, possible that the poor in the United States are very different in this respect from those in England.

Second, we presumably study other medical care systems to learn what we can from them. Many of our new developments in mental health, for example, followed practices first initiated in Europe and later imported to the United States. A comparative perspective gives us a better conception of the consequences of widely varying alternatives for structuring medical care.

The study of comparative medical systems suffers from the same basic problem as comparative studies in general—the substantial difficulties in specifying units that are both meaningful and comparable from one system to another. Most commonly, when we speak of comparative medical services we are thinking about rather large units that must exist in all medical systems because of the requirements necessary to implement existing knowledge and technology. For example, every medical system must have a mechanism for recruiting and training manpower and for allocating such manpower over a wide variety of medical functions. Also, every medical system must develop a pool of personnel that is available in some fashion as doctors of first contact, a way of organizing for the provision of intensive and technically sophisticated services, and a system of social and rehabilitation services surrounding the provision of medical care more narrowly conceived. Furthermore, every system must have a way of allocating and distributing hospitals, clinics, and medical manpower, and a set of rules or preferences as to which investments are more important than others. Or stated more simply, every medical system must have some form of general practice, some form of hospital system, and some form of organization for providing social and rehabilitation services; and the manner in which resources and talent are allocated to these sectors of care will depend on national values and perspectives.

These systems, however, need not be explicit. The American doctor's decision as to where he will locate his practice is no less planned than a distribution system which assigns doctors to particular areas of need. The unwillingness to impose a scheme for the distribution of new medical practices is as much a decision as the imposition of such a scheme, and it has measurable consequences. Similarly, the maintenance of an open system of medical training where any doctor can specialize is as much planned as a system which carefully regulates the number of specialists relative to the number of general practitioners. We should not be deceived by appearances; the major components of medical activity exist in all medical systems. Thus, when commentators lament that general practice is disappearing in the United States, what they really mean is that a particular form of providing general practice services is being abandoned. Every medical system must have some doctors who function as doctors of first contact and who screen and allocate patients to different parts of the medical care system; and, in this sense, general practice must always exist. A certain pattern of services, in meeting this function, may die out or may be radically altered, but there will always be some kind of practitioner who serves as a doctor of first contact and performs the selection function which is inherent in modern medical activity.

Just as there is confusion concerning the units of medical care systems, there is also confusion concerning meaningful dependent variables which are useful in evaluating how effectively different medical systems function. On the most simple level we can consider consumer and professional satisfaction. In comparative studies it is not difficult, for example, to obtain representative samples of users and providers and gauge their levels of satisfaction using comparable measures. We know, however, that consumers of medical care often have no basis for evaluating the services they use, and satisfaction may reflect in part the inability of the consumer to know the range of possible alternatives. Similarly, provider satisfaction may reflect the advantages the system offers professionals rather than the public generally. Perhaps the best way of evaluating the quality of services is through systematic auditing studies of medical care, which apply the same general standards to the care provided within different medical care systems. But even this is tricky, since doctors in different countries have varying notions of what constitutes a good service, and great care must be exercised in developing standards so that the traditions and fads of one system are not used in evaluating another. Moreover, economic standards must be taken into account. If quality of medical care is viewed from the perspective of an affluent country, it is somewhat different than that which should be applied to a poorer country. It may be reasonable to spend a few hundred dollars to do a careful preventive health examination when the consumer is affluent and when personnel are readily available, but such a work-up may be totally irresponsible when the consumer or the nation has limited economic resources. Medicine does not operate in a vacuum; and unnecessary costs for medical care may lead to the failure to meet other needs which affect health, welfare, and well-being.

Quality of care, moreover, is only one of many important issues pertinent to the evaluation of medical care systems. No matter what the quality of care, if it is inaccessible to needy groups it is of no value to them. Indeed, what is seen as highly sophisticated care from a medical educator's point of view may involve costs in resources and potentialities for distribution that are much higher than the gains obtained from a marginal improvement in quality. Any sophisticated evaluation of varying systems of medical care must consider the provision and distribution of services and the extent to which the population's minimal needs are effectively met. Since medical resources everywhere are limited, we must strive toward defining the mixture of quality and quantity that best serves the public interest.

Thus far I have been considering direct outputs of medical care systems, but there are various indirect measures which may ultimately have vast effects on the potential outputs. What is the rate of capital investment and replacement of facilities within a medical care system, and what are the incentives for continuing development and innovation? The consequences of such innovations may not immediately become evident, but over a long period such influences may very much affect the direction and vitality of medical care. Similar attention must be devoted to the question of manpower development and training.

Often analyses of medical care systems are concerned not with direct outputs but rather with the internal functioning of the system on the assumption that this is indicative of the quality of outputs that a system can provide. Thus it is possible to consider such issues as the rates of manpower loss, coordination of medical and social services, professional conflicts, and the like. A basic question here is whether medical services are organized and coordinated in a fashion that allows essential functions to be successfully implemented. These, of course, are not easy issues to attack, and I am not convinced that we have done very well in studying these.

Most commonly, analysts who attempt to generalize about relative outputs of medical care systems concern themselves with rates of mortality, morbidity, and medical utilization. These rates are tricky in that variations are as likely to be products of factors external to the medical care system as they are of the system itself. Most frequently, analysts focus on infant mortality as indicative of the quality of medical care distribution, but medical care is only one of many factors affecting the rates of death among infants. Similarly, overall mortality tells us less than we would like about the comparative quality of medical care. Many deaths have little to do with medical care, such as those from motor vehicle accidents. homicide, and the like. Although detailed mortality data may suggest deficiencies in medical services, interpretation of such data across national boundaries requires special caution.

Rates of medical utilization across cultures are also not fully comparable. Many services provided by doctors in one system may be provided by paramedical personnel in others, and while some countries still provide considerable domiciliary care in the case of serious illness and child-birth, others are much more dependent on the use of hospitals. In my estimation, *relative rates* of utilization are more informative in under-standing the functioning of medical systems than absolute rates. Rather than comparing absolute rates of utilization, we should be inquiring as to whether such rates within a medical care system are similar for the various social classes, or whether there are large gaps between the rich and the poor. Similarly, differences in the prevalence of disability and death among those with comparable diseases in different social groups in one society as compared with another may provide some understanding of the benefits and deficiencies of each system of medical care. It should be clear, however, that such observed differences may be attributable not to the system of medical services, but rather to other social conditions to which different subgroups are exposed affecting illness.

Having stated some of the problems and necessary cautions in cross-national comparisons, we now discuss, in the next chapter, the National Health Service of England and Wales and possible insights that it may provide for better understanding of the existent medical care crisis in the United States.

CHAPTER VIII

General Medical Practice in England and Wales: Its Organization and Future*

In 1965 the British Medical Guild, an organization developed by the British Medical Association, collected undated resignations of some 18,000 British general practitioners—the vast majority of all such practitioners working within the structure of the English National Health Service. These resignations were used to increase the strength of the general practitioners' position in negotiations with the Government for a new structure and system of remuneration for general practice. Although the Review Body on Doctors' and Dentists' Remuneration, in its 1966 report, concluded that the data available to them do "not establish that medical and dental earnings are as a whole substantially lower than they should be,"[1] they nevertheless awarded general practitioners an extraordinary large increase in remuneration. As the *London Times,* in an editorial on May 5, 1966, pointed out, despite the Government's income policies, an exception was to be made for doctors who "after an increase of about 12 per cent in 1963, fought for and got a further nine per cent just a year ago. Now they are to receive up to 16 per cent at once and the same again in a year's time." This extraordinary award, immediately accepted by the Government, was intended to meet what had been defined as a "state of crisis" in general practice—particularly the threat of growing emigration of doctors. In this paper I shall indicate the basis of my conclusion that the new income policy will do no more than encourage a respite in the altercation over medical care and that the basic difficulties of British

* Adapted from a paper published in the *New England Journal of Medicine,* 1968, 279:680–689, with permission of the *Journal.*

general practice remain.* I shall also consider the tremendous structural problems faced in attempts to alter present difficulties.

Stratification of British Medical Practitioners

Britain, like many European countries, maintains a separate role for general and hospital practitioners. Although all practitioners have the same basic medical education and develop similar values, some are channeled into exclusive hospital practice, and others are directed into practice in the community and excluded for the most part from hospital roles. By whatever criterion one wishes to impose—the complexity of medical work, level of remuneration or independence from the Government—it is clear and unequivocal that the hospital consultant occupies the upper tier on the medical hierarchy. Historically, the sharp division between generalists in the community and hospital doctors was encouraged by the general practitioners. As voluntary hospitals developed in England, and as the quality of their services became generally recognized, persons other than the impoverished came seeking medical care from hospital outpatient departments. The community practitioners vigorously resisted the extension of hospital-based services to paying patients and supported the doctrine of free care in hospitals for the needy, so as to make it less likely that hospitals would serve paying patients and thus compete with general practitioners for such patients.[2] Community practitioners supported the National Insurance Act of 1911, which provided wage earners with a general practice service that is the model for the service still existing today. This act ensured doctors a secure source of income and allowed them to refer their most difficult cases to hospital outpatient departments without any loss of income. Moreover, since hospital doctors still depended on community practitioners for private referrals, the circumstances required them to maintain a certain degree of civility toward practitioners.

The organization of the National Health Service in 1948 radically changed the dependence of the hospital doctor on referrals from general practitioners since hospital doctors themselves were to be paid on a

---

* The Review Body on Doctors' and Dentists' Remuneration has issued two additional reports since 1966, but these have not altered the basic income policy developed in that year. In its latest statement, issued on May 7, 1968, the Review Body defended its decision to recommend no further adjustments in remuneration at present in terms of the uncertainty of economic developments and national income policy. The *British Medical Journal* of May 11, 1968, in expressing its displeasure over the decision, notes some of the discrepancies in concern "about the burden of work in clinical practice" between the Review Body and the Royal Commission on Medical Education.

salaried basis. This new form of organization increased the likelihood that hospital doctors would more openly express their contempt for the limited capacities of the general practitioner and their disrespect for the level of medical work that characterized his responsibilities. Given the increasing development of medical technology and the growing importance of hospital care within the entire spectrum of medical practice, this more readily expressed attitude opened new wounds, and even if such attitudes were not openly expressed, general practitioners deeply felt their lower status. The general attitude of consultants, as perceived by the practitioners, was expressed by Lord Moran before the Pilkington Commission when the chairman indicated that it had been suggested that generalists and consultants were equal. Lord Moran emphatically denied this:

> Could anything be more absurd? I was Dean of St. Mary's Hospital Medical School for 25 years . . . all the people of outstanding merit, with few exceptions, aimed to get on the staff. There was no other aim, and it was a ladder off which some of them fell. How can you say that the people who get to the top of the ladder are the same people who fall off it? It seems to me so ludicrous.[3]

As Lord Moran pointed out, the general practitioner has in a sense fallen off the status ladder. Many doctors who do not qualify for hospital posts, however, have extensive hospital training comparable to board-eligible and board-certified specialists in the United States. In a study of a representative sample of general practitioners in England and Wales in 1965–66,* I found that 27 per cent reported four or more years of hospital training beyond medical school and 39 per cent reported at least three years of postgraduate training. These doctors, therefore, are often faced with a choice of general practice for which much of their specialty training appears superfluous, or they must seek opportunities outside the National Health Service. Since approximately only 3 per cent of the English population use private medical services, this medical sphere offers few real opportunities. Thus, doctors who wish to have alternatives must seek opportunities abroad.

* I obtained a representative sample of general practitioners by selecting random samples from each of the Executive Councils in England and Wales. Of the 1356 eligible respondents 60 per cent (813 doctors) completed a lengthy questionnaire, and 73 per cent (995 doctors) provided certain key information. Basic demographic data describing all general practitioners in England and Wales, as well as all the doctors originally designated in our sample, were provided by the Ministry of Health, thus allowing for an analysis of certain differences between the entire population of general practitioners, respondents to our survey and nonrespondents. Detailed analyses demonstrate that although our sample includes some over-representation of younger doctors and those practicing in groups, the basic characteristics of our respondents are very similar to those of all general practitioners in England and Wales. A discussion of detailed results from this survey is given elsewhere.[4]

Although it is difficult to develop precise figures, it is clear that the emigration of doctors from England and Wales has occurred at an alarming rate. Abel-Smith and Gales,[5] who have completed the most authoritative study on this issue, estimated that between January, 1955, and July, 1962, an average of 390 British-born and trained doctors left Britain each year and did not return. A recent study of doctors entering and leaving Great Britain in the three years ending September, 1965, reports a net loss of 1100 doctors born in the United Kingdom and Irish Republic.[6] However, a net gain in doctors born overseas appears to counterbalance this loss. These data suggest a replacement pattern where immigrating doctors from such countries as India and Pakistan replace British doctors who emigrated. It is not clear, however, whether incoming doctors assume medical tasks similar to those previously performed by migrating British doctors. Data presented by Abel-Smith and Gales[5] indicate that consultants rarely leave Britain, and only one quarter of the doctors who emigrated actually were general practitioners. The largest loss appears to come from hospital doctors in the grades of registrar, senior house officer and house officer—comparable for the most part to various levels of the residency in the United States. It appears clear that many of these doctors are unwilling to enter the limited general-practice role as it exists within the National Health Service. The most usual time of emigration appears to be between three and six years after registration. Abel-Smith and Gales,[5] in explaining their findings, note:

We could well appreciate the reluctance to enter general practice of those who had spent several years climbing the hierarchy which leads to consultant rank and saw or found no prospects ahead of them. It seemed to us understandable that they preferred to take their specialized skills to somewhere where they could use them rather than to enter the general field several years behind their contemporaries . . . Many of our respondents abroad who criticized the National Health Service saw general practice within it as a low status occupation. We do not know whether they had gained this attitude from the consultants at their teaching hospitals, from the focus of their medical education or from other sources. The separation of general practice in Britain from hospital practice was commented on adversely by many of our respondents.

In October, 1967, a Ministry of Health interview board visited several cities in North America and conferred with British-born doctors to study why they emigrated and the conditions under which they would return home.[7] Among the reasons cited for emigration were dissatisfaction with the terms and conditions of service, aspiration for a specialist career among those who either did not qualify in Britain or were reluctant to wait the required period for an available position, higher financial reward, available access to hospital facilities in North America and availability of academic positions and research facilities in the United States.

Influence of the International Medical-Care Market

The major countries to which British doctors migrate (Canada, the United States, Australia and New Zealand) face considerable demand for more medical manpower in the coming years. All these countries offer economic opportunities for medical practice that a public medical system in a country with England's wealth could not possibly match without grossly dislocating its priorities or distorting its sense of relative income distribution. Thus, it is difficult to see how any reasonable program in income terms can effectively alleviate the general practitioner's sense of relative deprivation. The average general practitioner does not compare himself with high-level civil servants but rather with his colleagues in other English-speaking countries and with consultants within the National Health Service. As the shortage of doctors has increased throughout the world, increased effort has been made to recruit British doctors, and it is possible, for example, to take the E.C.F.M.G. in Britain. British professional medical journals carry numerous advertisements from overseas offering the doctor higher income, better facilities and more medical responsibility than is available to him at home. Perhaps the most potent stimulant to the doctor's sense of deprivation results from the substantial emigration that has already occurred in that many doctors know friends, colleagues and classmates who are practicing abroad. As they hear news of the success and economic affluence of members of their own cohorts, they experience a deep sense of frustration and deprivation.

That the British Government cannot depend on such influences to subside is evident from an evaluation of the situation in the United States. Even with the use of conservative estimates, it is apparent that the number of new physicians to be educated in the coming decade and the likely increases in the productivity of the doctor will fall short of demand for medical services. Increased demand for medical services will develop as a consequence of a growing population and a higher average rate of utilization, attributable to changing behavior patterns, an aging population and new medical programs. Rashi Fein, of the Brookings Institution, estimates that demand for medical services by 1980 in comparison to 1965 will increase between 20 and 40 per cent.[8] Even on the assumption of an annual addition of 1600 foreign-trained physicians, and with the projected increases in the number of physicians American medical schools will

train taken into account, the United States will still have difficulty maintaining the present level of medical services. Given the likely circumstances, it seems reasonable to expect that the medical system of the
United States (and those of other countries as well) will exert even greater
pressure on the functioning of the National Health Service in the future
than in the past.

Effects of Growing Demand on the English National Health Service

The same factors increasing medical demand in the United States have
exerted similar pressures on the National Health Service. However, as
the number of patients and their rate of utilization have been increasing,
the number of general practitioners in relation to the population has
lagged, thus resulting in a higher patient load for the average doctor. In
1964, 1965 and 1966, for example, the actual number of doctors in general practice *decreased* by 505.[9] During 1966 there were 183 fewer than in
the previous year, although the population had increased by 300,000
during the year. The decrease in general practitioners was particularly
disturbing during the crisis of 1965–1966 since the pool system through
which they were paid was based on the number of practitioners rather
than on the amount of work. Although this aspect of the problem has
been remedied through the new remuneration scheme adopted in 1966,
the basic problem of high demand persists and may become considerably
worse in the future.*

A study in England and Wales disclosed that the very large demands
made on the general practitioner encouraged a pattern of work that was
personally frustrating and hardly conducive to providing a high quality
of patient care.[4] The average doctor responds to his growing practice and
to increasing demands on his time not by continually increasing his
workweek in comparison with those who have much smaller practices,
but by practicing at a different pace and style. He thus feels deprived not
only in terms of the hours he devotes to his patients but, more importantly, in terms of the amount of work and effort he must pack into this
period. Such a pattern of work requires doctors to practice on an as-
sembly-line basis, which diminishes the unique satisfactions possible in

---

* In its annual report published in July, 1967, the Ministry of Health reports the
average list size of general practitioners as 2453. Because of the unequal distribution of
doctors, there is variation in list size from one area to another, and in some parts of
England the average list size exceeds 3000 patients. A detailed analysis of the doctor's
workload and the way he distributes his time is given elsewhere.[4]

a general practice. If doctors' reports concerning their own behavior are accepted, spot diagnoses, inability to provide enough time for patients and failure to undertake an adequate examination or other necessary action are correlates of this pattern of practice. I do not mean to suggest that a similar form of practice is absent in the United States, but a major difference results from the British general practitioner's recognition that, unlike his American counterpart, he is not rewarded for the number of services that he provides.

The Royal Commission on Education, in its report of April, 1968, recognized the substantial manpower difficulties faced by the National Health Service.[10] They estimated that by 1975 Britain would be 11,000 doctors short of the number necessary to provide a satisfactory service on the present basis, and they foresaw even larger shortages in the future without vigorous efforts to expand places in existing medical schools and to develop new ones. To meet estimates of necessary manpower, medical graduates will have to increase from an estimated average of 3100 each year between 1965 and 1974 to 3850 a year during the period 1980–1984, and 4550 a year by 1990. The situation was viewed as serious enough to be called to the attention of the Ministry by the Commission in June, 1966, before its report had been completed, and some steps have already been taken. It is difficult to predict whether the Government will be sufficiently responsive to meet in a satisfactory way these projected needs. It is inevitable, however, that the burden on individual doctors will increase in the coming decade, and considerable gains in their productivity will be necessary to maintain the current level of services.

Changes in Medical Roles

The continuing advances in medical technology have greatly sharpened the distinction between more prestigious hospital work and the uncertainty and ambiguity of the role of the general practitioner. British experts on medical care often maintain that they do not wish to move in the direction of excessive specialization that they believe characterizes American medicine, and they speak proudly of the maintenance of their commitment to a general-practice service. Yet little progress has been made in clearly defining the relevance of the general practitioner's role in what has clearly become a new era in scientific medicine. Various committees have explored this question, but such attempts to define a coherent role for the general practitioner frequently strike the typical doctor as pious and unrealistic.

In October, 1963, a distinguished official committee, headed by Annis

Gillie, reported to the Minister on its two-year study of "The Field of Work of the Family Doctor."[11] The Committee argued that the general practitioner has a unique role in dealing with the social and psychologic problems of patients as well as serving as a "first line of defense in times of illness, disability and distress. . . ." Given the projected demand on the general practitioner's time and the lack of specification of the particular skills and technics through which this role can be realized, it is far from clear how his role should be structured or how he should be trained.

Medical education in Britain has been traditional in its approach, and it has been widely recognized that it does not prepare the student adequately for and does not encourage a favorable attitude toward general practice. The Royal Commission on Medical Education attacked this problem, in part, in its recommendation that the clinical undergraduate course be broadened in scope. The new program recommended gives much greater emphasis than before on the social and behavioral sciences and on encouraging a "holistic attitude towards patients." Although this goal is all to the good, it is not fully clear how such changes can lead to more effective functioning of general practitioners without radically altering the conditions under which they must work. The idea of a comprehensive approach to the patient inevitably leads to increased responsibility for the doctor, and this kind of program cannot easily be implemented concurrently with attempts to increase the doctor's productivity or the number of patients under his care.

Failure of Public Opinion

There is wide consensus among informed observers that the potentialities for an improved structure of general practice are not well developed within the National Health Service. The form of practice that prevails is still very similar to the panel that developed under the National Insurance Act of 1911. In the Review Body's report on remuneration in 1966 the need for more group practice was recognized, and an incentive system for group practice was developed through the provision of a basic practice allowance for doctors who work in groups.[1] However, the group-practice allowance is a very modest one, and almost half the general practitioners continue to work by themselves or with a single partner. Moreover, many of the partnerships and larger groups that have been developed have been organized for the purpose of sharing premises or for particular conveniences and advantages not clearly related to the quality of medical care provided. Group practice in a well organized medical sense is still relatively rare, and the common pattern is for doctors to work within poorly developed and inefficient premises with limited diagnostic facilities and ancillary help. Although studies auditing medical practice are rare, there is some evidence that the kinds of practice that exist are not conducive to care of high quality.[12] More than half the doctors canvassed in my study reported that a high standard of medical care was not realistic under present conditions of medical organization, and only about a third thought that good preventive care was possible. No one seriously contends that the general-practice service performs the role so idealistically described in some official British publications.

Although experts do not find general practice satisfactory, there is no evidence that this view is shared by the general populace. Indeed, there is an astonishing degree of satisfaction with medical care among consumers—particularly with general practice.[13] This is a consequence of the fact that most patients do not have a standard by which to measure their medical care, and there is widespread approval of the basic concept of providing free and equal access to medical care. By this criterion, the National Health Service has been extraordinarily successful. Unlike that in the United States, the consumption of medical services is not related to income.[13] The satisfaction of the public results in little political pressure on the government to make further investments in general practice as compared with such other priorities as housing, education and transportation.

Any dissatisfaction with health services expressed by the British public is frequently oriented toward the imposition of costs. Various surveys from time to time have shown prescription charges to be the focal point of more criticism than almost any other aspect of the service. The Labor Party, responding to its working-class constituency, supports the removal of cost barriers to medical care. The Conservatives, responding to their supporters, defend the imposition of such charges. In the midst of a vigorous dispute between general practitioners and the Government in 1964, when many defects in the Service were evident, the Labor Party in its election campaign promised to give priority to the removal of prescription charges, and it did so shortly after taking office.* Although politically popular, this action infuriated the doctors, who claimed that the removal of charges encouraged a frivolous attitude toward consultations.[14]

The satisfaction of the public with the state of medical affairs produces little pressure on the Cabinet and the Prime Minister to respond to the

---

* In imposing various measures to achieve economic stability during the period of devaluation of the pound, prescription charges were reinstated by the Labor Government.

Health Minister's proposals for increased allocations toward general practice. Since national planning takes place within a context of scarcity and competing demands, and since external pressures on the allocation process from other spheres are substantial, the lack of public clamor concerning the state of medical affairs does not produce a strong force to increase investments in medical care,[15] and Britain in recent years has been investing approximately 4 per cent of its gross national product in health services in comparison to the approximate 6 per cent characteristic of the United States.* There has been a clear failure to invest particularly in general practice, where it is difficult to provide evidence to support the contention that increased investment would have equal impact on health to competing public programs. The rebellion within the British Medical Association during the events leading up to 1965, the public clamor raised by the resignation threat and the emigration crisis produced such pressures during 1965, and these pressures caused the Government to accept the recommendations of the Review Body. But this settlement was a temporary expedient, and the Government achieved limited inducements for constructive change.

Proposals for Improving the Long-Term Condition of General Practice—Some Inherent Limitations

Even before 1948 there was considerable discussion of viable and effective alternatives to the prevailing structure of general practice, which was widely regarded as defective. It is ironic that little change has occurred, and it takes considerable optimism to anticipate that substantial change will take place in the future. When the national health program was being discussed, it was generally anticipated that health centers would be developed around the country and that these centers would serve as the focal point of an efficient and coordinated pattern of medical care. The failure to implement the health-center concept during the past 20 years was destructive to the development of a modern approach to the organization of general practice.

Health Centers. As far back as 1920 the Dawson Committee, established by the Ministry of Health, recommended general-practice and specialist health centers that were to work in a co-ordinated fashion.[16] Related ideas persisted and were prominent in the planning underlying the establishment of the Health Service. Indeed, under the act establishing the

---

* Since this paper was written, health care has become a larger component of the gross national product in both countries, but the differential remains.

Health Service, local authorities were supposed to build health centers for improving conditions in general practice and co-ordinating medical care.[17] These centers were seen as including any and all of the following services: general medical and dental services; pharmaceutical services; specialist and other services for outpatients; and local health-authority services and personnel.[18] Aneurin Bevan viewed the health center as one of the three main instruments of the Service, and before its inception, the Ministry referred to centers as the "key feature" of the new Health Service. Within this context it is indeed surprising that the Ministry did not implement this idea and later did much to impede it. By the end of 1959 there were only 23 health centers in England, Wales and Scotland, and some of these were truly health centers only in name.[16] In 1948, as soon as the Health Service was established, the Ministry excused local authorities from providing plans for such centers; when plans were presented, they were usually discouraged or rejected.[17]

Although many reasons have been offered, it is not fully clear why this idea that was the core of the new Health Service was so completely ignored. Eckstein gives the following explanation:

> It is clear that the Government had a change of heart on the Centres; but it is almost impossible to find a convincing reason for its changed attitudes . . . a decision not to go ahead with the Centres must have been made on general policy grounds. There is much circumstantial evidence to confirm this . . . most important of all, nothing really constructive was done by the Minister, despite parliamentary pressure, to see to it that sites and accommodations were reserved for the Centres in new housing estates and other building developments . . . In view of everything else, it is difficult to believe that this was just the result of an administrative mistake, particularly since the consequences of the mistake were pointed out to the Minister over and over again.[17]

Although there is no evidence of a specific cause for the Government's "change of heart," a variety of factors may have helped dampen enthusiasm for the implementation of health centers. It was apparent that the development of a national system of first-class health centers would be a costly project, and the Government was faced with a shortage of building materials and a variety of competing needs. Although the health centers were to be the responsibility of local government, the local authorities were in a poor condition financially and organizationally.[12] Moreover, the doctors were even more contemptuous and hostile toward local government than toward the Ministry of Health, and they looked with disfavor on giving up their personally owned premises to work within those owned by the authorities. Similarly, the British Medical Association viewed health centers as a possible threat to the independence of the doctor, and it provided little encouragement for the implementation of such forms of practice.[18] In the light of professional resistance and the lack of forceful public opinion on this matter, it is not difficult to see why the Government did not move ahead on the scheme. Having just completed a battle with general practitioners over the terms for their entry into the Health Service, the Government was well aware of the capriciousness of the doctors' rhetoric and politics. Finally, it should be noted that the health-center model was a radical departure from previous modes of organizing medical work. Although the Health Service involved other major departures from previous experience, as with the development of regional hospital boards and hospital management committees, these neither substantially affected the mode of the individual doctor's work nor aroused such fierce professional resistance.

As British medicine looks toward the future, the major solution that is persistently advanced is the implementation of the policy of developing health centers. The health center is viewed as a way of organizing general-practitioner services in a context where adequate diagnostic facilities and ancillary services are available and where the three aspects of the service (the general practitioner, the consultant specialist and the local authority health worker) can be integrated into a viable form of organization. Moreover, it is seen as a context that will reduce professional isolation among doctors, provide reasonable opportunities for the maintenance of professional skills and help increase the individual doctor's efficiency and productivity. Thus far, health centers have differed widely in their organization, as well as in size, availability of facilities, and the provision of care:

At one relatively remote centre there are good diagnostic facilities and consultant sessions, and at another neither of these is provided, since the district hospital is around the corner. At one centre some patients are initially seen by a nurse, and at another the doctors make it a rule to speak personally to every patient who telephones. At yet another centre a pilot scheme for reducing visiting by bringing the patient to the centre is to be tried.[19]

Although there were only 38 health centers operating in England and Wales at the end of 1966 (excluding establishments developed before 1948), further development was encouraged in April, 1967, when the Ministry of Health offered advice to local authorities on the planning and submission of proposals for new health facilities. This Ministry statement appears to give priority to health centers over other forms of new general-practice facilities, although through the National Health Service Act of 1966 the Government also set up an independent corporation to help doctors finance their own practice premises. As of December, 1967, 180 health centers were being planned or built,[19] and it is estimated that 284 new ones will be built by 1976.[18] Health-center developments will receive further encouragement from the report of the Royal Commission on Medical Education, which states that health centers are the most obvious setting for the future of general practice, and that the most usual form of practice in future years will consist of groups of 12 or more doctors working with the assistance of nurses, other ancillary personnel and computer aids. The Commission recognizes the inadequacy of the organization of present centers, but takes an optimistic view of their future evolution.

In most of the centres so far established, however, the general practitioners practice as individuals or in two or more groups which are largely independent of each other. We think such arrangements represent only one stage in a continuing evolutionary process, and that eventually all the general practitioners and the local health authority staff working in the centre will be linked together and will often become a single team.[10]

Given the history of health centers in Britain, it is necessary to consider the factors that might impede the successful implementation of the goals defined as so important by the Royal Commission.

Although more doctors appear to be oriented to the idea of health centers than before, old difficulties continue. Britain continues to face serious economic problems and many competing priorities for public funds. Similarly, old suspicions persist, and there is no evidence of widespread receptivity to health centers. Even if one assumed the development of 300 to 500 new health centers by 1975, with 10 to 15 doctors each, such centers would only include a modest proportion of British general practitioners. But even this goal appears dubious, given the general state of opinion among general practitioners. The 1965–1966 survey of general practitioners referred to above[4] found that doctors still give health centers very low priority in relation to other remedies that they propose, and they show little receptivity to closer cooperation with the local authorities. Moreover, unlike most expert observers in the medical-care field, these doctors attribute little importance to increasing access to diagnostic facilities, maintaining adequate premises or improving professional contacts with colleagues relative to such matters as increased remuneration. If my analysis is correct, the doctors focus their discontent on the money issue, thus tending to minimize the importance of changing the conditions that produce their hostility and discontent.

The tremendous hostility toward the Government and governmental controls still pervades the point of view of many doctors. Ironically enough, the Ministry of Health intervenes in the affairs of general practice to an extraordinarily limited extent, although there may be a tendency to overburden the doctor with requirements concerning certification of patients' illness. But, for the most part, doctors are left to pursue their work with little interference or dictation. The Ministry does audit the average cost of prescriptions written by doctors, and when they far exceed the norm, such doctors may be visited by a regional medical officer, who encourages them to consider costs. In 1965, for example, only 999 such visits were made for more than 20,000 practitioners, and an additional 160 visits were made to discuss particular prescriptions that were viewed as extraordinary in some fashion. However, during the same year only four practitioners had remuneration withheld because of excessive prescribing.[20] Although disciplinary procedures exist within the National Health Service, they tend to protect the doctor amply,[21] and doctors are exposed to sanctions only after having been found guilty by colleagues of having committed such gross improprieties as sexual exploitation of patients, drunkenness on duty or refusal to attend a sick patient in need. Yet doctors show tremendous hostility toward any attempt to audit their work or to establish disciplinary procedures no matter how benign the procedures or how substantial their protections. In the survey[4] only a third of the doctors regarded it as proper for the Ministry of Health to attempt to influence prescribing habits of doctors, and only one tenth thought it would be proper for them to concern themselves with referral habits (which they do not presently do). It is an interesting fact that one quarter of the doctors did not agree that it was proper for the Ministry of Health to attempt to evaluate the quality of care provided in general practice. Although specific information on this point was not obtained in the survey, it is my impression, on the basis of conversations with a large number of general practitioners, that a major factor influencing attitudes toward health centers is a fear among many that this would lead to greater visibility and supervision of their work.

The Clinical Assistantship and Other Hospital Appointments. To alleviate the need for middle-level staff in hospitals, the Ministry of Health suggested that general practitioners have part-time employment in hospitals as clinical assistants. The clinical assistant was to serve as an aid to consultants in the outpatient department by assuming responsibility for particular sessions. Although this work might involve some complex medical problems, and might allow doctors opportunities to pursue special interests, the clinical assistant has only limited status in the hospital and cannot admit his own patients to beds under his jurisdiction. A fair number of doctors have found such appointments helpful and stimulating, and this has led some analysts to suggest that opportunities for clinical assistants should be extended to give more general practitioners a place in hospitals. The Commission on Medical Education also views this concept as a reasonable one in integrating the work of hospitals with the work of the general practitioner, and indicates that such appointments will help break down the distinction between the two branches of the National Health Service. Yet the survey in 1965–1966[4] showed no significant differences in level of satisfaction between doctors who had such appointments and those who did not. If this finding is an accurate one, it is difficult to see how the clinical assistantship will materially affect the doctor's situation.

It is not too difficult to understand the failure of the clinical assistantship to have more effect. For some doctors who aspire to improve their skills, who have specific medical interests they would like to develop further and who find a friendly and compatible situation to work within, such opportunities may substantially increase professional gratifications. But the lower status of the clinical assistantship places an insecure practitioner in a situation where he may feel slighted and exploited. It is not unusual for doctors holding such appointments to perceive an attitude among more prestigious hospital staff that makes them conscious of being in the "lowly" role of the student. At least when a doctor remains within his practice he is not exposed face to face with the fact or suggestion that he is one who has "fallen off the ladder."

It appears clear that nominal appointments to hospital staffs will not retard the malaise of the general practitioner, although such appointments provide possibilities of alleviating his professional isolation. In contrast, it is equally clear not only that the kind of hospital affiliation common in the United States and Canada lacks feasibility from an organizational and historical point of view, but also the pattern itself may be undesirable in that it encourages doctors to undertake medical procedures beyond their competence and training. The role of general practitioners in surgical work, for example, would be undesirable and, indeed, this is a pattern that good American hospitals are trying to remedy.

Of the many discussions of the role of the British general practitioner in hospital care, perhaps the most reasonable proposals are those suggested by Professor McKeown,[22] who believes that "consultant practice should be restricted to services which require both referral and specialization as conditions of expert service; it should not be based on broad age periods such as childhood and advanced age, where the patient is able to make his way directly to the appropriate medical attendant." He suggests that general practice should be stratified into four services in which the practitioner would accept comprehensive responsibility including community and hospital practice: obstetrics, pediatrics, adult medicine and geriatrics. In short, the specialist would serve as a "real consultant" on difficult medical problems when he took charge, but he would not necessarily take over all medical care provided within hospitals.

Although Professor McKeown's proposals have many appealing aspects, they offer various difficult problems. The organization of practice on the basis of the life cycle and on continuing care from one doctor within each of the life stages is based in part on the assumption of a stationary population. But geographic mobility in Britain will increase in the future, and it is difficult to see how the principle of continuity of care can be maintained under his scheme. Moreover, it is probable that practices covering some age groups will be considerably more appealing than others to doctors, and it is likely that a status hierarchy would develop within general practice and areas such as geriatrics would suffer vast shortages of medical manpower. Perhaps the most important barrier of all—even if the scheme was fully desirable—is the response of the medical elite, who are a powerful interest group and who will not accede quietly to a proposal that will substantially shrink the consultant ranks. Even if a slow contraction of consultants was agreed to, it is not clear how the joint responsibility in hospitals between consultants and general practitioners could be worked out. It is unlikely that the consultants would ever agree to an arrangement that allows the larger number of general practitioners to encroach on their authority and position. If the authority of the consultant is fully protected, however, he may dominate the general practitioner in the hospital in a fashion that would only draw more sharply the status division among doctors. England is very clearly a country in which status divisions have special importance, and this is a pattern which gives every indication of continuing to exist for a long time to come.

The Future of General Practice

As one looks ahead it is important to consider whether general practice, as it is now thought of, has any future. The British have maintained that it does, and a group of eminent general practitioners within the College of General Practitioners have made the following argument in support of general practice:

Those who visit countries where the family doctor has disappeared find that the first effect is a complete loss of the services of a personal doctor who looks on his patient as an individual in the context of a family and the community; the patient then becomes uncertain and confused in his relations with the medical service.

The second effect is that care provided by specialists does not include the broader outlook and perspectives of the general practitioner and, with it, the abilities to protect and guide the patient through the medical jungle.

The third effect is that the front-line of medical care is pushed right back to the doors of the hospitals; medical care becomes an expensive and impersonal matter, creating fresh problems for hospitals, doctors and patients alike. We can briefly state that the *Roles of the General Practitioner* include those of a personal, family and community doctor; of protector of his patients from wrong or unnecessary hospitalization, protector of hospitals of the wrong types of cases, and protector of the community by saving money; of coordinator of all available medical and social services; and of manipulator of the patient's personal, social and medical environments, whether in the family, at work or elsewhere.[23]

Given the heavy patient demands on the British doctor's time and the inefficient organization of his practice, the general practitioner often fails to perform properly even the most primary aspects of his role: screening patients for serious physical disorders; providing continuing care for disabled patients outside the hospital; routine screening procedures for preventive purposes; and psychosocial care. Although doctors at the time of the survey may have exaggerated the difficulties of performing these functions—in the light of the prevailing political climate—general information on the Health Service suggests that these perceptions are not too unreal. Only about two fifths of the doctors thought that the conditions of general practice made it realistic to expect them to screen out patients with serious physical disorders, to provide follow-up care for psychiatric patients after discharge from the hospital, or to undertake routine screening through cervical smears; only about a third of the doctors considered it realistic to provide psychosocial care, and it is a relatively rare doctor who will give many patients the opportunity "to talk on for a half hour to get things off his chest," or who will ordinarily spend as much as half an hour to explore the patient's social and emotional background. Given these facts, it is difficult to see how the doctor can reasonably conform to the idealistic expectations of him.

In sum, there is a very large gap between official conceptions of what the general practitioner can and should do and what is reasonable under the prevailing conditions of practice.[24] Despite its obvious defects, however, the National Health Service has made remarkable progress in ensuring the availability of medical care to the population in terms of need rather than in terms of the ability to pay, and there is no question that this has had a significant effect on the quality of care received by the working man. Although the United States, the most affluent of all countries, invests a larger proportion of its gross national product than Britain in the provision of medical services, it continues to have a substantially higher rate of infant mortality.[25] The utilization of medical services in Britain, unlike that in the United States, is not correlated with income, and the mortality rates among the rich and the poor are more equal in Britain than in the United States.[26] I believe that it is facts of this kind that raise serious questions in the minds of many experts about whether a vast investment in improving the system of general practice will be repaid sufficiently in lower mortality and morbidity in comparison with investments in housing, transportation, schools and other programs aimed at improving the environment. In an economy of scarcity this is always a salient question, and the evidence for a concerted governmental effort in general practice as compared with these other areas is hardly impressive. Given the traditions and politics of medicine in Britain, it is difficult to see why the Government should be motivated to undertake this task.

The Royal Commission on Medical Education recognized some of the basic difficulties in the organization of general practice, and a strategy aimed at breaking down the hierarchical relations among doctors is suggested. Most controversial among their suggestions is the following recommendation:

. . . the general professional training required for prospective general practitioners after the intern year should, like that for other specialties, be of three years' duration and that two years' further professional training and experience should be required before vocational registration in this field. We believe that the introduction of a training scheme for general practice on the lines we have proposed would greatly enhance the attractiveness of general practice as a career. . . .[10]

The difficulties with the recommendations of the Royal Commission are exemplified by the contradictions inherent in them. Britain faces a growing shortage of medical manpower (particularly in general practice), but a longer and more intensive period of training for general practitioners is considered necessary. Great need exists to increase the individual doctor's efficiency and productivity in the face of growing medical demand, but it is asserted that doctors must provide a more comprehensive service, applying behavioral and social knowledge as well as medical science. These are all laudable goals of course, but they do not all flow from the same form of medical organization.[27]

It is thus my conclusion that, despite the present awareness of the inadequacies of the organization of general practice in Britain, prospects for a vastly improved system of general practice in the near future are dim. No doubt various correctives will be applied when political pressures mount, but the conservatism of medical institutions and the apathy of public opinion will be slow to change. Unless economic conditions substantially improve or attitudes among doctors radically alter, it appears that pressures of emigration will inevitably mount and erode the gains from decisions to increase medical-school places and the production of doctors. Britain may be able to replace its own migrants with colored doctors from abroad, but such a pattern not only encourages medical shortages in underdoctored countries but also adds strain to the growing racial difficulties in Britain.

It would be unwise to underestimate the influence of the Royal Commission on Medical Education or the ability of the Government to improve the condition of general practice truly if it is determined to do so. The diagnosis is clear even if the solutions are as yet untested. Britain, however, is a traditional society, and the forms of medical practice and medical attitudes that exist have deep historical roots. Implementing the necessary modifications of medical practice would be task enough; to do so successfully in an environment of vast economic difficulties, important competing social needs, entrenched traditions and vested interests, vigorous international competition for medical manpower and the absence of strong public pressures would be extraordinary indeed.

Postscript

Several years have passed since I wrote this essay on the future of general practice in England and Wales, and its republication allows me, in retrospect, to consider again my conclusion that the prospects for a vastly improved system of general practice in the near future are dim. Although I have not had an opportunity to obtain additional primary data since 1966, I did have an opportunity to return for several weeks in 1969 and visit with various informed observers of medical developments. I have also continued to follow developments through British publications and particularly the wealth of information on the National Health Service provided annually by the Department of Health and Social Security.

Since the essay was written, there has been considerable ferment in the National Health Service. Most dramatic has been the continuing discussion of the possible reorganization of the System,[28] which would basically involve an integration of services provided by general practitioners, hospitals, and local authorities through decentralizing the management of the Service among area health authorities responsible for population groups between 200,000 and 1,300,000. The lack of coordination of the three aspects of the Service, which have long origins, has been a persistent problem in the effective provision of health care services, and it is significant that responsible officials are now making serious efforts to remedy this problem. It is very difficult to see, however, how the types of changes in management proposed can effectively come to terms with the complexity of the difficulties toward which they are directed. Administrative changes will have to be far-reaching if they are to affect significantly the entrenched patterns presently existing. However, developments along these lines merit continued watching.*

There are some observers in England who feel strongly that the situation in general practice has improved significantly since 1966 when I did my study of British general practitioners. They point particularly to the development of health centers, a reversal in the decreasing number of general practitioners, and lesser acrimony within the medical profession generally. Although it is true that the new forms of reimbursement developed within the agreement reached in 1966 did help alleviate some of the bitter dissatisfaction then evident among general practitioners, disputes have continued to develop from time to time concerning remuneration since then, and there is little reason not to anticipate more such disputes in the future. The form of capitation and associated payments now used, however, are more closely linked to the actual work doctors do and thus arouse less dissatisfaction than before. Moreover, incentive payments for continuing education have had an important impact on the number of postgraduate courses general practitioners now take, and probably contribute indirectly to the quality of care in general practice.

The major issue, of course, is the extent to which the existing workload and pattern of practice is consistent with the noble definition of the doctor's functions and the degree to which more efficient and effective forms of delivering primary care services have been achieved. Here the data do not support the apparent enthusiasm.[29] In 1966, average list size for general practitioners was 2453; it increased to 2495 in 1969, and then dropped to 2478 in 1970. In short, the average patient load has increased rather than decreased since my study was completed. As for health centers, it is clear that the government is finally seriously encouraging their development, but the process is a slow one. As of 1970, there is a total of 191 such centers with an additional hundred presently being built. Approximately 2000 general practitioners (10 per cent) now partly practice in such premises, but the average size of such centers tends to be small, 5.6 doctors. In short, many of the health centers are not major variants of preexisting forms of practice. Although some British observers are impressed by the extent of group practice, the fact remains that approx-

* For a recent review of the continuing discussion and its changing emphases, see S. M. Shortell and G. Gibson, 1971, "The British National Health Service: Issues of Reorganization." *Health Services Research*, 6:316–336; also see D. Mechanic, 1972, "Rhetoric and Reality in Health Services Research." *Health Services Research*, 7:61–65.

imately 70 per cent of British general practitioners continue to practice by themselves or in two or three man partnerships.

Thus, in retrospect, I have little reason to believe that conditions in general practice have shifted in any significant way in recent years. If the Government persists with health center development, and makes efforts to reduce the patient loads of general practitioners, and to better integrate their services with hospital and local authority functions, then real possibilities for improvement in care will exist. But at the present time, much of this remains in the talking stage, and many of the basic problems that have plagued the National Health Service since its inception still continue to exist.

Notes

1. Great Britain, Review Body on Doctors' and Dentists' Remuneration. (1966). *Seventh Report.* Cmnd. 2992. London: Her Majesty's Stationery Office.

2. Abel-Smith, B. (1964). *The Hospitals, 1800–1948: A Study in Social Administration in England and Wales.* London: Heinemann.

3. Ferris, P. (1965). *The Doctors.* London: Gallancz.

4. Mechanic, D. (1968). "General Practice in England and Wales: Results from a Survey of a National Sample of General Practitioners." *Medical Care,* **6:**245–260.

5. Abel-Smith, B. and K. Gales (1964). *British Doctors at Home and Abroad.* London: Bell.

6. Ash, R., and H. D. Mitchell (1968). "Doctor Migration 1962–1964: With Addendum for 1964–1965 from Ministry of Health." *British Medical Journal,* **1:**569–572.

7. Report and Recommendations of Ministry of Health Interview Board (1968). "Emigration of British Doctors to United States of America and Canada." *British Medical Journal,* **1:**45–48.

8. Fein, R. (1967). *The Doctor Shortage: An Economic Diagnosis.* Washington: The Brookings Institute.

9. Great Britain, Ministry of Health (1964). *Annual Report,* Cmnd. 2688; (1965), *Annual Report,* Cmnd. 3039; (1966), *Annual Report,* Cmnd. 3326. London: Her Majesty's Stationery Office.

10. Great Britain, Royal Commission on Medical Education (1968). *1965–1968 Report.* Cmnd. 3569. London: Her Majesty's Stationery Office.

11. Great Britain, Ministry of Health (1963). *The Field Work of the Family Doctor.* London: Her Majesty's Stationery Office.

12. Forsyth, D. (1966). *Doctors and State Medicine: A Study of the British Health Service.* Philadelphia: Lippincott.

13. Cartwright, A. (1967). *Patients and Their Doctors: A Study of General Practice.* London: Routledge.

14. Mechanic, D., and R. Faich (1970). "Doctors in Revolt: Crisis in the British National Health Service." *Medical Care,* **8:**442–455.

15. Eckstein, H. H. (1960). *Pressure Group Politics: The Case of the British Medical Association.* Stanford, Calif.: Stanford University Press.

16. Stevens, R. (1966). *Medical Practice in Modern England: The Impact of Specialization and State Medicine.* New Haven: Yale University Press.

17. Eckstein, H. H. (1964). *The English Health Service: Its Origins, Structure, and Achievements.* Cambridge: Harvard University Press.

18. Ryan, M. (1968). "Health Centre Policy in England and Wales." *British Journal of Sociology,* 19:34–46.

19. British Medical Journal (1967). "Health Centre Explosion." Leading Article. *British Medical Journal,* 4:759.

20. Great Britain, Ministry of Health (1965). *Annual Report,* Cmnd. 3039. London: Her Majesty's Stationery Office.

21. Curran, W. J. (1966). "Legal Regulation and Quality Control of Medical Practice Under British Health Service." *New England Journal of Medicine,* 274:547–557.

22. McKeown, T. (1965). *Medicine in Modern Society: Medical Planning Based on Evaluation of Medical Achievement.* London: George Allen and Unwin.

23. College of General Practitioners, London (1965). *Report of a Symposium on the Art and the Science of General Practice.* Torquay: Devonshire Press.

24. Mechanic, D. (1968). *Medical Sociology: A Selective View:* New York: Free Press.

25. National Center for Health Statistics (1965). *Infant and Perinatal Mortality in the United States.* PHS Publication No. 1000, Series 3, No. 4. Washington: U. S. Government Printing Office.

26. Moriyama, I. M., and L. Guralnick (1965). "Occupational and Social Class Differences in Mortality." In Milbank Memorial Fund: *Trends and Differentials in Mortality.* Papers Presented at the 1955 Annual Conference of the Fund. New York: Milbank Memorial Fund.

27. Mechanic, D. (1967). "Changing Structure of Medical Practice." *Law and Contemporary Problems,* 32:707–730.

28. Department of Health and Social Security (1970). *The Future Structure of the National Health Service.* London: Her Majesty's Stationery Office.

29. Department of Health and Social Security (1971). *1970 Annual Report.* Cmnd. 4714. London: Her Majesty's Stationery Office.

CHAPTER IX

General Medical Practice: Some Comparisons Between the Work of Primary Care Physicians in the United States and England and Wales*

A major factor in the ferment concerning medical care has been the increasing inaccessibility of the general physician. It has been well established that in recent decades the proportion of physicians in primary medical care (including general practitioners, internists, and pediatricians) relative to all physicians has been declining,[1] and consumers frequently complain about the difficulty of finding a primary physician, unwillingness of the doctor to make home calls, and impersonality in health care. It is fully apparent that modifications in the delivery of health services must deal with present difficulties if they are to be reasonably responsive to consumer needs and expectations.

In contrast, the National Health Service of England and Wales has made a concerted attempt to maintain the structure of primary care through its system of general practice. Approximately 40 per cent of all English doctors are general practitioners and maintain community practices averaging about 2500 patients. These doctors practice largely outside the hospital, although a significant proportion of them have access to beds for obstetrics.[2] Difficulties in general practice in England have been described in the previous chapter, but available evidence also suggests considerable satisfaction among British consumers with general practice and good accessibility to care.[3]

---

* Adapted from a research report to appear in *Medical Care*, 1973.

In both countries there is currently considerable agonizing over the responsibilities of the primary care physician and the types of training that best prepare him for the problems encountered in general practice. There are major differences of perspective among commentators, some of whom are concerned with how to bring the scientific expertise and the latest technology of the teaching hospital to bear on the community practice of medicine, others who feel that the models of practice taught are inappropriate to the needs and proper approach of a generalist practicing in the community. Implicit in the attempts to encourage health center practice in Britain and health maintenance organizations in the United States is a desire to deal with a greater proportion of medical problems within the context of ambulatory care, making appropriate use of existing technical and ancillary resources. But the proper standards for such practice are themselves in flux, and are likely to undergo considerable modification in the coming years. This chapter presents data showing some of the similarities and variations among English and American primary care physicians.

Sources of Data

In 1966, a random sample of general practitioners in England and Wales was selected for the investigation by the Ministry of Health, and each doctor received a long questionnaire. After from one to three communications, 60 per cent of the doctors (813) had returned completed questionnaires. On the fourth approach a much shorter questionnaire was sent, and an additional 13 per cent responded, yielding a total response rate of 73 per cent (995 doctors) for many key items. Basic demographic data about all general practitioners in England and Wales, as well as all of the doctors designated in our sample, were provided by the Ministry of Health. Detailed analyses of the characteristics of the sample in comparison to the population, between responders and nonresponders, and between early and later responders are reported elsewhere.[4] Although the sample obtained had some overrepresentation of younger doctors and those in larger groups, for the most part the respondents were very similar in demographic characteristics to all general practitioners in England and Wales.

While the general practitioner is a structured position in the National Health Service, there is no comparable position in the United States. One way of obtaining a comparable group is to define primary care physicians as doctors of first contact, that is, office-based doctors that are likely to offer general services on a community basis. Ordinarily, this would include general practitioners, internists, and pediatricians. It is arguable as to whether obstetricians should be included in this definition, but since British general practitioners do a considerable amount of obstetrics, it seemed reasonable to include office-based obstetricians in the population. With the assistance of the American Medical Association, a random sample of office-based general practitioners, internists, pediatricians, and obstetricians was selected with different sampling ratios among group and nongroup practitioners classified by their primary activity code. The population from which the sample was drawn included 82,271 nongroup practitioners and 12,772 group practitioners. Among the nongroup population, 56 per cent were general practitioners, 21 per cent internists, 14 per cent pediatricians and 9 per cent obstetricians. Among group practitioners, comparable percentages were 37, 32, 15, and 16. A questionnaire similar to but shorter than the British questionnaire was sent to each member of our sample between the period October, 1970 to March, 1971. After five approaches, 1458 physicians (66 per cent of our sample) returned completed questionnaires.

The American Medical Association provided a tape containing information on the entire sample from their Physicians' Records Information System. In a preliminary analysis, comparing the data describing physicians who responded to our survey with the total sample on such attributes as year of graduation, sex, state within which the doctor practices, birthdate, license year, National Board year, amount of postgraduate education, source of professional income, present employment, government service, specialty boards, and memberships in specialty societies, no differences of significance were obtained. In no case did any category vary by more than 2 or 3 per cent in comparing those who responded with the entire sample.

A somewhat sharper picture of possible biases emerges in comparing the minority who did not respond to the survey with those who did. Here we find that nonrespondents include a higher proportion of older doctors (23 per cent 61 years or older), those who graduated from medical school in 1935 or earlier (20 per cent), and those who were licensed to practice in 1940 or before (23 per cent). The comparable figures among respondents were 16 per cent, 13 per cent, and 18 per cent. Nonrespondents were more likely to be in individual fee for service practice (53 per cent) than respondents (44 per cent) and also were more likely to be on full-time salaries (4 per cent versus 2 per cent). Nonrespondents were also less likely to have their specialty boards (23 per cent) than respondents (33 per cent) and were less likely to belong to at least one specialty society (49 per cent versus 34 per cent). This selective tendency relative to specialty boards and specialty societies is most pronounced among pediatricians. In sum, although the respondents are characteristic of the entire sample, there was some selective response to the survey. It is noteworthy that the character of this selectivity is similar to that obtained in the British sample. Since we have differentially sampled nongroup and group physicians in the United States, data for these categories will be presented separately.

Before presenting our comparative data, some cautions should be noted. Both surveys depend entirely on doctors' reports of various behaviors and activities, and for the most part, independent data to assess the accuracy of these reports are not available. Moreover, respondents may frequently answer questions in a fashion which presents them in a favorable light, and they may knowingly and unknowingly distort or exaggerate their responses to promote particular positions. The data from British general practitioners were collected in the midst of a remuneration dispute and the data from American physicians were collected during a time when there has been considerable discussion of the adequacy of medical organization and medical care. Also, there is a differential of more than four years between the two surveys. Finally, although both surveys elicited response rates higher than usual in such surveys of physicians, a significant number of doctors in both samples did not return questionnaires. Although we have attempted to ascertain the impact of nonresponse on various kinds of information available on all physicians, it is impossible to make such estimates for many items of importance for which data are unavailable.

Some Comparative Data

Among the British general practitioners we studied, 19 per cent were solo practitioners, 52 per cent were in two or three man partnerships, 16 per cent were in four man partnerships, and 11 per cent were in larger groups. Among American primary care physicians in office-based practice, 13 per cent were in groups as their primary activity. Of the remaining 87 per cent, 51 per cent were in solo practice, 36 per cent were in partnerships, 11 per cent shared facilities with other doctors but maintained independent practices, and 2 per cent had other arrangements. In both countries, solo practice and small partnerships constitute clearly the dominant forms of delivering primary medical services.

Since the roles of British G.P.'s and American primary care physicians vary substantially, we shall concentrate on those aspects common to both. American doctors report spending much more time seeing patients in their offices relative to British doctors and much less time visiting patients in their homes. We asked doctors in both samples to report the amount of time they had spent the day prior to completing our questionnaire seeing patients at their office or, if the prior day had been atypical, during the most recent typical day. Only 6 per cent of British G.P.'s reported spending six or more hours seeing patients at their offices in comparison to 67 per cent of nongroup and 70 per cent of group physicians in the American sample. In contrast, only 15 per cent of British doctors reported spending less than two hours on home calls as compared with 92 per cent of nongroup and 99 per cent of group physicians in the United States. More than half of the British doctors spend from two to four hours for home calls, and 32 per cent spent more than four hours on this activity.

As an examination of Table 1 shows, the vast majority of American doctors made no home calls at all, varying from 52 per cent of nongroup G.P.'s to 100 per cent of group obstetricians. But even among G.P.'s there is little home visiting; only 9 per cent of nongroup G.P.'s and 3 per cent of group G.P.'s made three or more home calls. In contrast, two-fifths of the British G.P.'s reported 15 or more home calls during the previous day, and only 6 per cent reported less than 5. We asked similar questions about office consultations and home calls in respect to "a typical day" with comparable results. The most extraordinary aspect of these data concerns the very large number of patients that British G.P.'s manage to see within the limited time they spend in surgery.

American doctors, in contrast to their British counterparts, also have a great deal of contact with patients through hospital rounds and telephone consultations. Among nongroup physicians, two-fifths reported visiting less than 5 hospital patients during the previous day, two-fifths reported making between 5 and 10 visits, and one-fifth reported 11 or more such visits. The comparable percentages for group practitioners were 36 per cent, 41 per cent and 23 per cent. Internists saw the most patients on hospital rounds (28 per cent of nongroup and 37 per cent of group internists saw 11 or more such patients) and pediatricians saw the least (8 per cent of nongroup pediatricians and 5 per cent of group pediatricians saw 11 or more). One-fifth of general practitioners saw a comparable number of patients on hospital rounds. Relevant to telephone conversations with patients, three-fifths of the nongroup physicians and one-half of the group physicians reported 10 or more such conversations. Pediatricians clearly reported the most such telephone consultations; 84 per cent of the nongroup pediatricians and 64 per cent of the group pediatricians reported 10 or more such consultations during the previous day.

Table 1 Number of Reported Patient Visits in Office and Home during Previous Day among British General Practitioners and among Varying Types of United States Primary Care Physicians (Per Cent)

	British General Practitioners (N = 813)[a]	General Practitioners Nongroup (N = 599)[a]	General Practitioners Group (N = 111)[a]	Internists Nongroup (N = 231)[a]	Internists Group (N = 91)[a]	Pediatricians Nongroup (N = 136)[a]	Pediatricians Group (N = 43)[a]	Obstetricians Nongroup (N = 150)[a]	Obstetricians Group (N = 58)[a]
Number of patients seen during previous day at office									
0–10	} 5	6	6	21	16	2	5	8	7
11–19		10	5	42	49	9	12	15	12
20–29	12	27	32	24	29	30	36	42	39
30–36	21	23	21	9	5	22	21	20	29
37–43	13	14	16	1	1	13	17	10	7
44–50	20	8	10	1	—	13	2	3	3
51–64	17	8	6	} 1	—	5	7	} 2	} 2
65 or more	12	4	3		—	6	—		
Number of home calls during previous day									
None		52	75	70	82	81	95	96	100
1		26	15	18	11	11	3	1	—
2		13	7	8	5	5	3	—	—
3		5	1	3	1	1	—	1	—
4 or more		4	2	1	1	1	—	3	—

[a] The sample sizes shown here and in subsequent tables, unless otherwise specified, constitute the full sample available in the analysis. Percentages are calculated only for doctors responding to the specific question, and thus sample size may vary slightly from the base and from one question to another. Percentages do not always equal 100 per cent due to rounding errors.

Approximately one-third of the doctors reported seeing patients in other contexts, but for the most part the number of patients seen was very small.

We asked each of the doctors in our American sample to give us three estimates for the number of hours they work during a typical week. We then cumulated the time reported in each of these three questions to form an estimate of reported typical workweek, and these data are shown in Table 2. The figures reported cannot be taken on face value without independent validation, and these estimates are at best "rough"; nevertheless, they can be indicative of various trends and variations among the specialties and types of practice. Except for the general practitioners, nongroup practitioners tend to report longer workweeks, with nongroup internists most likely to report a workweek exceeding 60 hours. This is attributable in part to the tendency of internists to report more time on various aspects of continuing education.

Table 3 reports estimates based on time budgets provided for the previous day by British and American doctors. The items used in the two countries vary, but estimates based on five selected items among the American doctors are roughly equivalent to the British reports. This comparison underestimates the time British doctors spend on telephone work which is small relative to the American situation and underestimates the time American physicians spend on surgery and in delivering babies. The data suggest that a somewhat higher proportion of American doctors report working longer hours on the previous day, although the differences are not particularly large. The proportion of doctors that reported working 12 hours or more during the previous day is highest among nongroup practitioners, but there are only small reported differences between American group practitioners and British G.P.'s. These data suggest that American physicians work somewhat longer hours than British G.P.'s, but that both groups report relatively long days. The major differences appear not so much in the length of the workday, as in the character of daily activities.

Practice Orientations among British and United States Primary Care Physicians

One way of assessing, indirectly, the character of the doctor's approach to the patient is to describe his use of diagnostic facilities and his social orientation to medical care. We asked United States respondents to report whether they had used each of 14 diagnostic procedures in the previous two weeks, 13 of which were identical to those we presented to our British

Table 2 Reported Time Expenditures for a "Typical Week" among United States Primary Care Physicians (Per Cent)

	General Practitioners		Internists		Pediatricians		Obstetricians	
	Nongroup (N = 599)	Group (N = 111)	Nongroup (N = 231)	Group (N = 91)	Nongroup (N = 136)	Group (N = 43)	Nongroup (N = 150)	Group (N = 58)
Hours spent during a typical week seeing patients								
Less than 40	29	17	17	22	20	24	41	32
40–49	19	33	27	29	27	33	24	32
50–59	24	24	27	33	25	24	15	21
60 or more	29	27	29	16	28	19	20	16
Additional hours during a typical week devoted to practice management (excluding direct patient contact)								
2 or less	29	41	23	46	28	65	35	45
3–5	32	31	35	22	34	21	33	36
6–10	26	21	30	21	28	9	18	14
11 or more	14	6	12	10	9	5	14	5

Table 2 (*Continued*)

	General Practitioners		Internists		Pediatricians		Obstetricians	
	Nongroup (N = 599)	Group (N = 111)	Nongroup (N = 231)	Group (N = 91)	Nongroup (N = 136)	Group (N = 43)	Nongroup (N = 150)	Group (N = 58)
Additional hours on activities related to practice such as attending meetings, medical reading, etc.								
2 or less	31	35	19	18	19	19	29	28
3–5	35	31	39	31	42	46	37	33
6–10	28	27	28	40	34	28	26	22
11 or more	7	7	13	11	5	7	8	17
Total reported hours spent during a typical week (sum of three above categories)								
Less than 40	10	6	6	9	7	18	25	12
40–49	14	17	11	13	16	14	15	24
50–59	26	28	26	40	27	32	21	29
60–69	22	26	28	20	28	21	14	17
70 or more	28	23	30	18	23	14	26	17

151

Table 3 Reported Time Budgets for the Previous Working Day among British and United States Primary Care Physicians (Per Cent)

	British General Practitioners[a] (Specified Items)[b] (N = 772)	United States Primary Care Physicians			
		Nongroup (First Five Items)[c] (N = 1148)	Group (First Five Items)[c] (N = 310)	Nongroup (All Items)[d] (N = 1148)	Group (All Items)[d] (N = 310)
Less than 6 hours	4	3	4	2	1
6 hours or more but less than 8 hours	12	10	9	3	3
8 hours or more but less than 10 hours	42	26	33	13	16
10 hours or more but less than 12 hours	29	34	37	33	37
12 hours or more	14	26	18	49	44

[a] Part of our analysis of British doctors is based on a data tape that excluded 41 doctors because they failed to respond to 10 per cent or more of our questions. In remaining cases, where data on a particular question were missing, the respondent was assigned to the mean response of those replying to the question. The demographic profile of this sample was almost identical to the profile of all respondents.

[b] Items include seeing patients at surgery, domiciliary visits and travel, other work relevant travel, administrative and paper work, and hospital work.

[c] Items include seeing patients at your office, talking with patients or other doctors on phone, house calls and related travel, hospital rounds and related travel, and administrative and paper work.

[d] Includes five items above and also doing surgery, delivering babies, continuing education, and other professional duties.

sample. As an examination of Table 4 shows, in every case American doctors were more likely to use these procedures than their British counterparts. As might be expected, internists and general practitioners, on the average, were more likely to use these procedures than obstetricians and pediatricians. American doctors in group practice are more likely to use each of these diagnostic procedures regardless of speciality, although this factor only accounts for modest differences. Having 14 procedures and 4 subgroups of doctors allows 56 comparisons between nongroup and group practitioners. In 48 of these comparisons, doctors in group practice were more likely to use the given procedure, although the average difference between solo and group practitioners was only 7 percentage

Table 4   Reported Use of Various Diagnostic Procedures among British and United States Primary Care Physicians (Per Cent)

| | Reported Use in Previous Two Weeks | | |
| | British General Practitioners ($N = 813$) | United States Primary Care Physicians | |
Procedure		Nongroup ($N = 1148$)	Group ($N = 310$)
Full-size chest x-rays	67	91	94
Bone and joint x-rays	57	81	79
Bacteriologic examination of urine	57	78	91
Glucose tolerance tests	15	65	68
Erythrocyte sedimentation rate	48	67	74
Blood sugar	21	90	92
Prothrombin activity	20	64	66
Serum cholesterol	15	71	73
Blood culture	4	35	40
Liver function tests	16	67	75
Serum electrolytes	10	71	77
Radioactive iodine uptake	3	29	32
Protein-bound iodine	[a]	71	75
Electrocardiogram	15	83	84
Hemoglobin	80	[a]	[a]
Red blood cell count	70	[a]	[a]
White blood cell count	67	[a]	[a]
Routine urinalysis	53	[a]	[a]

[a] Not asked.

points. Significant deviations by specialty included the tendency of obstetricians to be less likely to use full-size chest x-rays, bone or joint x-rays, erythrocyte sedimentation rate, prothrombin activity, serum cholesterol, blood culture, liver function tests, radioactive iodine uptake and electrocardiogram; the tendency of pediatricians to be less likely to use glucose tolerance, blood sugar, prothrombin activity, serum cholesterol, liver function tests, radioactive iodine uptake, protein bound iodine and electrocardiograms; and the tendency for general practitioners to be less likely to use blood cultures.

American doctors are clearly dependent on the clinical laboratory to a point which some commentators regard as excessive, while it is generally agreed that the average primary care physician in Britain does not do sufficient laboratory work. Younger British doctors and those in group practice are more likely to use diagnostic aids, and some recent data on doctors practicing in health centers reported by Kern[5] show very strong evidence of increased use. Kern's data includes many younger doctors who tend to be more likely to use diagnostic aids, but even this sample has a lower rate of diagnostic use than either American G.P.'s or internists. It should be noted, however, that a good deal of the diagnostic work which characterizes American practice is performed in British hospital out-patient departments, where patients are readily referred by general practitioners.

Table 5 also provides some comparative data on the performance of various tasks. There are only 4 items in the British and American surveys where the questions were sufficiently similar to argue for comparability (tape sprains, open abcesses, excise simple cysts, and suture lacerations). These are all relatively simple procedures which one might expect a primary care physician to perform. Relevant to three of these procedures, British G.P.'s are comparable to American G.P.'s and pediatricians. There is more variability in reports of excising simple cysts, where both American G.P.'s and obstetricians are relatively likely to perform the procedure, and pediatricians and internists relatively unlikely. British G.P.'s fall between these two groupings. Cartwright[6] has queried British doctors about other procedures, and has found only small proportions performing them: administering intravenous fluids (37 per cent), aspirating chest (22 per cent), injecting piles (19 per cent), cauterising cervix (17 per cent), reducing simple limb fractures (15 per cent), lumbar puncture (7 per cent), sigmoidoscopy (3 per cent), electrocardiography (3 per cent), ligating varicose veins (3 per cent), estimating hemoglobin with a hemoglobinometer (27 per cent), and use of a laryngoscope (35 per cent). An exception was doing a vaginal exam with a speculum which was reported by 88 per cent of the British G.P.'s. These data support the general impression of observers that British G.P.'s function as generalists but in a relatively restricted manner. In contrast, American general practitioners have a much wider range of practice. The fact that more than a third of American generalists report doing major general surgery, suggests that this may have some disadvantages.

The data presented in Tables 4 and 5 show considerable variability in the work of G.P.'s, internists, pediatricians and obstetricians. To some extent such differences reflect expected varying case mix, but they also suggest that the tendency to classify all these types as primary care physicians in assessing physician distribution may be somewhat misleading. These types of practitioners are usually categorized together with the implication that they perform as generalists and maintain a very wide scope of practice. But these data suggest that a large proportion of such practices are more restricted than generally believed.

Table 6 provides some fragmentary data on the doctors' social orienta-

Table 5 Comparisons of Various Aspects of the Work of Primary Care Physicians in Britain and in the United States (Per Cent)

| | | Kern Data[a] | United States Primary Care Physicians | | | | | | | |
| | British General Practitioners (N = 772) | British GP's in Health Centers (N = 95) | General Practitioners | | Internists | | Pediatricians | | Obstetricians | |
Aspects of Work			Nongroup (N = 599)	Group (N = 111)	Nongroup (N = 231)	Group (N = 91)	Nongroup (N = 136)	Group (N = 43)	Nongroup (N = 150)	Group (N = 58)
Use of Diagnostic procedures during previous two weeks[b]										
5 or less	70	⎱24	8	6	3	—	29	32	46	29
6–7	15	⎰	9	2	5	—	26	20	21	26
8–9	6	19	20	12	15	7	25	20	17	29
10–12	7	⎱57	52	66	56	66	20	22	14	16
13	1	⎰	10	14	22	28	1	7	1	—

British General Practitioners

	Cartwright Survey, 1963[c] (N = 157)	Cartwright Survey, 1967[d] (N = 442)

	Cartwright 1963 (N = 157)	Cartwright 1967 (N = 442)	US GP Nongroup	US GP Group	Internists Nongroup	Internists Group	Pediatricians Nongroup	Pediatricians Group	Obstetricians Nongroup	Obstetricians Group
Reports uses of following procedures on occasion or more frequently[k]										
"Tape" (strap)[f] sprains	91	98	86	88	56	42	78	71	16	12

155

Table 5 (Continued)

156

Reports uses of following procedures on occasion or more frequently[k]	British General Practitioners		United States Primary Care Physicians							
			General Practitioners		Internists		Pediatricians		Obstetricians	
	Cartwright Survey, 1963[c] (N = 157)	Cartwright Survey, 1967[d] (N = 442)	Nongroup (N = 599)	Group (N = 111)	Nongroup (N = 231)	Group (N = 91)	Nongroup (N = 136)	Group (N = 43)	Nongroup (N = 150)	Group (N = 58)
Excise simple cysts	62	62	94	90	20	11	28	19	87	93
Open abcesses	89	94	99	95	56	46	92	73	97	95
Suture lacerations (stitch cuts)	93	94	98	95	37	31	85	80	62	65
Do proctoscopic or sigmoidoscopic exam[g]	3	e	83	86	89	91	40	39	43	33
Take and interpret your own electrocardiograms (perform electrocardiography)	3	e	69	81	98	97	24	43	76	16
Do vaginal exam with a speculum	e	88	99	98	96	92	30	39	99	100
Use a laryngoscope	e	35	48	62	30	27	58	71	20	26
Do uncomplicated obstetrics	25[h]	20[j]	59	58	—	—	3	—	97	100
Do well-baby care	e	e	91	83	7	1	97	100	14	11
Do simple psychotherapy	22[i]	e	96	99	95	93	93	95	88	93
Do pap smears	e	e	98	94	94	92	7	5	99	100
Set simple fractures	e	e	80	77	6	3	50	32	5	2

Table 5 (*Continued*)

Reports uses of following procedures on occasion or more frequently[k]	British General Practitioners		United States Primary Care Physicians							
	Cartwright Survey, 1963[c] (N = 157)	Cartwright Survey, 1967[d] (N = 442)	General Practitioners		Internists		Pediatricians		Obstetricians	
			Nongroup (N = 599)	Group (N = 111)	Nongroup (N = 231)	Group (N = 91)	Nongroup (N = 136)	Group (N = 43)	Nongroup (N = 150)	Group (N = 58)
Do major general surgery	e	c	35	37	1	—	5	—	74	74
Take and interpret selected x-rays in your office	e	e	57	87	53	73	31	64	17	41

[a] Kern5 obtained data from 96 of a sample of 140 general practitioners in 24 health centers in England, Wales, and Scotland. The study was restricted to centers housing at least four general practitioners in communities of 50,000 or less.

[b] This scale includes only those diagnostic procedures included in the questionnaires in both countries.

[c] A representative two-stage sample of 195 general practitioners of whom 157 responded. See Cartwright.6

[d] Patients interviewed in 12 areas of England and Wales named their doctors, resulting in 552 names. Of those who were sent questionnaires, 442 responded. See Cartwright.3

[e] Question not asked.

[f] Wording on some of the items varied. British wording given in parentheses.

[g] British doctors were only asked about proctoscopic examinations.

[h] These data come from my survey and are in response to the question, "Do you do domiciliary obstetrics?"

[i] These data are from my survey and are in response to the question, "Do you do any regular psychotherapy with patients?" This question obviously has different meaning than the one posed to American physicians.

[j] This is the estimated proportion of doctors with 50 or more obstetric cases in previous 12 months. See Cartwright.3

[k] The data are reported using identical categories in my survey and in Cartwright (1967). In Cartwright (1965) data are reported as the "proportions who said they carry out these procedures."

tions, their satisfaction, and degree of frustration. These measures appear to have validity, and they are discussed in greater detail elsewhere.[4] Contrary to general belief, these data support the notion that American doctors are more socially oriented to medical care than their British counterparts who are also less satisfied and more frustrated. These data must be viewed with some caution since the social orientation questions all involved items as to whether it is appropriate for persons with varying kinds of problems to seek the assistance of physicians. British doctors tend to have very heavy workloads, and since they are paid on a capitation system they have little incentive to encourage "marginal" consultations. In contrast, in the American case there is usually an economic incentive for additional patient visits. However, there were only trivial differences between American group and· nongroup physicians despite the fact that one-third to one-half of group physicians reported receiving salaries as the major component of their remuneration, while nongroup physicians depended largely on fee for service.

As an examination of Table 6 also shows, American doctors express less frustration, as reflected in their estimates of trivial and inappropriate consultations, than their British counterparts, and also report considerably greater satisfaction. The British data reflecting dissatisfaction may be somewhat exaggerated by the political dispute over remuneration and terms of service that were concurrent with the survey, but it is unlikely that these events could account for the magnitude of observed differences. In both countries doctors were most dissatisfied about time—being able to devote sufficient time to each patient, total amount of time devoted to one's practice, and the limited leisure time available. But unlike British general practitioners, American doctors are far more satisfied with their income, status, incentives, and professional arrangements. Some improve-

---

[a] The items used are the propriety of consulting the doctor for family financial troubles, disobedience of children, marital difficulties, handling behavior in a relative such as drunkenness, children's poor school performance, birth control advice, problems with drinking too much, general feelings of unhappiness, anxieties about child care and obesity. Also included was a correlated question: "Some medical commentators have recently argued that there is a growing tendency for people to bring less serious disorders to doctors and more readily seek help for problems in their family lives. In general do you feel that this is a good or bad trend, given present conditions of medical practice?"

[b] There was a significant variation in the way the question was worded in the two countries. In the British case, the question asked was "In general, how satisfied are you with general practice?" In the American case, the question referred to "your practice." We gathered considerable data on satisfaction, and we have examined the internal consistency of these data. We feel confident that these two questions are reasonably comparable.

Table 6 Comparison of British and United States Primary Care Physicians on Measures of "Social Orientations to Medical Care," "Frustration," and "Satisfaction" (Per Cent)

	British General Practitioners (N = 772)	United States Primary Care Physicians			
		General Practitioners		All Nongroup (N = 1148)	All Group (N = 310)
		Nongroup (N = 599)	Group (N = 111)		
Social orientations to medical care[a]					
High (scores of 1 to 3)	24	43	47	38	40
Medium high (scores 4–5)	39	38	38	38	35
Medium low (scores of 6–7)	27	16	14	19	19
Low (scores of 8 or 9)	10	4	1	6	5
Index of frustration; per cent of patient visits estimated as trivial, unnecessary, or inappropriate					
Less than 10 per cent	12	33	28	36	36
10 per cent or more but less than 25 per cent	29	35	36	35	35
25 per cent or more but less than 50 per cent	35	23	24	22	19
50 per cent or more	24	9	13	7	10
Satisfaction[b]					
Very satisfied	10	53	56	51	52
Fairly satisfied	41	42	41	44	43
Not very satisfied	35	4	3	4	4
Quite dissatisfied	14	—	—	1	—

ments have been made in remuneration and other conditions of work since the British survey was completed.

One aspect of the British pattern of general practice that has frequently been commented upon is the professional isolation of the general practitioner from his peers. We asked doctors in both countries a very similar question regarding the frequency with which they seek advice from other medical men concerning some aspect of their practice. The question asked of American doctors was somewhat more rigorous in its criterion, since it referred to *specifically* contacting other doctors to seek advice in comparison to the British version which asked "How frequently do you seek advice . . . ?" Yet despite this, American doctors report that they much more frequently seek such advice, with 43 per cent of the nongroup practitioners and 56 per cent of the group practitioners indicating that they seek such advice several times a week, in contrast to only 16 per cent of the British doctors.

It is possible that this type of contact might be influenced by friendship patterns and social customs generally rather than the way in which professional practice is structured. We also asked two identical questions of doctors in both countries concerning social contacts and friendships among doctors. In both cases, as Table 7 shows, the distributions were very similar suggesting that the patterns of professional advice seeking probably cannot be attributed to different types of social relationships in the two countries.

Attitudes toward Medical Practice and Government

In both countries we asked doctors a series of attitudinal questions concerning government involvement in medical affairs, the role of self-sacrifice in being a doctor, and uncertainty in carrying on a general practice. Table 8 provides data on those items which are to some extent comparable. There was only one item where we asked a clearly comparable question concerning the role of government, and this statement dealt with whether it is proper for government physicians to attempt to evaluate the quality of care in general practice. About three-quarters of the British doctors agreed that this was proper, but only 26 per cent of American nongroup practitioners, and 35 per cent of group practitioners agreed. Although this is only a single item, it does suggest considerably more receptivity to government auditing among British general practitioners than among their American counterparts. As the data in Table 9 relevant to controls show, the vast majority of American doctors approve of peer review of medical work in the hospital, but their enthusiasm is

Table 7 Professional and Social Contacts among Primary Care Physicians in Britain and the United States (Per Cent)

Measures of Contact	British General Practitioners (N = 772)	United States Primary Care Physicians	
		Nongroup (N = 1148)	Group (N = 310)
Frequency of seeking advice from other medical men concerning some aspect of practice[a]			
Several times a week	16	43	56
Every week or so	28	21	19
Couple times a month	17	12	8
A few times a year or less	40	24	17
Frequency of social contact with other physicians in homes			
Every week or so or more	17	10	11
A couple of times a month	19	23	24
A few times a year	43	45	50
Hardly ever	21	22	15
Number of three closest friends who are doctors			
None	24	27	23
One	35	36	37
Two or three	41	37	40

[a] A slight wording difference is discussed in the text.

much dampened when the review is to be carried out by physicians from outside their own community. These data suggest that American doctors remain quite suspicious of controls by government, or even physician groups outside their immediate community. Pediatricians and internists are least resistant toward outside controls.

In respect to attitudes toward sacrifice, we found no consistent differences between British and American doctors. Among American physicians, doctors in group practice were less likely to endorse sacrificing attitudes, but such differences were relatively modest and have limited practical significance. The third set of items concerned uncertainty about the nature of knowledge underlying decisions that the general practitioner has to make. In my observations of British doctors, I was impressed that such uncertainties were widely prevalent and contributed to the crisis in role definition of the general practitioner. There was only

Table 8 Attitudes of Primary Care Physicians in Britain and the United States toward Various Aspects of Medical Practice (Per Cent)

Per Cent Agreeing on Various Attitudes	British General Practitioners (N = 772)	United States Primary Care Physicians							
		General Practitioners		Internists		Pediatricians		Obstetricians	
		Nongroup (N = 599)	Group (N = 111)	Nongroup (N = 231)	Group (N = 91)	Nongroup (N = 136)	Group (N = 43)	Nongroup (N = 150)	Group (N = 58)
Government auditing									
It is quite proper for government physicians (the N.H.S.)[a] to attempt to evaluate the quality of care patients receive (provided in general practice)	74	20	30	34	41	38	41	29	29
Sacrificing orientation									
One should not become a doctor unless he is willing to work long and irregular hours	76	88	76	89	78	83	76	89	88

Table 8 (*Continued*)

Per Cent Agreeing on Various Attitudes	British General Practitioners (N = 772)	United States Primary Care Physicians							
		General Practitioners		Internists		Pediatricians		Obstetricians	
		Nongroup (N = 599)	Group (N = 111)	Nongroup (N = 231)	Group (N = 91)	Nongroup (N = 136)	Group (N = 43)	Nongroup (N = 150)	Group (N = 58)
One should not become a doctor unless he is willing to sacrifice his own needs to those of the general welfare	67	56	37	58	42	50	51	51	54
Uncertainty in medical decision making In general practice, one's decisions often are not based on well-established knowledge	58	28	21	45	54	38	38	46	53

163

Table 8 (*Continued*)

Per Cent Agreeing on Various Attitudes	British General Practitioners (N = 772)	United States Primary Care Physicians							
		General Practitioners		Internists		Pediatricians		Obstetricians	
		Nongroup (N = 599)	Group (N = 111)	Nongroup (N = 231)	Group (N = 91)	Nongroup (N = 136)	Group (N = 43)	Nongroup (N = 150)	Group (N = 58)
Given the conditions of general practice, the doctor is not really in a position to make many of the assessments he is called upon to make	b	19	20	33	40	35	33	38	43
Given the conditions of general practice, the doctor isn't really in a position to make the evaluations necessary for issuing medical certificates	41	b	b	b	b	b	b	b	b

a Differences in wording on the British questions are noted by parentheses.
b Question not asked.

one instance where the identical question was asked in both countries, and this item concerned whether general practice decisions are based upon well established knowledge. On this item, British general practitioners express much greater uncertainty than American general practitioners but, in general, American internists and obstetricians respond very much as the British doctors do. The American pediatricians fall between these two extremes. The American general practitioners also express less uncertainty than other American subgroups on a question concerning the doctor's certainty in making many of the assessments for which he is called upon.

In considering these responses, we should note that the questions were addressed to "general practice" and thus general practitioners were probably responding more in terms of their conceptions of their own practices than the other subgroups. American general practitioners seem to have made a better adaptation to feelings of uncertainty than their British counterparts and this is probably due to the wider scope of their practice, their greater dependence on modern technology and laboratory aids, and their closer tie to hospital work. From the point of view of physicians with more restricted practices, however, general practice appears more vague and ill-defined.

Table 9 shows physicians to be relatively evenly divided on many of the major innovations currently under discussion. These attitudinal items are of a very general nature, and doctors may generally approve of an innovation until it encroaches on his practice or demands that he change his accustomed habits; and, similarly, there are data that indicate that doctors' cooperation with a new program may be relatively independent of their initial attitude toward it.[7] These attitudes, however, suggest trends which are reviewed within the context of other findings in the discussion that follows.

Discussion and Conclusions

The types of data presented in this chapter are descriptive rather than evaluative and implications for public policy do not naturally flow from them. Nor do they pertain directly to the major problems we confront in maintaining primary health care services, in excessive specialization and subspecialization, in the maldistribution of physicians and in maintaining coordinated and comprehensive health care services. Moreover they speak to doctors' orientations and responses and not to those of their clients, and the interests of these two groups are clearly different. However, when viewed in a larger context, these data provide some apprecia-

Table 9 Attitudes of United States Primary Care Physicians toward New Features of the Organization of Medical Care (Per Cent)

Proportion Responding that They Strongly Approve or Moderately Approve	General Practitioners Nongroup (N = 599)	Group (N = 111)	Internists Nongroup (N = 231)	Group (N = 91)	Pediatricians Nongroup (N = 136)	Group (N = 43)	Obstetricians Nongroup (N = 150)	Group (N = 58)
Financing								
Concept of government financing of medical care as in the Medicaid program in your state	38	44	44	57	45	51	39	51
Federal financing of medical care through some system of National Health Insurance	32	44	41	51	43	54	39	41
Practice organization and innovations								
Community health centers such as those established by the Office of Economic Opportunity	52	59	69	78	68	80	60	66

Table 9 (Continued)

Proportion Responding that They Strongly Approve or Moderately Approve	General Practitioners		Internists		Pediatricians		Obstetricians	
	Nongroup (N = 599)	Group (N = 111)	Nongroup (N = 231)	Group (N = 91)	Nongroup (N = 136)	Group (N = 43)	Nongroup (N = 150)	Group (N = 58)
Prepaid group practice such as the Kaiser-Permanente Plan or the Health Insurance Plan of New York	40	61	54	65	61	86	45	76
Doctors working on a salaried basis	37	54	50	57	54	68	39	66
Controls over medical work								
Peer review of medical work in the hospital	83	90	88	96	93	100	85	90
Peer review of medical work in the doctor's office	44	57	67	77	69	78	54	64
Review of hospital work by physicians from outside one's community	35	44	54	57	51	60	44	34

Table 9 (*Continued*)

Proportion Responding that They Strongly Approve or Moderately Approve	General Practitioners		Internists		Pediatricians		Obstetricians	
	Nongroup (N = 599)	Group (N = 111)	Nongroup (N = 231)	Group (N = 91)	Nongroup (N = 136)	Group (N = 43)	Nongroup (N = 150)	Group (N = 58)
New practitioners								
The use of specially trained physician's assistants who work under the doctor's supervision in his practice	78	85	79	87	82	93	74	88
The training of non-M.D. associates who work independently to some extent in under-doctored areas	51	72	62	75	63	68	55	65
Multiphasic health testing								
Multiphasic health screening as part of a doctor's or clinic's practice	75	79	79	82	80	86	73	81
Autonomous programs of Multiphasic Automated Health Testing	60	70	57	63	64	69	61	68

tion of the advantages and difficulties of primary care practice in the two countries.

Unlike Britain, which directs doctors into general medical practice through organizational means, the American system presently has no mechanism to keep physicians in primary medical care. Our data suggest, however, that it may be incorrect to regard internists and pediatricians as modern replacements of traditional practitioners in that the scope and character of their practice diverges markedly in many respects from the more traditional doctor. If the trend should continue, and we have every reason to believe it will, then the distress of patients concerning the availability of a comprehensive family physician is likely to continue well into the future. Those American doctors who continue to maintain a practice of wide scope appear to function with greater gratification than their British counterparts, who have a much narrower general orientation which seems to exaggerate the disparity between the scientific orientation of medical schools and their own daily practice. They express greater uncertainty about what they are doing, more disillusionment with their role and they seem more isolated from the mainstream of medicine than is true of their American counterparts.

It appears that the British general practitioner still offers certain advantages that seem to be disappearing in the United States. Within the limits we have described, British G.P.'s take on a wide variety of routine functions which patients expect doctors to perform, and which account for much of the demand on the doctor's time. Our data indicate that an American patient, with his own internist or pediatrician, has no assurance that such routine functions will be performed by his own doctor if needed. Simple procedures such as suturing lacerations, excising simple cysts, taping strains and the like may be referred to the local emergency room or some other doctor. Similarly, it seems regrettable that the physician home visit is now defunct in the United States. Certainly, given the shortage of physician manpower, the costs of medical care, and the expense of educating new physicians, it would be wasteful to attempt to replicate the high prevalence of home visiting characteristic of the British situation, and even there home visiting is decreasing with time. But it is also difficult to believe that the current situation where home visiting has become a rarity is a particularly desirable pattern. The primary care physician can learn a great deal about a patient and his difficulties by visiting the home from time to time. Yet it seems unlikely that the current trend can be turned back and, given the pressures on medical care, it seems apparent that alternatives will be necessary.

If, indeed, primary care physicians of the future are to be internists and pediatricians, and perhaps some family doctors as well, then it would be prudent to encourage such physicians to enlarge the scope of their practices so that they can encompass routine problems of care as well as those more complicated. It seems apparent that one way of doing this is to make use of trained assistants and technicians who can expertly carry out certain procedures that the doctor is unwilling to do himself. These procedures would include handling simple trauma, dealing with problems of behavior and child care, simple surgery, health education, and the like. It is reasonably clear from our data that physicians support the use of such assistants, but thus far there is no evidence that they are widely or effectively used. Nurse practitioners and others might also be helpful in reviving the institution of home visiting which, if well organized, can contribute to a more comprehensive pattern of primary care than is now evident. Such goals as increasing the scope and comprehensiveness of practice perhaps may best be fulfilled within the context of prepaid group practice, and certainly such practices facilitate the effective use of technology and ancillary workers, but at least one major study has suggested that such practices may be less responsive to the social and psychological aspects of the doctor-patient relationship.[8]

Although we have not examined such issues as the doctor-patient relationship directly, the data we have provide a mixed picture in respect to the issue of the relative merits of group versus nongroup practice. Nongroup doctors are more likely to make homecalls, however few, but there are no differences between group and nongroup doctors in their orientations to medicine. Doctors in groups appear to do somewhat more diagnostic work, have more professional contact with colleagues and are generally more receptive to a variety of innovations in practice organization (see Table 9). We have no way of assessing to what extent these differences are a product of group practice, or the result of a selection process in which persons with certain characteristics have chosen one or the other type of activity. Although some have suggested that group practice is less satisfying than an independent one, our data suggest that at least those doctors already in group practice are no less satisfied than their counterparts in nongroup practice.

Although our data are rather gross relative to time budgets, they suggest that nongroup practitioners work longer hours than those in groups. Given the extremely long hours worked by physicians, this is a mixed blessing, but these data do support Bailey's concern[9,10] that group practice may lead to a more limited work week, thus minimizing already scarce physician manhours. Of course, our data do not exclude the possibility that physicians who are somewhat less oriented to long workweeks are presently selected into group practice, or that incentives can be developed to increase the workweek among group practitioners if this was seen as desirable.

In sum, our data indicate that primary medical practice in the United States and Britain are radically different types of practice (see Chapter 10), and that within the United States the concept of the primary care physician involves varied orientations and patterns. There is little doubt that an effective system of health care services depends on a viable system of delivering and coordinating primary care, and it is clear that we still have much work to do in developing viable future models of primary health services that make use of modern developments in medical technology and knowledge, but that are also responsive to the needs and human dilemmas of those who seek the care of a physician.

Notes

1. Fein, R. (1967). *The Doctor Shortage: An Economic Analysis.* Washington: The Brookings Institute.
2. Mechanic, D. (1968). "General Practice in England and Wales: Results from a Survey of a National Sample of General Practitioners." *Medical Care,* 6:245–260.
3. Cartwright, A. (1967). *Patients and Their Doctors: A Study of General Practice.* London: Routledge and Kegan Paul.
4. Faich, R. (1969). "Social and Structural Factors Affecting Work Satisfaction." Dissertation in the Department of Sociology, University of Wisconsin.
5. Kern, D. "Survey of Communication Patterns Between General Practitioners and Consultants: A Preliminary Report." Unpublished Manuscript, Harvard Medical School.
6. Cartwright, A. (1965). "General Practice in 1963: Its Conditions, Contents and Satisfactions." *Medical Care,* 3:69–87.
7. Colombotos, J. (1971). "Physicians' Responses to Changes in Health Care: Some Projections." *Inquiry,* 8:20–26.
8. Freidson, E. (1961). *Patients' Views of Medical Practice.* New York: Russell Sage Foundation.
9. Bailey, R. (1970). "Economies of Scale in Medical Practice." In H. E. Klarman, (ed.), *Empirical Studies in Health Economics.* Baltimore: Johns Hopkins Press.
10. Bailey, R. (1970). "Philosophy, Faith, Fact and Fiction in the Production of Medical Services." *Inquiry,* 7:37–53.

CHAPTER X

Practice Orientations among General Medical Practitioners in England and Wales*

The appropriate role of the general practitioner is a major issue within the context of modern medical care. With the development of advanced technology and specialized knowledge, there has been some movement in all medical systems away from general practice as the common mode of meeting the medical needs of the population. In the United States, where the proliferation of medical specialization has been pronounced, there is growing skepticism concerning the viability of general practice. Most medical students in the United States now specialize, and few choose an unrestricted general practice following the completion of their training.

In contrast, the English National Health Service through its structure has continued to support a general practice approach. Implicit in this approach is the concept of a family doctor who not only meets the more routine medical needs of the population but who also is concerned with the wider family and community ramifications of illness, who views the problem of disease in a broad social context, and who takes a preventive approach to the patient.[1-3]

Although ideal descriptions of general practice involve many aspects, at least two dimensions run through all discussions of the proper role of the general practitioner. First, his medical competence is assumed; i.e., he is expected to have sufficient scientific know-how to locate cases requiring more detailed appraisal and care and to refer them to an appropriate consultant. Moreover, he is expected on his own to diagnose and treat more common acute disorders and to manage the care of many chronic

---

* Adapted from a paper published in *Medical Care*, 1970, 8:15–25, with permission of the Lippincott Company.

patients. Second, it is assumed that the general practitioner will have a wide scope of concern, involving himself not only with the patient's illness but with the implications of health and disease for work, family life, and the patient's general welfare. In short, the general practitioner is also expected to exercise a social orientation that views *dis-ease* in its wider community context. The purpose of this report is to examine the characteristics of doctors and the modes in which they practice that can be compared to these ideals.

Measures of Practice Orientations

In a general survey it is impossible to measure directly the quality of general practice. In this study, we have attempted to assess indirectly and crudely the practice orientations of general practitioners. In doing this, we have tried to measure two components of their practice—the use of diagnostic and laboratory aids, and the degree of the doctor's acceptance of a social role.

Diagnostic Use. In this analysis, the assumption is made that the extent of the doctor's use of diagnostic and laboratory aids reflects his scientific and technical orientation to medical practice. Although the indiscriminate and improper use of laboratory aids reflects poor scientific practice, it is reasonable to expect in the British situation, where the use of diagnostic and laboratory aids is modest, that the level of use roughly depicts the doctor's orientation to medicine as a technical activity. We thus asked respondents if they used each of the following procedures during the previous two weeks: full size chest x-rays, bone and joint x-rays, bacteriologic examination of the urine, glucose tolerance tests, hemoglobin, white blood count, red blood count, routine urinalysis, erythrocyte sedimentation rate, blood sugar, prothrombin activity, serum cholesterol, blood culture, liver function test, serum electrolytes, B.M.R., CSF micro and culture and chemistry, radioactive iodine, and electrocardiogram. Of the 19 possible procedures, 19 per cent of respondents reported using three or less, 45 per cent reported using four to seven, 21 per cent reported using eight or nine, and 16 per cent reported using ten or more.* We cannot assume that the answers to this question accurately portray behavior during the two-week period in question; all we need assume is that the answers in general reflect the extent of use of these procedures.

Social Orientations to Medicine. We roughly depict the general prac-

* Because of rounding errors, percentages do not always equal one hundred. Thus, slight variations in the total percentage of doctors having various characteristics will occur in subsequent analysis.

titioner's social orientation through responses to two questions. The first question asks the doctor whether he believes it is proper for patients to consult their G.P. for each of the following problems: family financial troubles, disobedience of children, marital difficulties, how to handle behavior such as drunkenness in a relative, children's poor school performance, birth control advice, problems with drinking too much, general feelings of unhappiness, anxieties about child care, and obesity. Respondents were given the options of "yes," "sometimes," and "no" for each item. The second question, correlated with the first, was: "Some medical commentators have recently argued that there is a growing tendency for people to bring less serious disorders to doctors and more readily seek help for problems in their family lives. In general do you feel that this is a good or bad trend, given present conditions of medical practice?" Doctors were given the options of responding that it was a "very good," "good," "rather disturbing," and "very disturbing" trend. The question included the phrase "present conditions of medical practice" because we wished to separate those who endorse the idea in general from those who feel it is a good trend even under the conditions of limited medical manpower. Each doctor in the sample received a score on social orientations based on their responses to the two questions.

Results

It is commonly believed that a technical and a social orientation are not fully compatible; thus, the first issue we face is the relationship between these two orientations. An examination of Table 1 shows that this

Table 1   The Relationship between Diagnostic Use and a Social Orientation to Medicine Among 772 British General Practitioners

Social Orientation to Medicine	Report of Number of Procedures Used During the Previous Two Weeks							
	5 or less		6 or 7		8 or 9		10 or more	
	%	N	%	N	%	N	%	N
High (scores of 1–3)	23	(57)	26	(60)	18	(29)	36	(43)
Medium high (scores of 4–5)	34	(87)	42	(98)	46	(74)	32	(39)
Medium low (scores of 6–7)	27	(68)	24	(57)	31	(50)	24	(29)
Low (scores of 8 or 9)	16	(41)	09	(21)	06	(9)	08	(10)
Total	100	(253)	101	(236)	101	(162)	100	(121)

contention is not supported. Indeed, doctors who use the smallest number of procedures are overrepresented among those with the lowest social orientation scores, and the group with the highest use of procedures has the largest proportion of doctors with high social orientation scores. Overall, the relationship between these two variables is a very modest one, indicating considerable independence between these two orientations.

Table 2 presents data relating various factors to the use of diagnostic and laboratory procedures. As an examination of the table will show, those who use more procedures, in contrast to those using less, have practices in smaller communities, and they are more likely to have direct access to N.H.S. beds and hospital appointments. Such doctors, with higher use of procedures, also have a tendency to organize their practices differently. They are more likely to be part of larger groups or to have partners, to use an appointment system, to take supplementary course work, and to do some regular psychotherapy. These doctors include more younger practitioners and less older ones, and they are more likely to be members of the Royal College of General Practitioners. On the average, they devote more time to their practices than doctors using fewer procedures, they have more private patients, and they read more professional journals, although these differences tend to be small. Finally, they tend to view a smaller proportion of their patients' consultations as trivial, inappropriate, or unnecessary, and are more satisfied with their access to medical facilities.

Table 3 presents some findings concerning factors associated with a social orientation to medicine. As one might reasonably expect, doctors who are higher on the social orientation variable are more likely to report that they seek out patient problems, that it is the doctor's responsibility to manage psychiatric patients, and that they do psychotherapy. Such doctors also, as one might expect, report less of their case load as trivial, unnecessary, or inappropriate. Although social orientation is not clearly related to access to N.H.S. beds, those who fall lowest on social orientation have considerably less access to beds. Those with a high social orientation score are more likely to be members of the Royal College of General Practitioners, to have taken supplementary course work during the five years previous to the survey, to have had some special training in psychiatry, social medicine, or the behavioral sciences, and to have more contact with other doctors relating to professional matters.

Doctors who report a high social orientation to medicine tend to be much higher than other doctors on most of our measures of satisfaction, and they appear to take a more favorable attitude toward general practice and the health service in general. They tend more than other doctors to believe that it is possible to practice high quality medicine under present

Table 2 Factors Associated with Use of Diagnostic and Laboratory Procedures (Per Cent)

Aspects of Doctors and Their Practices	Report of Number of Procedures Used During the Previous Two Weeks				
	5 or less (N = 253)	6 or 7 (N = 236)	8 or 9 (N = 162)	10 or more (N = 121)	r^a
(a) Practices in a community of:					
Less than 25,000 population (N = 233)	23	30	35	40	
25,000 to 99,999 population (N = 276)	30	37	38	40	−22
100,000 or more population (N = 263)	47	32	27	20	
(b) 40 years of age or less (N = 272)	25	34	48	41	
41–55 years of age (N = 378)	53	50	43	49	−20
56 years of age or older (N = 122)	22	17	09	10	
(c) Has direct access to N.H.S. beds (N = 420)	43	53	60	74	−22
(d) Has an appointment on staff of N.H.S. hospital (N = 269)	23	34	41	51	−21
(e) Uses an appointment system (N = 261)	20	29	52	46	−23
(f) Has taken supplementary course work in past five years (N = 507)	55	65	80	71	17
(g) Member of the Royal College of General Practitioners (N = 216)	19	27	35	39	−17
(h) Solo practice (N = 160)	27	22	14	13	
Two or three partners (N = 533)	64	69	75	71	16
Four or more partners (N = 79)	08	09	10	16	

176

Table 2 (*Continued*)

Aspects of Doctors and Their Practices	Report of Number of Procedures Used During the Previous Two Weeks				r^a
	5 or less (N = 253)	6 or 7 (N = 236)	8 or 9 (N = 162)	10 or more (N = 121)	
(i) Above median category in total practice time spent during day previous to interview (N = 332)	42	45	48	50	16
(j) Median category or above in satisfaction with access to medical facilities (N = 427)	48	56	58	66	−18
(k) Reports 26 or more private patients (N = 148)	14	22	18	26	15
(l) Does some regular psychotherapy (N = 172)	17	19	29	34	−14
(m) Reports reading three or more professional journals (N = 229)	24	32	35	36	13
(n) Reports that 50 per cent or more of surgery consultations are for trivial, unnecessary, or inappropriate reasons (N = 187)	30	26	15	19	10

a Product moment correlation coefficient for use of diagnostic procedures and measure of the independent variable. All r's reported are statistically significant at the .05 level.

177

Table 3 Factors Associated with Social Orientation to Medicine (Per Cent)

Aspects of Doctors and Their Practices	Scores on Social Orientation to Medicine Index				
	High (Scores of 1–3) (N = 189)	Medium high (Scores of 4–5) (N = 298)	Medium low (Scores of 6–7) (N = 204)	Low (Scores of 8–9) (N = 81)	r^a
(a) Has direct access to N.H.S. beds (N = 420)	60	54	56	38	10
(b) Reports that 50 per cent or more of surgery consultations are for trivial, unnecessary, or inappropriate reasons (N = 187)	10	22	29	52	−34
(c) Reports that he seeks patient's problems and provides supportive treatment regardless of whether patient asks for help (N = 465)	75	64	49	37	−26
(d) Agrees that in all cases it is the G.P.'s responsibility to manage psychiatric patients released from the hospital (N = 264)	43	36	28	23	24
(e) Does some regular psychotherapy (N = 172)	32	24	15	10	18
(f) Member of the Royal College of General Practitioners (N = 216)	36	27	25	19	−17
(g) Has taken supplementary course work in past 5 years (N = 507)	72	69	64	44	−14

178

Table 3 (*Continued*)

Aspects of Doctors and Their Practices	Scores on Social Orientation to Medicine Index				r^a
	High (Scores of 1–3) (N = 189)	Medium high (Scores of 4–5) (N = 298)	Medium low (Scores of 6–7) (N = 204)	Low (Scores of 8–9) (N = 81)	
(h) Above median category on contact with other doctors on professional matters (N = 333)	62	42	43	28	−12
(i) Has any training following medical school relating to social and family medicine, psychiatry, or behavioral sciences (N = 189)	30	27	22	12	−11
(j) General satisfaction with general practice—above median category (N = 362)	62	48	38	30	26
(k) Median category or above in belief that high quality practice is possible under present conditions (N = 436)	66	60	50	36	−20
(l) Above median category on willingness to sacrifice own interests scale (N = 307)	46	41	39	23	−12
(m) Above median category on willingness to accept authority of Health Ministry (N = 248)	38	31	31	25	−17

a Product moment correlation coefficient for social orientation to medicine score and measure of the independent variable. All r's reported are statistically significant at the .05 level.

179

conditions of practice. They are somewhat more positive toward health ministry standards and controls. Doctors low on social orientation are less likely to accept the view that doctors must sacrifice their own interests relative to those of patients.

Since the assumption of the paper is that it is essential that doctors maintain scientific and social orientations simultaneously, Table 4 combines these two variables. In each case, we have dichotomized each distribution at the median category. Doctors who report using eight or more procedures are classified as high diagnostic use, while those using seven or less are classified as low diagnostic use. Similarly, doctors with a social orientation score of 1–4 are classified as high social orientation, while those with scores of 5–9 are classified as low social orientation. Combining these two categorizations yields four groups with the following number of cases: low social orientation-low diagnostic use ($N = 275$); low social orientation-high diagnostic use ($N = 149$); high social orientation-low diagnostic use ($N = 214$); and high social orientation-high diagnostic use ($N = 134$). For convenience we shall label them as withdrawers, technicians, counselors, and moderns.

As an examination of Table 4 will show, there is a tendency for results reported previously to persist without very large interactions between diagnostic use and social orientations. There were, however, some interactions of considerable interest. Cartwright[4] has shown that doctors' reports of the proportion of their practices concerned with trivial and inappropriate complaints is indicative of a wide range of other responses. While 38 per cent of withdrawers in our sample reported that 50 per cent or more of their patients presented trivial, unnecessary, or inappropriate complaints, only 10 per cent of moderns gave a similar response. Another indication of a modern orientation was the practice of some psychotherapy; while approximately two fifths of the moderns reported doing some psychotherapy, only from 14–23 per cent of the other groups reported doing as much. One of the most impressive findings is the high proportion of members of the Royal College of General Practitioners in the modern group—44 per cent. Only 21 per cent of the withdrawers were members of the College. Although very few of the doctors in our sample were members of the Royal Society of Medicine, more than half of these doctors were in the modern group. Another indication of orientation was the reading of *Lancet,* a highly sophisticated journal dealing with medical issues of general interest. Only 77 doctors indicated that they either read *Lancet* selectively or in whole. While 19 per cent of moderns reported reading this journal, only 6 per cent of withdrawers, 8 per cent of counselors, and 11 per cent of technicians gave a similar report.

It is interesting to note that 37 per cent of technicians and moderns

Table 4 Factors Associated with General Practice Orientations (Per Cent)

Aspects of Doctors and Their Practices	Withdrawers (N = 275)	Technicians (N = 149)	Counselors (N = 214)	Moderns (N = 134)
(a) Has direct access to N.H.S. beds (N = 420)	45	65	52	66
(b) Hospital appointment (N = 269)	28	25	25	23
(c) Reports that 50 per cent or more of surgery consultations are for trivial, unnecessary, or inappropriate reasons (N = 187)	38	24	16	10
(d) Reports that he seeks patient's problems and provides supportive treatment regardless of whether patient asks for help (N = 465)	51	51	68	77
(e) Agrees that in all cases it is the G.P.'s responsibility to manage psychiatric patients released from the hospital (N = 269)	25	38	37	43
(f) Does some regular psychotherapy (N = 172)	14	21	23	39
(g) Solo practice (N = 160)	24	13	26	15
Two or three partners (N = 533)	68	72	65	75
Four or more partners (N = 79)	09	15	09	10
(h) Reports 26 or more private patients (N = 148)	16	17	20	26
(i) Above median category in total practice time spent during day previous to interview (N = 332)	38	53	40	48
(j) Uses an appointment system (N = 261)	23	52	26	48
(k) Member of the Royal College of General Practitioners (N = 216)	21	30	26	44
(l) Overall satisfaction with general practice (N = 362)	38	40	53	56

Table 4 (Continued)

Aspects of Doctors and Their Practices	Withdrawers (N = 275)	Technicians (N = 149)	Counselors (N = 214)	Moderns (N = 134)
(m) 40 years of age or less (N = 272)	35	52	22	38
41–55 years of age (N = 378)	48	43	55	48
56 years of age or older (N = 122)	17	05	22	14
(n) Has taken supplementary course work in past five years (N = 507)	58	72	61	81
(o) Above median category on contact with other doctors on professional matters (N = 333)	33	55	44	49
(p) Median category or above in belief that high quality practice is possible under present conditions (N = 436)	51	53	60	66
(q) Has any training following medical school relating to social and family medicine, psychiatry, or behavioral science (N = 189)	17	28	24	35
(r) Reports reading three or more professional journals (N = 229)	24	34	29	37
(s) Above median category on willingness to sacrifice own interests scale (N = 307)	35	42	43	41
(t) Above median category on willingness to accept authority of Health Ministry (N = 248)	31	29	36	33
(u) Practices in a community of:				
Less than 25,000 population (N = 233)	24	37	29	37
25,000 to 99,999 population (N = 276)	36	38	31	41
100,000 or more population (N = 263)	40	26	40	22
(v) Median category or above in satisfaction with access to medical facilities (N = 427)	49	56	56	55

are found in communities of less than 25,000 population, in contrast to 24 per cent of withdrawers and 29 per cent of counselors. In contrast, 40 per cent of withdrawers and counselors are found in areas of 100,000 or more of population as compared with 26 per cent of technicians and 22 per cent of moderns. Although access to N.H.S. beds and hospital appointments are greater in smaller communities, diagnostic use is not associated with hospital appointments, although it is with access to N.H.S. beds. With the concentration of hospitals and consultants in larger urban areas, doctors in such areas apparently are more likely to depend on the hospital to do much of the diagnostic work.

Discussion

Overall, we have not been particularly successful in accounting for differences in practice orientations among doctors. It is quite clear that the dominant orientation among younger doctors is the technical role, while older doctors are overrepresented among the counselors. The modern orientation—the one we have defined as the most desirable one—corresponds fairly closely to the age distribution of the entire sample of doctors. Both technicians and moderns tend to predominate in communities of less than 100,000 population in contrast to counselors and withdrawers, two fifths of whom are located in areas of more than 100,000 population. One wonders whether the presence of large hospitals close by in more urbanized areas—particularly teaching hospitals—discourages doctors from assuming a wider medical responsibility for their patients. Moderns and technicians are more likely to have access to hospital beds than counselors and withdrawers, and these are more readily available in smaller community hospitals than in the major urban hospitals.

By most definitions of modernity, technicians and moderns appear more advanced in their practices than counselors and withdrawers. They are both more likely than counselors and withdrawers to be part of a partnership or group practice, to have an appointment system, to take supplementary course work, to have contact with other doctors on professional matters, and to do more professional reading. One of the most impressive findings was the extent to which moderns held membership in the Royal College of General Practitioners. When the data were collected, special qualifications were not required for membership, yet more than twice as many moderns in contrast to withdrawers held such membership, and moderns were also much more likely to be members than either technicians or counselors. Whether the educational program and values of the College influence the way doctors practice, or whether doctors who are more committed to certain ways of practicing select themselves into membership, cannot be answered by our data. It seems reasonable to expect, however, that the educational program of the College, which emphasizes many of the aspects of practice associated with modernity, has some effect on doctors.

An issue of some concern is the relatively large number of younger doctors in the technician group. These doctors who are less committed to the social aspects of practice appear to be in many respects as disgruntled as the withdrawers. On most measures of dissatisfaction, for example, they rate as a relatively unhappy group. More than twice as many technicians as moderns feel that 50 per cent or more of their surgery consultations are for trivial and unnecessary reasons, and many of the patients they are likely to see in general practice require other than a traditional technical approach. It is interesting to note that the technicians have not had, on the average, less training specific to social science and psychiatry than other groups, and indeed they appear to be comparable to the other types in their acknowledgment of the G.P.'s responsibility for managing psychiatric patients released from the hospital. In a sense, this too is a technical task requiring special skills and knowledge of drugs. It is primarily the more common psychologic and social complaints of patients that they seem to frown on treating.

The issue remains as to what other factors might contribute to practice orientations since we found that much of the variance remains unexplained. Part of this is due to measurement error, but it is also likely that the value orientations and personality characteristics of doctors also play some part in defining how doctors orient themselves to their practices and how they deal with their daily tasks.

Notes

1. College of General Practitioners, London (1965). *Report of A Symposium on the Art and the Science of General Practice.* Torquay: Devonshire Press.
2. Great Britain, Royal Commission on Medical Education (1968). *1965–1968 Report.* London: Her Majesty's Stationery Office.
3. Great Britain, Ministry of Health (1963). *The Field of Work of the Family Doctor.* London: Her Majesty's Stationery Office.
4. Cartwright, A. (1967). *Patients and Their Doctors: A Study of General Practice.* London: Routledge.

CHAPTER XI

The English National Health Service: Some Comparisons with the United States*

There is now wide appreciation, in large part as a result of experience with Medicare and Medicaid, that continuing investment in medical care without associated change in the structure and functioning of medical institutions is relatively ineffective; and much attention needs to be paid to the kinds of incentives that must be tied to new investments in the health field. In thinking through such questions, it is often valuable to have a contrasting experience that helps direct the kinds of questions we ask and the kinds of considerations we take into account. This article attempts to develop issues concerning the future delivery of health care in the United States by using the English National Health Service as a contrast.

In developing this contrasting perspective, considerable caution is necessary. Medical systems arise from particular historical circumstances and are part of a country's developing culture. Although the National Health Service officially originated in 1948, its roots are centuries old.[1] The creature of 1948 was basically a consolidation of long-existing components. For example, the general practice pattern—with doctors paid on a capitation basis for patients on their panels—dates back at least to the National Insurance Act of 1911, when such a system was provided for wage earners but not their families. The voluntary hospitals in Britain have very old origins, and the closed staffs, characteristic of most European hospitals, are traditional. Similarly, although the existing organization and stratification of the health professions may have

* Adapted from a paper published in the *Journal of Health and Social Behavior*, 1971, **12**:18–29, with permission of the American Sociological Association.

been solidified through the establishment of the National Health Service, the division of functions was clear well before that time, as was the traditional separation of the medical services provided by general practitioners, hospitals, and local authorities.

There is every reason to believe that the future pattern of health services in the United States will in large part reflect present traditions and professional patterns of organization; and although significant changes will occur in the organization of medical services, it is highly unlikely that we will seek the specific solutions characteristic of the British experience. But the British experience is particularly interesting because it provides some appreciation of the outcomes possible under varying national investment, professional organization, division of functions, and instruments for establishing national priorities.

It might be useful to begin with some rather general conclusions about the British experience that will be considered in greater detail later. Despite a variety of persistent problems, the National Health Service demonstrates the possibility of providing a "reasonable" level of medical care to an entire population in terms of need rather than the ability to pay. This has been accomplished with a very modest national investment varying from 4 to 5 per cent of Britain's gross national product. To the extent that public health indicators such as mortality and morbidity can be taken as partly indicative of the effectiveness of health services, one can find little to fault the effectiveness of the system. There is no doubt about the popularity of the National Health Service among the British population, and the overall quality of hospital care and the performance of consultants are highly evaluated by medical observers. Unlike the United States, the British have continued to make an organizational commitment to primary care services through the system of general practitioners, but until recently they were reluctant to invest substantial funds in this aspect of the Service. It is generally conceded that general practice has been the weakest link in the system, and it is clear that although consumers prefer the general practitioner, it is the GP who has been the most disenchanted and most vociferous critic of the National Health Service. Despite its weaknesses, however, the general practice system offers patients easy access to a doctor without serious barriers. In short, the British experience demonstrates that with planning and coordination, limited resources and facilities can be used reasonably efficiently to achieve a level of care that is in large part responsive to the needs of the population. Having said this much, we must now backtrack to consider specifically varying aspects of the delivery of medical care, compare our experience with the British, and explore what elements available in the British experience may be modifiable and adaptable to our own system of care.

Some Basic Comparative Facts

The American means of delivering medical care is considerably more expensive than the British investment, on both an absolute and a relative basis. Even in relative terms the American investment is approximately two-fifths higher than British expenditures. This is reflected in available manpower and facilities as well as in other ways. First, the United States has relatively more doctors than the British. The resulting availability of medical care, however, is difficult to calculate because of the varying allocation of physician functions in the two countries and the larger proportion of medical manpower in research, teaching, and administration in the United States.

While a decreasing proportion of American physicians has been involved in primary care (GP's, internists, and pediatricians),[2] the British have made a serious attempt to preserve the primary care structure through their organized system of general practice. In Britain about 40 per cent of the doctors are general practitioners, and of these, about half have limited access to hospital beds primarily for obstetrics.[3] Average patient load is approximately 2500 patients,[4] but there are significant variations from doctor to doctor. The remainder of British physicians work mostly in hospitals, approximately one-third of the fulltime equivalents occupying positions as consultants.[4] The proportion of consultants in hospitals is somewhat higher than this, but many consultants have some private practice and choose to accept less than the full number of sessions. Most of the remaining hospital doctors are registrars at various grades (roughly equivalent to residents at various levels in the United States).

The overall situation can to some extent be illustrated by comparing the approaches to surgery in the two countries.[5] Roughly speaking, the British—relative to their population—have half the number of surgeons we have, and they do approximately half the surgery. The relative rates of surgery, however, vary widely from procedure to procedure. British surgeons are much less likely to undertake less urgent procedures and those of questionable efficacy. For example, the rate of tonsillectomy in Britain is approximately one-half that in the United States; however, British surgeons are more than twice as likely as American surgeons to do an adenoidectomy without a tonsillectomy. The rates of surgery in the two countries show little difference on such procedures as thyroidectomy, appendectomy, and operations of the eye. Rather substantial differences exist on such procedures as hysterectomy, inguinal herniorrhaphy, hemorrhoidectomy, and cholecystectomy.

Expert observers agree that there is much unnecessary surgery in the United States, as in the case, for example, of tonsillectomy,[6] but it is also clear that necessary but nonacute surgery in Britain may involve long delays. In assessing the relative quality of surgery in Britain, most expert observers agree that their surgical consultants are of high quality. The statement by Bunker[5] is relatively typical:

> If the qualifications of the surgeon are considered a valid index of quality of care, the quality of surgery in England and Wales must be considered superior to that in the United States. Virtually all surgery in England and Wales is performed by consultant specialists and senior registrars, or by house officers under their direct supervision. Furthermore, there are at least twice as many candidates as there are positions, thus providing an additional degree of quality selection. In comparison to the strict state control in England and Wales, regulation of surgery in the United States occurs at the local level or not at all. Individual hospitals may require board certification, or equivalent training, but many do not. Of the 68,000 physicians listed in full-time or private practice of surgery, less than two thirds are certified by a surgical board or are fellows of the American College of Surgeons.

It is frequently alleged that because of the small number of surgeons in England, necessary surgical procedures are unreasonably delayed. At least one study comparing hospital admissions in Arbroath, Scotland, and Waterville, Maine, showed similar waiting times,[7] but there are few data that allow comparison of surgical waiting time in the two countries. The British annually publish data on the waiting list for various parts of the Service,[4] but it is known that these lists are inflated by multiple listings and by persons who expedited their care through private practice. In any case, it is instructive to inspect those areas where waiting lists appear excessive. One measure of this might be the size of the waiting list on a particular service relative to the total number of discharges and deaths during the year for that service. For the overall surgical services for the year 1968, the total waiting list at the end of the year was one-fifth of the total discharges and deaths on all surgical services. This is in contrast to the medical departments, where the waiting list was less than one per cent of total discharges and deaths.[4] It is clear, however, that if one looks at the various surgical departments, there are wide variations in the waiting list that reflect priorities. The two areas where the waiting list is largest are plastic surgery and tonsillectomy and adenoidectomy, where the waiting lists are 63 per cent and 49 per cent, respectively, of total discharges and deaths for those services. Other areas where the waiting list is more than 25 per cent of total discharges and deaths include other ear, nose, and throat areas (29 per cent), ophthalmology (27 per cent), and dental surgery (25 per cent). Waiting lists in such areas as thoracic surgery, neurosurgery, and radiotherapy are less than 10 per cent of total discharges and deaths. In the two largest departments, general surgery and gynecology, the waiting lists are, respectively, 16 per cent and 19 per cent of total discharges and deaths.

Rates of admission to hospitals are considerably lower in England than in the United States, but average length of stay is significantly higher than in American hospitals.[8,9] Averages here are highly deceptive, since variations among hospitals are extremely large in both countries.[10,11] It is reasonably clear, however, that the structure of the National Health Service, in part, explains both these variations. The British continue to encourage home care in a variety of ways, and they depend to some extent on domiciliary obstetrics, involving approximately one-fifth of all births. Also, general practitioners who require assistance in managing a sick patient may request a consultation from the domiciliary specialist service, and during 1968 more than 315,000 such consultations were provided.[4] Furthermore, under normal circumstances GP's do not admit patients to hospitals, but refer the patient to a consultant who assesses the need for hospitalization. Such hospital doctors impose a somewhat higher criterion for hospital admission than would an American physician who can admit his own patient. It is clear, then, that in Britain patients are less readily admitted to hospitals than in the United States, and consequently those who are admitted tend to have more serious problems, which probably contributes to the average length of stay. Also, the sharp division between medical care given by the general practitioner and services provided by the consultant staff and other hospital doctors often involves a break in the continuity of care and a tendency to work up the patient on admission as if no information at all were available. Furthermore, shortages in nursing staff and in other ancillary services create a backup that may lengthen the average stay. Average length of stay in British hospitals tends to be similar to that in VA hospitals in the United States, and these two hospital systems share several characteristics. A comparative study of such hospitals might yield interesting results.

In developing some ideas as to what we might learn from the British in the area of medical care organization, we will discuss briefly each of the following items: (1) relative mortality; (2) distribution of services; (3) distribution of medical manpower; (4) patient satisfaction; (5) abuse of medical services; (6) physician satisfaction; (7) continuity of care; (8) quality of controls over professional work; (9) financial investment; (10) special services such as mental health care; and (11) capacity for innovation and change. These are but a limited number of dimensions around which such a discussion can be oriented.

Relative Mortality. England has lower infant and adult mortality rates than the United States,[12,13] but one must be careful in attributing such differences to the organization of health services as we usually think of them. Mortality is more closely related to the character of life and the quality of the environment than it is to the specific administration of medical services.[14] In making comparisons, one must take into account the heterogeneous nature of the American population group, the wide variations that exist between the poor and those who are better off, and special risks characteristic of the culture, such as the rate of fatalities from motor vehicle accidents, the high rate of homicide, and the like. There is no evidence that relative differences in longevity in the two countries are attributable to differences in medical care. In the case of infant mortality, there is more substantial reason for believing that the quality of prenatal and infant care services has some relationship to rates of death. In contrast to potential—as measured by rates of infant mortality achieved by countries such as Holland, the Scandinavian nations, and even some of the Eastern European nations that have underdeveloped medical services, but ones more socially organized than our own—American mortality among infants is much higher than it should be.[15] To some extent, English experience is instructive. Going back to the Maternity and Child Welfare Act of 1918, the English have given special attention to expectant and nursing mothers and children under five years of age. This Act stimulated maternity and child welfare centers, home visiting, improved nutrition, and a variety of other valuable services. The easy accessibility to prenatal and child care, as well as other health measures instituted by the Ministry of Health and the local health authorities, contributed significantly to the reduction of infant mortality.[15] Much of infant mortality is a product of the quality of the infant's environment, and health measures that optimize conditions for childbirth and infant development are required on a social scale.

Distribution of Services and Medical Manpower. The utilization of medical services in the United States has been higher among upper-status groups than among lower-status groups.[14] No such relationship appears to exist in England, where economic barriers to medical care have been eliminated.[16] Certainly, one of the most impressive accomplishments of the National Health Service has been to provide care in relation to need rather than in response to the ability to pay. No doubt the wealthy, if they wish, can purchase amenities not easily available from the Health Service, and even the Health Service provides somewhat greater amenities in Southern England than in other areas of the country such as in the industrial North and Wales. However, these are rather minor aspects of the whole, and the outstanding fact is that the distribution of manpower and facilities that has been achieved is truly impressive.

The distribution of medical resources is accomplished in a variety of ways. A country that determines the need for facilities on the basis of central planning has considerable control over their distribution, although even this process is influenced by the strength with which different groups make their needs felt.[17-19] The distribution of manpower is somewhat more difficult, since democratic nations are always cautious in imposing personal controls on behavior. At the level of the hospital, distribution of doctors poses no serious problems. The number of hospital vacancies in the country is limited, and if hospital doctors wish positions, they must go where work is available. This principle operates most effectively at the level of the consultantships, which are coveted positions, and less effectively at the registrar grades and in relation to nursing services. The largest problems exist at the level of general medical practice, and because there is no unified structure of practice, it is diffcult to control individual behavior of general practitioners. The English to some extent achieve redistribution through two mechanisms: (1) by providing an additional income increment for practicing in an area designated as underdoctored, and (2) by designating certain areas as closed to new practices and screening entry into others that are described as intermediate areas. In 1968 the average number of patients per doctor in designated areas (underdoctored) was 2819; in contrast, the average patient load in restricted areas was 1811.[4] The English, however, use such mechanisms rather conservatively.[20] The allowance for locating a practice in underdoctored areas is small, and the areas restricted to new practices in 1968 covered only 7 per cent of the English population.[4] Thus, British GP's continue to have considerable latitude in choosing practice locations, although it is more difficult to build a practice quickly in areas with more doctors. Overall, the system works fairly well; even these very modest mechanisms have contributed to a relatively good spread of doctors, although some problems in distribution persist. England, however, in comparison to the United States, is small and more urbanized, and comparable incentives that have been developed privately by some communities in the United States have not been particularly effective. Communities have offered doctors rent-free facilities, guaranteed incomes, and the like, but these have not had a major impact on the distribution of doctors. It is clear that the distribution of doctors in the United States will continue to be one of the most difficult problems in the delivery of medical care. Barring some form of coercion, which is unlikely, the approach to this problem will have to be complex and multifaceted.

Patient Satisfaction. Every recent survey of the British population shows enormous consumer satisfactions with the National Health Service.[16] Although patients in all countries are reluctant to report dissatisfaction with their physicians, it is clear that patient complaints concerning costs, impersonality of medical care, and difficulty in getting in touch with one's doctor are more evident in the United States. Informed criticism among medical care experts, journalists, and persons involved in the health field is also more apparent in the United States. Whatever the deficiencies in English general practice—and there are many—it is clear that the English highly value the easy direct access to and continuing relationship with a primary medical practitioner, and a large majority of the people prefer their general practitioners to hospital specialists.[16]

An indirect way of measuring dissatisfaction is to gauge the extent to which patients seek care outside their usual source. Private practice has always existed in England, but no more than 3 to 5 per cent of the population use such practitioners.[21] General practitioners in the Health Service are allowed to pursue private practice, but most are unable to attract significant numbers of private patients. On the contrary, older GP's have the most private patients—many of the patients having been with these doctors prior to 1948. There is little evidence that doctors entering the National Health Service after 1948 have been able to attract any substantial number of private patients.[22] To some extent, growing malpractice litigation in the United States reflects patient dissatisfaction with medical care. There is reason to believe that malpractice suits are more likely to arise under circumstances where personalized aspects of health services have broken down,[23] although the rate of litigation is also a product of changing cultural attitudes about initiating legal action.

Abuse of Medical Services. It is commonly believed in this country that British patients abuse the National Health Service. Dissatisfied GP's in England frequently complain of patients who come for reasons they feel to be trivial and unnecessary.[24] Obviously, some abuse exists in all systems of care, and the appropriate question is whether it becomes excessive when economic barriers to medical care are removed.

Although detailed utilization data are not available, the information that exists shows average utilization of the British general practitioner to be similar to average doctor visits in the United States.[16, 25] Given these facts, it is difficult to maintain that the National Health Service encourages excessive abuse. Since British doctors appear to complain more about such consultations than their American counterparts, some other explanation must exist. One possibility is that British doctors who are remunerated on a capitation basis resent "trivial consultations" more than doctors who receive a fee for service. Indeed, American doctors under some circumstances may have some incentive for encouraging such consultations, while British doctors who define a consultation as trivial can only view it as a nuisance. In a study of English general practitioners,

I found that very busy doctors who see many patients within short spans of time are more likely than others to define a large proportion of the patients they see as presenting trivial and unnecessary complaints.[24,26] It appears that doctors who practice on an assembly line basis become upset by patients who have difficult psychological or psychosocial problems that cannot be dealt with relatively quickly and that consume a great deal of time. It appears that seeing such consultations as trivial reflects a certain kind of practice that cannot cope with larger concerns of patients, and where the doctor experiences frustration in attempting to see all the patients who wish his advice.

As for the abuse of hospitals, it is clear that client control is much more powerful in the United States than in Britain. Since access to a hospital in Britain is largely controlled by special hospital doctors, patients have relatively little influence on such decisions.[27] In the United States, where the medical decision resides with the patient's usual doctor, and where the doctor has little formal responsibility to the hospital, patients can be more influential in making their wishes felt.[28] The structure of insurance and medical organization in the United States does not encourage cost consciousness on the part of either the patient or his doctor and may result in excessive use of the hospital. Moreover, hospitalization may be convenient for the doctor and may facilitate the best utilization of his time.

Physician Satisfaction. One of the major criticisms of the National Health Service is that the conditions of work are dissatisfying to physicians, and that this results in significant emigration. Such criticisms are valid to some extent, but they are usually overstated. For the most part, consultants in the British system are extremely satisfied with their conditions of work, and it is relatively rare to hear complaints from this group. Basic remuneration is reasonably good, and doctors may also undertake private practice. Moreover, incentives for good practice are encouraged through a system of merit awards that provides varying increments of additional remuneration to physicians and surgeons who have achieved some distinction in their field.[20] The highest level of such awards approximately doubles the consultant's total remuneration from the Health Service, but lesser awards are also available for younger men and those with lesser accomplishments. In 1968, 3102 consultants were receiving awards, approximately one-third of the total.[4]

There has been significant dissatisfaction among general practitioners through the years, attributable partly to difficulties in the remuneration system, the growing burdens of general practice with larger numbers of patients, and the general practitioner's uncertain status.[19] These problems have deep roots and probably cannot be effectively remedied without significant changes in medical education, the facilities for general medical practice, and, most important, a reduction in the number of patients for whom the doctor must assume responsibility. The dissatisfaction is probably in part inherent in the maintenance of a clearly stratified two-tier system of medical care where general practitioners come to be looked upon as failures in the medical world.[18] One possible remedy prescribed by the Royal Commission on Medical Education[29] is the development of a specialty in general practice, but it is not fully clear that such a program can mitigate dissatisfaction without substantial alteration in the value structure of medicine.

Through emigration Britain has in recent years lost a large number of doctors, as well as many other highly trained and qualified technical personnel who can obtain better remuneration and working conditions in other English-speaking countries. It is clear, however, that the major group of doctors emigrating have been those with substantial hospital training who cannot obtain consultant positions in British hospitals.[30] Such highly trained doctors aspire to a higher level of technical practice than general practice offers, and seek opportunities outside the country. Given the shortage of doctors in English-speaking countries and the manner in which the English have chosen to organize their health services, this may be a necessary cost for a country with limited economic resources. Improving the conditions of work for general practitioners and changing the value system of medical practitioners will help alleviate the problem, but some loss of doctors is part of the general movement of highly qualified scientific talent to contexts that can provide greater opportunities to pursue one's work with minimal limitations on facilities and autonomy.

Continuity of Care. Both the United States and Britain face problems in providing continuity of care that result from the growing complexity and specialization of health care in general. But the character of each medical form of organization results in varying discontinuities. With growing specialization in the United States, many patients do not have a single doctor who knows them and their family. They may choose a different physician depending on the nature of the problem, and thus their basic care tends to become fragmented. In contrast, the British maintain considerable continuity at the general practice level, with the same doctor often providing general medical, pediatric, obstetrical, and less complicated psychiatric care.[8] Once hospitalization is required, however, the American doctor frequently retains the care of the patient and uses knowledge he has obtained at some earlier point. The stratification between general practice and hospital care characteristic of British medicine, on the other hand, creates a discontinuity between the general practitioner's service and hospital care. In England, once the patient is referred to a hospital, the patient's GP no longer has any responsibility for his care, and the primary care physician provides very little input to the patient's continuing care. Communication is often also poor when the patient returns to his general practitioner, and these sharp breaks between the hospital and the community detract from good comprehensive care.[31] In both systems general social services and ancillary health services tend to be relatively isolated from the rest of the health system, and overall coordination presents significant difficulties. The British are structurally in a better position to achieve effective coordination, but traditional patterns of separation between the three parts of the health service have considerable momentum.[32]

Effective Controls. There is increasing concern in both the United States and Britain with the modes of organization most conducive to high quality care. Both nations appear to be moving toward similar types of approach in the area of formal and informal controls. One way in which the British control the quality of hospital work is through a highly rigorous selection process: Persons who receive consultant appointments are carefully screened, and other hospital doctors work under their supervision. Although such selection is not characteristic of American medicine, it is clear that hospitals are increasingly concerned about the qualifications of their staff, and that in the better hospitals minimum standards for hospital privileges on various services are being established. American hospitals have review procedures that allow the work of doctors to be monitored; if utilized fully, such procedures have considerable potential. The British have no such procedures, but have in recent years been discussing the adoption of the hospital committee review system to their context.

For the most part, the work of general practitioners receives little monitoring, but the American system that brings the GP into hospitals allows his work to be more visible and provides some potential opportunity for his practices to be influenced. The British GP is very largely isolated from colleague control, and this no doubt gives relatively little opportunity for corrective feedback.[3] The government does to some extent monitor unusual prescriptions, but the impact of this on quality care is relatively small, and the motivation for monitoring is primarily from the point of view of cost.

Financial Investment. It is difficult to compare countries like England and the United States, which have such varying resources and modes of allocation, but some general observations are worth noting. In Britain expenditures for health care are made centrally, and the allocation process is relatively tidy. Since decision making is centralized within the government, expenditures for health care are subject to the usual political pressures and the establishment of priorities among varying national needs. In contrast, expenditures in the United States result from government investments, consumer expenditures, and private philanthropy. Although American financing is more untidy—and to some extent inefficient—the multiple providers of funds may contribute some vitality and growth to the health field;[9] but under some circumstances it can also result in considerable inflation.[33] In the United States the total government investment approximates two-fifths of the medical care dollar, but even these funds are contributed by a variety of agencies and programs with different objectives. Thus, the state of financing is unlikely to be the product of any single set of decisions, although such major programs as Medicare or Medicaid have a pervasive influence on the overall flow of events.

Certainly the evidence shows that the health sector in America has grown more rapidly than in Britain in both an absolute and relative sense. How one weighs such growth against the costs is, of course, a value question. Obviously, such investments must be considered within the entire context of needs and priorities that different nations have established, and we cannot assume that the same pattern of expenditure is equally desirable in situations that vary in terms of needs and resources.

Special Services Relevant to Rehabilitation. The effectiveness of a health system must be judged not only by traditional medical functions, but also by the larger spectrum of supporting medical and health services. How a medical system copes with disability and establishes its rehabilitation functions is central to the effectiveness of the health services system. The United States has examples of marvelous utilization of rehabilitation potential, but the question to be posed concerns the effective implementation of rehabilitation capacities on a wide scale.

By far, the largest problem in the rehabilitation area is the field of mental disorders. Since cures are presently unavailable, the system must function by maintaining, sustaining, and rehabilitating patients within the context of their condition. Overall, it seems clear that the British have been more effective in marshaling their resources for this effort, and hospital psychiatry in Britain appears to be superior to typical mental hospital care in the United States. Moreover, the British have moved more rapidly and vigorously than we into such areas as community care, sheltered workshops, work rehabilitation, and the like. In recent years large investments in the United States for community mental health centers have improved the overall situation, but hospital psychiatry for the most disabled patients is less professional than in Britain.[34]

Although the rehabilitation field is too complex and diverse to summarize grandly, one has the distinct impression from visiting facilities in both countries that the British place a higher value on rehabilitation and are more willing to devote their efforts to helping persons live within the limits of their illness. The emphasis on these human values is epitomized by legislation that requires employers to hire a certain proportion of disabled persons as part of their work force. Employers who have too few such employees are expected to give preference in hiring to the disabled. The system does not always work quite this way in reality, but it is clear that such legislation embodies values more strongly held in Britain than in the United States and reflects their approach to health care generally.

Capacity for Innovation and Change. The potential for change and development, like other dimensions, reflects the way in which services are organized. In American medicine tremendous energy is devoted to innovation—particularly of a scientific and technical character—and such change occurs rapidly and with relatively little resistance. The problem is not encouraging innovation, but institutionalizing it throughout the professions and health institutions as a whole. Although technical innovations diffuse relatively rapidly, there is considerable resistance to social innovations, and usually such innovations are rarely implemented across the board.[35] In Britain the system tends to be somewhat more sluggish and resistant to change, but it is much easier to implement change throughout the entire health structure. For example, the growth of community care in Britain, although somewhat uneven, never quite created the difficulties characteristic of the American situation.[36] It appears as if American medicine may offer more fertile ground for a variety of ideas for innovation and change, but when a solid one comes along, the British are more able to implement it on a widespread basis.

It should be clear from the foregoing discussion that the two systems of medical care we have been comparing operate with different traditions and under varying incentives and restraints. It is worth repeating, in retrospect, an earlier caution that systems of care arise out of particular historical circumstances, and comparisons across cultures can be fraught with danger. But it is also becoming increasingly apparent that systems of medical care organized on the basis of varying ideologies are confronting similar technological and organizational problems, and that they appear to be moving toward rather common responses that reflect the nature of the problems more than the nature of the ideologies. The British system demonstrates how a rather modest medical structure can cope with difficult and persistent problems that also plague us. Although it would be dangerous to generalize from Britain to the United States, and often the observations in this article have been based on fragmentary and incomplete data involving issues yet to be fully resolved, a prudent approach requires that we look at how other nations and systems have coped with problems for which we seek solutions, as a background for instituting change within our own context. In this effort, I believe, we have much to learn from the British that may be valuable to us as we approach our present crisis in health care.

Notes

1. Abel-Smith, B. (1964). *The Hospitals: 1800–1948*. London: Heinemann.
2. Fein, R. (1967). *The Doctor Shortage: An Economic Analysis*. Washington: The Brookings Institute.
3. Mechanic, D. (1968). "General Practice in England and Wales: Results from a Survey of a National Sample of General Practitioners." *Medical Care*, 6:245–260.
4. Department of Health and Social Security (1969). *1968 Annual Report*. Cmnd. 4100. London: Her Majesty's Stationery Office.
5. Bunker, J. P. (1970). "Surgical Manpower: A Comparison of Operations and Surgeons in the United States and England and Wales." *New England Journal of Medicine*, 282:135–144.
6. Bolande, R. P. (1969). "Ritualistic Surgery—Circumcision and Tonsillectomy." *New England Journal of Medicine*, 280:591–596.
7. Simpson, J., et al. (1968). *Custom and Practice in Medical Care: A Comparative Study of Two Hospitals in Arbroath, Scotland, United Kingdom, and Waterville, Maine, U.S.A.* London: Oxford University Press.
8. Fry, J. (1969). *Medicine in Three Societies*. New York: American Elsevier.
9. Anderson, O. (1963). "Health Service Systems in the United States and Other Countries—Critical Comparisons." *New England Journal of Medicine*, 269:839–843.
10. Somers, H. M., and A. R. Somers (1967). *Medicare and the Hospitals: Issues and Prospects*. Washington: The Brookings Institute.
11. Revans, R. W. (1964). *Standards for Morale: Cause and Effect in Hospitals*. New York: Oxford University Press.
12. National Center for Health Statistics (1967). *International Comparison of Perinatal and Infant Mortality: The United States and Six West European Countries*. PHS Series 3, No. 6. Washington: U. S. Government Printing Office.
13. Rutstein, D. (1967). *The Coming Revolution in Medicine*. Cambridge: MIT Press.
14. Mechanic, D. (1968). *Medical Sociology: A Selective View*. New York: Free Press.
15. National Center for Health Statistics (1968). *Infant and Perinatal Mortality in England and Wales*. PHS Series 3, No. 12. Washington: U. S. Government Printing Office.
16. Cartwright, A. (1967). *Patients and Their Doctors: A Study of General Practice*. London: Routledge and Kegan Paul.
17. Eckstein, H. (1960). *Pressure Group Politics: The Case of the British Medical Association*. Stanford: Stanford University Press.
18. Mechanic, D. (1968). "General Medical Practice in England and Wales: Its Organization and Future." *New England Journal of Medicine*, 279:680–689.
19. Mechanic, D., and R. Faich (1970). "Doctors in Revolt: The Crisis in the English National Health Service." *Medical Care*, 8:442–455.
20. Stevens, R. (1966). *Medical Practice in Modern England*. New Haven: Yale University Press.

21. Mencher, S. (1967). *Private Practice in Britain: The Relationship of Private Medical Care to the National Health Service.* Occasional Papers on Social Administration No. 24. London: Bell and Sons.

22. Mechanic, D. (1970). "Private Practice Among General Practitioners in the English National Health Service." *Medical Care,* 8:324–332.

23. Blum, R. (1960). *The Management of the Doctor-Patient Relationship.* New York: McGraw-Hill.

24. Mechanic, D. (1970). "Correlates of Frustration Among British General Practitioners." *Journal of Health and Social Behavior,* 11:87–104.

25. Eckstein, H. (1964). *The English Health Service: Its Origins, Structure and Achievements.* Cambridge: Harvard University Press.

26. Mechanic, D. (1970). "Practice Orientations Among General Medical Practitioners in England and Wales." *Medical Care,* 8:15–25.

27. Cartwright, A. (1964). *Human Relations and Hospital Care.* London: Routledge and Kegan Paul.

28. Freidson, E. (1970). *Profession of Medicine: A Study of the Sociology of Applied Knowledge.* New York: Dodd, Mead.

29. Royal Commission on Medical Education (1968). *1965–1968 Report.* Cmnd. 3569. London: Her Majesty's Stationery Office.

30. Abel-Smith, B., and K. Gales. (1964). *British Doctors at Home and Abroad.* Occasional Papers on Social Administration No. 8. Hertfordshire: Codicote Press.

31. Forsyth, G., and R. F. Logan (1968). *Gateway or Dividing Line: A Study of Hospital Out-Patients in the 1960's.* New York: Oxford University Press.

32. McKeown, T. (1965). *Medicine in Modern Society.* London: Allen and Unwin.

33. U. S. Senate, Committee on Finance (1970). *Medicare and Medicaid: Problems, Issues, and Alternatives.* Washington: U. S. Government Printing Office.

34. Mechanic, D. (1969). *Mental Health and Social Policy.* Englewood Cliffs: Prentice-Hall.

35. Banfield, E. C., and J. Q. Wilson (1963). *City Politics.* New York: Vintage.

36. Connery, R. (1968). *Politics of Mental Health: Organizing Community Health in Metropolitan Areas.* New York: Columbia University Press.

PART FOUR

SPECIAL ISSUES
IN HEALTH CARE

CHAPTER XII

Response Factors in Illness: The Study of Illness Behavior*

Medicine has three principal tasks—to understand how particular symptoms, syndromes, or disease entities arise either in individuals or among groups of individuals; to recognize and cure these or to shorten their course and minimize any residual impairment; and to promote living conditions in human populations which eliminate hazards to health and thus prevent the occurrence of disease. Each task can only be pursued with maximal effectiveness if the *integral* importance of social and psychological, as well as biological factors, is appreciated.

Much medical activity—whether in research, clinical practice, or preventive work—requires an understanding of the cultural and social pressures which influence an individual's recognition that he needs advice, his decision whether to seek it, his choice of counsellor, his cooperation in carrying out any measures that are suggested and his willingness to remain in contact should there be any recommendation that further supervision is needed. Unless our knowledge of these processes is taken into account in training doctors, dealing with patients and designing sociomedical services, we shall continue to make grave errors in all three fields.

In this essay, I shall consider only one aspect of these problems: that concerning response factors in illness. Although there is a good deal to learn in this area, considerable knowledge is already available.

Data about illness, whether clinical or epidemiological, usually contain two kinds of information: one on the state of the patient (for example, a description of symptoms or dysfunctions); and the other on his reactions to his condition. The physician's diagnosis is influenced by each of these

---

* Adapted from a paper published in *Social Psychiatry*, 1966, 1:11–20, with permission of Springer-Verlag.

kinds of information. He obtains data from physical examination and laboratory studies and also from a clinical history, which usually includes the patient's reactions to his condition. Within the traditional medical model, the patient lodges a complaint and the physician attempts to account for, explain, or find justification for it through his investigation. Logically, if not empirically, the diagnostic situation involves two sets of facts: historical data and symptoms reported by the patient or other informants about his condition, and data obtained by the physician through a systematic examination for abnormal signs and through laboratory investigation if necessary. Thus it is logically possible for physicians to hypothesize that some patients are hypochondriacs or malingerers if they note substantial discrepancies between the patient's complaints and other findings elicited through an independent investigation of the complaints.

However, it is often very difficult in the process of medical (and particularly of psychiatric) diagnosis to make an objective and independent examination of the patient's state of health. So much depends upon information provided and processed by the patient and other informants, and colored by their needs and reactions, that the study of these responses becomes a central concern of medicine itself. It is these "secondary" psychological and social processes, as contrasted with the "primary" biological ones usually considered by doctors, that I refer to under the heading of "illness behavior." The term "illness" has always been used in two ways in medicine. On the one hand it has referred to a limited scientific concept (with which I am not here specifically concerned) and, on the other, to any condition which causes, or might usefully cause, an individual to seek advice from a doctor. "Illness Behavior" is any behavior relevant to the second, more general, interpretation. It is therefore necessary to consider what goes on even before a person sees a doctor. I also wish, in this paper, to illustrate how the importance of "reaction" components in illness has been independently recognized and explored in a number of different areas of medical and sociomedical investigation.

On the most simple and obvious level, the extent to which symptoms are differentially perceived, evaluated and acted (or not acted) upon by different kinds of people and in different social situations is obvious. Whether because of earlier experiences with illness, because of differential training in respect to symptoms, or because of different biological sensitivities, some persons make light of symptoms, shrug them off, and avoid seeking medical care. Others will respond to little pain and discomfort by readily seeking care, by releasing themselves from work and other obligations, and by becoming dependent on others.[1] Thus, the study of illness behavior involves the study of attentiveness to pain and symptomatology, the examination of processes affecting how pain and symptoms are defined, accorded significance and socially labelled, and the consideration of the extent to which help is sought, change in life regimen affected, and claims on others made.

The study of illness behavior by its very nature requires an epidemiological model. Since illness behavior affects the utilization of medical care, choice of paths to possible advisors, and responses to illness in general, the selection of patients who seek help from general practitioners, from clinics, or even from hospitals is usually biased. Groups of patients with a particular disease, selected from such populations, will usually be biased compared with those in the general population with the same disease, but untreated, and this is particularly true for illnesses of high prevalence which are easily recognized by the public and known to have a benign course.[2] Approximately, only one in three persons who report illnesses in a household interview seek a physician's advice, and in any given month only nine of 750 persons who report illnesses will be hospitalized.[3]

Different patterns of illness behavior may be viewed from at least three general perspectives. First, such patterns of behavior may be seen as a product of cultural and social conditioning, since they may be experienced and enacted naturally in the social contexts within which they appear relevant. Secondly, illness behavior may be seen as part of a coping repertoire—as an attempt to make an unstable, challenging situation more manageable for the person who is encountering difficulty. Thirdly, illness behavior may be analyzed in terms of its advantages for the patient in seeking and obtaining attention, sympathy and material gain.

Illness Behavior as a Culturally and Socially Learned Response

Cultures are so recognizably different that variations in illness behavior in different societies hardly need demonstration. The idea implicit in much of the anthropological work is that primitive conceptions of illness are part of a learned cultural complex, and are functionally associated with other aspects of cultural response to environmental threat. Some of the earlier investigations of illness behavior in America were based on the same idea—that different patterns of response to illness are culturally conditioned and functionally relevant. Thus Koos[4] observed that upper class persons were more likely than lower class persons to view themselves as ill when they had particular symptoms and when they were questioned about specific symptoms, they reported more frequently than lower class persons that they would seek the doctor's advice. Illness responses were described in this study as part of a constellation of needs including those associated with work, family and finances. Saunders[5] described in some detail the differences between "Anglos" and Spanish-speaking persons in the American Southwest in attitudes and responses toward illness and in the use of medical facilities. Whereas the Anglos preferred modern medical science and hospitalization for many illnesses, the Spanish-speaking people were more likely to rely on folk medicine and family care and support which was more consistent with their cultural conceptions. More recently, Clark[6] has described how Mexican-Americans view various life situations and symptoms as health problems in contrast to physicians who do not view these problems with similar seriousness and alarm. Other problems among these people which are ignored and undefined are seen by physicians as serious health problems. Similar observations have been made concerning various American Indian groups, and in a variety of other cultural contexts.

The role of cultural differences in illness behavior was nicely described by Zborowski[7] who, in a study of ethnic reactions to pain in a New York City hospital, observed that while Jewish and Italian patients responded to pain in an emotional fashion, tending to exaggerate pain experiences, "Old Americans" tend to be more stoical and "objective," and Irish more frequently denied pain. Zborowski also noted a difference in the attitude underlying Italian and Jewish concern about pain. While the Italian subjects primarily sought relief from pain and were relatively satisfied when such relief was obtained, the Jewish subjects were mainly concerned with the meaning and significance of their pain, and the consequences of pain for their future welfare and health. In trying to explain these cultural differences, Zborowski reports that Jewish and Italian patients related how their mothers showed overprotective and overconcerned attitudes about the child's health, and participation in sports, and how they were constantly warned of the advisability of avoiding colds, fights, and other threatening situations. Zborowski reports that:

> Crying in complaint is responded to by parents with sympathy, concern and help. By their overprotective and worried attitude they foster complaining and tears. The child learns to pay attention to each painful experience and to look for help and sympathy which are readily given to him. In Jewish families, where not only a slight sensation of pain but also each deviation from the child's normal behavior is looked on as a sign of illness, the child is prone to acquire anxieties with regard to the meaning and significance of these manifestations.

Although Zborowski presents something of a caricature, it is clear that he views the etiology of these behavioral patterns and attitudes as inherent in the familial response to the child's health and illnesses.

Zborowski's observations concerning ethnic differences in illness behavior have been supported in a variety of other studies. Croog[8] administered the Cornell Medical Index to two thousand randomly chosen army inductees. He found that Italian and Jewish respondents reported the greatest number of symptoms of illness. He further found that although the Italian response was associated with low educational status, reports of symptoms among Jewish respondents were not affected by the educational variable. Mechanic,[9] studying 1300 students at two American universities, found that Jewish students reported higher illness behavior patterns than either Protestant or Catholic students. Since income was also found to be related to illness behavior reports, and since Jewish students were also more likely to be represented in the higher income groups, the analysis was repeated, controlling income. The differences in illness behavior reports between Jewish and other students were only significant for the high income group. Mechanic also attempted to test the hypothesis that use of medical services was an alternative among several possible modes of dealing with stress, and that the difference in reports of illness behavior between Jewish students and Catholic and Protestant students could be explained by the relatively limited involvement in religious activities among Jewish students. This hypothesis was not confirmed. The observed difference in illness behavior patterns has persisted in other studies. Segal,[10] in a study of student clinic facilities, found that Jewish students used such facilities somewhat more than Catholic or Protestant students. Similarly, several studies of the use of psychiatric facilities have shown a higher receptivity and utilization rate among Jewish subjects.[11-14]

Suchman[15] in a recent study of 5340 persons in different ethnic groups in New York City found that the more ethnocentric and socially cohesive groups included more persons who knew little about disease, who were skeptical toward professional medical care, and who were dependent during illness. He found that the Jewish respondents were more likely to report a high or moderate pattern of "preventive medical behavior" and "acceptance of the sick role" as compared with respondents from the other groups studied, but that they were not particularly different from other groups on the scale dealing with dependency during illness.

The studies described above suggest considerable consistency in ethnic variations in illness behavior. Although such trends are clear, the variation within groups is much greater than it is between groups. In any case, it is important to note that illness behavior patterns can have both healthy and unhealthy consequences. For example, the traditional concern about health among Jewish persons—especially the health of children—can under some circumstances lead to overconcern and can encourage doubts and anxiety. Such concern and attention can also encourage a high standard of infant rearing and caring as suggested by an early study of infant mortality among immigrants to America which showed that although the Jewish group was foreign born, had just as many children, and had an income which was much lower than that of native-born whites, this group had the lowest rate of infant mortality of all the groups studied, including the native-white population.[16]

Although it is fairly clear that culturally learned differences in illness behavior are important to some extent, such differences explain only a small proportion of the total variation in behavior. Moreover, the contribution of other factors is not well understood. Mechanic,[17] in a study of 350 mother-child pairs attempted to investigate the relationship between maternal attitudes and maternal illness behavior, and between these and the illness behavior of their children. The sample chosen from a relatively homogeneous population in the Midwest of America did not include any substantial ethnic diversity. Data were obtained from both mother and child independently, as well as from teachers, school records, and a daily illness log maintained by the mother. Mechanic found that the mothers' attitudes toward illness and illness behavior were rather poor predictors of the attitudes of their children. Maternal attitudes however played a more important role in determining whether medical aid would be sought for the child when ill.

In this study of the illness behavior of children, the two best predictors of children's reports of "fear of getting hurt" and "attention to pain" were the child's age and sex. Boys were more stoical than girls, and older children were more stoical than younger children. These findings support the idea that age and sex role learning is important in illness behavior and attitudes toward health risks. The results are consistent also with a number of other observations such as the higher utilization of medical facilities among women compared with men,[18] and the higher rate of accidents among boys compared with girls of the same age. Similarly, in another study of reported responses to illness, Mechanic[19] found that respondents expected women to be less stoical than men when ill.

In summary, it seems fair to conclude that cultural and social conditioning play an important though not an exclusive role in patterns of illness behavior, and that ethnic membership, peer pressures, and age-sex role learning to some extent influence attitudes towards risks and towards the significance of common threats.

Links between Reaction Pattern and Physiological Response

It is interesting to note that, in general, observations from field studies concerning ethnic differences in the perception of pain have withstood not only repeated study, but also more detailed scrutiny under laboratory conditions. Sternbach and Tursky,[20] for example, brought Irish, Jewish, Italian and "Yankee" housewives into a psycho-physiological laboratory where they administered pain by electric shock, recording skin potential responses. Their findings tend to support some of the observations made by Zborowski. They found, for example, that Italian women showed significantly lower upper thresholds for shock, and fewer of them would accept the full range of shock stimulation used in the experiment. The investigators believe that this response is consistent with the Italian tendency to focus on the immediacy of the pain itself as compared with the future orientation of the Jewish response tendency. Similarly, they believe that the finding that "Yankee" housewives had a faster and more complete adaptation of the diphasic palmar skin potential has an attitudinal correlate to their "matter of fact" orientation to pain. As they note: "This is illustrated by our Yankee subjects' modal attitude toward traumata, as they verbalized it in their interviews: 'You take things in your stride.' No such action-oriented, adapting phrase was used by the members of the other groups. The similarly undemonstrative Irish subjects may 'keep a tight upper lip' but 'fear the worst,' a noxious stimulus being a burden to be endured and suffered in silence."

However, we must be careful in generalizing conclusions from laboratory pain situations to pathological pain experiences. Henry Beecher,[21] an eminent researcher and Anesthetist-in-Chief at the Massachusetts General Hospital, has reported the failure of fifteen research groups to establish any dependable effects of even large doses of morphine on pain of experimental origin in man, although the effect of morphine on pathological pain is substantial. He has found it necessary to distinguish between pain as an *original sensation* and pain as a *psychic reaction*. As Beecher notes, one of the difficulties with most forms of laboratory pain is that they minimize the psychic reaction which plays an essential role in pain associated with illness. For example, in a comparative study of pain, he asked a group of wounded soldiers and a group of male civilian patients undergoing major surgery the same questions about their desire for pain medication. While only one-third of the soldiers wanted medication to relieve their pain, 80 per cent of the civilians wanted such pain relief although they were suffering from far less tissue trauma. He explains the variation in terms of differing definitions of pain in the two circumstances. The soldier's wound, Beecher explains, was an escape from the battlefield and the possibility of being killed; to the civilian surgical pain was viewed as a depressing, calamitous event. Beecher reports that the civilian group reported strikingly more frequent and severe pain and he concludes that there is no simple, direct relationship between the wound *per se* and the pain experienced. He further concludes that morphine primarily acts on the reactive component of the pain experience, largely through a process of "mental clouding."

The reactive or definitional component in illness has long been recognized as a significant aspect not only in defining the condition but also in the patient's response to treatment. Physicians working with the severely ill are often impressed by the attitudinal component and its influence on the patient's condition. In its extreme form, physicians have commented on the importance of the patient's "will to live" although it has been difficult to quantify this phenomenon or to present clear evidence in support of its importance. At best, we have anecdotal reports of preparation for death and actual death following witchcraft, and some physiological explanations have been offered to explain the mechanisms involved in such impressive happenings.[22] But if we are to integrate such events with our common conceptual schemes we require a better understanding of such phenomena as they occur in more subtle but more observable forms.

Models for the experimental study of the psychophysiology of stress that more closely take into account the reactive or definitional components are beginning to be developed. It has long been recognized that difficult life circumstances or experimentally constructed "stress situations" lead to varied physiological and social responses. It is believed that these differences are due to subjects' differing definitions and capacities to cope with these stimuli, and genetic differences. Until recently, psychophysiological investigations have not taken into consideration differing definitions of experimental "stressors" and the differing capacities of subjects to deal with them. Recently, Lazarus and his colleagues[23] have developed a method for inducing different psychological sets in subjects who are viewing the same threatening films, and they have demonstrated the importance of the definitional set in the reactions of subjects to the experimental films. They as well as others have also observed that, as subjects are exposed over many trials to the threatening films, they appear to develop orientations or adaptations which allow them to experience the same stimulus more calmly. In sum, the reactive component is obviously important and manipulation of "reactive sets" in experiments appear to affect physiological response.

The definitional components in response to difficult circumstances have also been observed in natural situations where physiological response has been studied. Friedman[24,25] and his colleagues in making observations of parents anticipating the death of their children who were suffering from neoplastic diseases found that urinary 17-hydroxycorticosteroid levels in parents would vary from one parent to another, and from one period in the child's illness to another. The period of highest "distress" as measured physiologically occurred for most parents well before the death of the child, the most common situation being when the child was put on the critical list for the first time. For some of the parents the death of the child seemed to be a relief, and it appears as if they had already worked through a substantial part of their grief prior to the death of the child. Other parents, however, who maintained hope despite evidence to the contrary, and who showed little marked acceleration in 17-hydroxy-corticosteroid levels at crucial points during the illness, seemed to experience a marked acceleration after the child died. The study illustrates both the tremendous variability in response to difficult circumstances, and the probable link between coping reactions and physiological responses under "stress."

Illness Behavior as a Coping Response to Situational Difficulties

The idea that illness is "stressful" and that it may engender further life difficulties is sufficiently obvious to require no elaboration. What is interesting to the behavioral scientist, however, is the tremendous variability in response to what is presumably the same illness condition. While one person will hardly acknowledge a condition and refuse to allow it to alter his life, another with a more mild form of the same condition will display profound social and psychological disabilities.

An emotional component has often been seen in the etiology or precipitation of illness.[26-30] What is often less appreciated is the importance of life difficulties in influencing illness behavior. Indeed, it appears from a careful scrutiny of psychosomatic evidence that "distress" is often more influential in its effects on seeking help and on the expression of illness, than it is on the actual occurrence of the condition. Balint[31] has argued, for example, that the presentation of somatic complaints often masks an underlying emotional problem which is frequently the major reason why the individual has sought advice. Certainly, what little evidence we have on this point suggests that a complaint of trivial illness may be one way of seeking reassurance and support through a recognized and socially acceptable relationship when it is difficult for the patient to present the underlying problem in an undisguised form. In such circumstances the real problem may not even be consciously recognized.* The emphasis Balint places on emotional factors in the utilization of the general prac-

* For a more detailed discussion of this point, see D. Mechanic, 1972, "Social Psychologic Factors Affecting the Presentation of Bodily Complaints." *New England Journal of Medicine*, **286:**1132–1139.

titioner appears, nevertheless, to be oversimplified since it fails to take into account the more complex relationship between life difficulties and social and cultural patterns.

Mechanic and Volkart[32] have attempted to examine this problem through an investigation of more than 600 students at a major university. One of the major concerns of the study was the relationship between measures of "stress," and measures of illness behavior, and their joint effect on the use of medical facilities. Analysis of the data showed that perceived stress (as measured by indices of loneliness and nervousness) and illness behavior (as measured by several hypothetical items concerning the use of medical facilities) were clearly related to the use of a college health service during a one year period. Among students with a high inclination to use medical facilities and high "stress," 73 per cent were frequent users of medical services (three or more times during the year), while among the low inclination–low "stress" group, only 30 per cent were frequent users of such services. Our attention, however, centered on the interaction between our measure of "stress" on the one hand, and illness behavior on the other, in encouraging a person to present a complaint. When illness behavior patterns were statistically controlled, we found that the influence of "stress" was somewhat different among persons with a high receptivity to medical services than among those who were less inclined to favor medical services. In the high inclination group, "stress" was a rather significant influence in bringing people to the physician. Thus among those with high "stress," 73 per cent used facilities frequently, while only 46 per cent did so among those with low "stress." Although the same trend was observed among those who were less inclined to seek advice from a doctor, the relationship was substantially smaller, and not statistically significant. Thus our data support the interpretation that "stress" leads to an attempt to cope; those who are inclined to adopt the patient role tend to adopt this particular method of coping more frequently than those who are not so inclined.

As I have already noted, the reactive component in illness is clearly relevant to treatment response. Beecher,[21] for example, has collected considerable data to show that the effectiveness of a placebo is very much greater when the patient is distressed than when he is not. Placebos, for example, have very little effect on relieving pain inflicted in the laboratory but they are impressive in relieving pain following surgery. Beecher has accumulated data from several laboratories which show placebos effective in relieving pain of angina pectoris, seasickness, headache, cough, and so on. In reviewing fifteen studies totalling 1082 patients he found an average of 35.2 (plus or minus 2.2) per cent relieved by placebo. In contrast, Beecher calculates the effectiveness of placebos in relieving experimentally contrived pain as 3.2 per cent; thus the placebo is ten times as effective in relieving pain of pathological origin (where distress is an important factor) than it is in relieving pain of experimentally contrived origin.

Studies in social psychology have shown that under situations that are difficult, usual habits and problem-solving patterns may be disrupted and behavior may become disorganized. Under these conditions the directions which coping attempts take depend on the one hand on external influences and stimuli which serve to define circumstances and their meaning, and on the other on past experience and preparation. We will discuss each of these in turn.

In a recent ingenious experiment, Schachter and Singer[33] have shown how external cues influence behavior and feeling states under conditions of altered physiology. They demonstrated that whether subjects experienced anger or euphoria when injected with epinephrine was dependent on whether they had (1) an *appropriate explanation* for their altered physiological state and (2) *directive external cues*. When the individual had an appropriate explanation for his feelings, he had little need for evaluating himself in terms of environmental stimuli and was not very much affected by them. However, when individuals had no immediate explanation for their altered feelings, external cues became important and, in the experimental situation, determined the emotional state. The same type of altered physiological experience was variously interpreted as happiness or anger depending on cues determined by stooges of the experimenter who were playing the role of subjects. Thus we see that, when persons lose their bearings, environmental cues play an important part in helping the person make sense of his subjective state. Placebos may determine cues in a similar way during illness.

Several studies similarly reflect the importance of cultural and developmental experiences in reactions to threatening circumstances. Schachter,[34] in another set of impressive experimental studies, showed that first-born and only children were more likely to affiliate when threatened in adult life than other adults. Schachter believes that the attention given to the first child, and the inexperience of parents, is likely to instil a greater dependence on others in first and only born children as compared with later born children. Although birth order has not been studied directly in illness behavior studies, several other investigations support the idea that past experience, habits, and social values help define—consciously and unconsciously—the alternatives that will be utilized in challenging circumstances.

Phillips,[35] for example, in a recent study has shown that attitudes of self-reliance and health values both affect the willingness of people to report that they would seek help when ill. Many studies of delay in treatment reflect the same tendency for delay to be related to a constellation of ingrained sociomedical habits[36] which tend to be typical—at least in the United States—of the lower socioeconomic groups. Suchman[15] found, for example, that both individual medical orientation (an index based on knowledge about disease, on skepticism about medical care, and on dependency in illness) and social group organization (an index based on ethnic exclusiveness, friendship solidarity, and family orientation to tradition and authority) were related to socioeconomic status. A "parochial" as compared with a "cosmopolitan" social structure and a "popular" as compared with a "scientific" orientation to medicine were both linked with lower socioeconomic status. Similarly, persons of higher socioeconomic status were more likely to buy health insurance, to get a periodic medical check-up, to receive polio immunization, to eat a balanced diet, and they more frequently had eye examinations and dental care.

Under conditions of manageable difficulties, persons have a tendency to normalize or ignore symptoms that do not become too severe. For example in our study discussed earlier[37] we found that when illness is of a kind that is common and familiar, and the course of the illness is predictable, the presentation of the illness for medical scrutiny is substantially related to the inclination to use medical services as measured by hypothetical illness situations. As symptoms become more atypical, less familiar, and less predictable in their course, the role of social and situational factors in bringing a person for medical attention becomes less important. Similarly, Scheff and Silverman,[11] in a study of the use of a college psychiatric clinic, found social and demographic factors to be better predictors of the use of such facilities than the "seriousness" of the patient's condition. However, when they stratified their psychiatric cases into those more serious and those less serious, it became clear that while social and demographic factors were crucial in the presentation of "moderate psychiatric problems," they were relatively unimportant in predicting use of such facilities among those with "severe psychiatric problems."

If we are to make progress in the study of illness behavior, it becomes necessary to move beyond gross cultural and social differences in illness patterns toward the development of a social-psychological model which gives a clear conception of the processes involved when someone seeks help. From our various studies, we are able to suggest a working model which describes some of the contingencies relevant to illness behavior.[38] Seven groups of variables appear to be particularly important: (I) the number and persistence of symptoms; (II) the individual's ability to recognize symptoms; (III) the perceived seriousness of symptoms; (IV) the extent of social and physical disability resulting from the symptoms; (V) the cultural background of the defining person, group or agency in terms of the emphasis on tolerance, stoicism, etc.; (VI) available information and medical knowledge, and (VII) the availability of sources of help and their social and physical accessibility. Here we include not only physical distance and costs of time, money and effort, but also such costs as "fear," stigma, social distance, feelings of humiliation, and the like.

When we inspect these seven groups of variables, it becomes clear that what may appear salient to the definer may not appear relevant to the physician. For example, the recognizability of symptoms is not necessarily correlated with medical views of their seriousness. Similarly, some symptoms which are, for example, disfiguring or disruptive or which bring about work disability may be self-limited and medically trivial while other symptoms (such as signs of cancer) may have no disruptive effects at all. Yet one of the major cues patients use in deciding to seek help is the disruption of their activities. Illness behavior and the decision to seek medical advice frequently involves, from the patient's point of view, a rational attempt to make sense of his problem and cope with it within the limits of his intelligence and his social and cultural understandings.

Zola[39] has attempted to delineate five timing "triggers" in patient's decision to seek medical care. The first pattern he calls "interpersonal crisis" where the situation calls attention to the symptoms and causes the patient to dwell on them. The second "trigger" he calls "social interference"; in this situation the symptoms do not change, but come to threaten a valued social activity. The third "trigger"—"the presence of sanctioning"—involves others telling him to seek care. Fourthly, Zola discusses "perceived threat" and, finally, "nature and quality of the symptoms." The latter "trigger" involves similarity of symptoms to previous ones or to those of friends, and the like. Zola reports the impression that these "triggers" have different effects in various social strata and ethnic groups.

The difficulty in preventive medicine is that commonsense models of health and coping with disease do not necessarily conform to scientific models, yet it is usually commonsense models that determine the use of medical facilities. Similarly, a frequent problem faced by the physician in providing care is the failure of the patient to conform to medical advice and most typically this occurs when the patient fails to take his drugs or return for follow-up because, subjectively, he feels well. From the patient's commonsense perspective, to stop medication or cancel a follow-up visit when he is feeling well is logical.

Illness Behavior as an Attempt to Seek Secondary Advantages

Since illness is recognized as an acceptable cause for withdrawing from certain role obligations, social responsibilities, and expectations, persons may be drawn to the patient role in order to obtain secondary advantages, to make claims on others for care and attention, and to provide an acceptable reason for social failure. Thus, individuals may be motivated to adopt the "sick role,"[40] and others may be anxious to accord people the status of sickness in order to avoid embarrassment and social difficulties. The interpenetration between medical and other social institutions is quite complex, and often these relationships are not fully appreciated.

In the final analysis, illness and social disability are socially defined and somewhat arbitrary.[41] The problem of mental subnormality, for example, is a greater problem in a highly developed industrial nation requiring a high level of skills than it is in a communal agrarian community; and if we had no schools most of the mildly subnormal would be unrecognized and undefined. Similarly, the extent to which people are to be held accountable for fulfilling responsibilities regardless of health status involves a compromise between personal and community needs. The need to minimize the consequences of ill health as a practical or a humanitarian gesture is theoretically only one value to be weighed against other personal and social goals, and the limits and scope of the definition of illness may serve different needs and different agencies, depending on social, political, and historical contingencies.

Since a discussion of problems of the definition of "illness," as distinct from "illness behavior," will take us too far afield, I will not develop the topic here.[42] It should, however, be noted that the concept of illness can be used to support humanitarian values in the face of moral and legal sanctions.[43] Thus, illness concepts are used to overcome restrictive laws on abortion, or on criminal responsibility, as an excuse for academic failure, and so on. On other occasions, the concept of illness may be used to discredit peoples' views and actions, and to undermine their integrity. The use of illness labels may differ depending on who controls medical institutions, and the goals they are meant to serve.[44] Medical independence of political control is of obvious importance here as is the necessity for medical decisions affecting the community to be reviewed by expert laymen. In a free society the value and functions of medicine have primary relevance from a social standpoint in that they can enhance or retard the ability of the individual to fulfil personal and social choices. Physicians, on the whole, have been very successful in protecting medical systems from external manipulation for non-medical purposes. For the most part, even in this complicated age, the doctor serves as the patient's agent, and often even as his advocate.

As society becomes more humanitarian, and as illness becomes not only an excuse for social failure and neglect of social responsibilities but also cause, in and of itself, for monetary and social compensation, the relationship between illness as a physical state and as a secondary coping technique becomes even more difficult. It is fairly obvious that under some circumstances desire for compensation for injury and disability may encourage persons to exaggerate their inabilities to perform routine tasks, and discourage attempts to cope with the disability.

Discussion: Implications of Illness Behavior for Medical Care

The value of a medical perspective which takes into account illness behavior can be illustrated by a study at the Massachusetts General Hospital.[45] The hypothesis was that the patient's cultural background would influence how the patient presented his symptoms, and thus, how the doctor evaluated them. The analysis was undertaken because the investigator had the impression that more Italian than Irish or Anglo-Saxon patients were being labelled as psychiatric problems although there was no objective difference in the extent to which members in these groups reported psychosocial problems. Zola selected a group of 29 patients who presented themselves at the Medical and Ear, Nose and Throat clinics, but for whom no medical disease was found. There was good reason to believe that these groups of patients did not differ in the extent of their life difficulties. But it was clear that their mode of cultural expression was very different. Italians are more emotional in the presentation of symptoms, and give more attention and expression to pain. Zola found that psychogenesis was implied in the medical reports of 11 of the 12 Italian cases, and only in four of the thirteen remaining cases. Although this was not a well controlled study, the results strongly suggest that the patient's cultural mode of expression affected how the doctor viewed him and how he was medically evaluated.

The place of illness behavior is particularly important in disorders that are largely diagnosed through behavioral manifestations and the patient's social history. For it is particularly difficult to separate symptoms from subcultural patterns of expression and affect, and different behavioral patterns among the various social strata. Similarly, it is in such disorders that symptoms and etiological factors are more frequently confused with factors which may differentially lead to social intervention and the seeking of care.

The provision of care depends to a considerable extent on the social and cultural processes that lead particular people to define themselves as requiring care, or that lead others to define them as targets for community action. Many factors unrelated to the severity of illness and incapacity may assist in the selection of patients for care, while other persons requiring attention to a greater extent go unnoticed.

We all recognize that there are many persons in the general population who require care and treatment and who can benefit by it but do not come to the attention of care facilities. Conversely, there are some who have developed an overdependence on the physician, psychiatrist, or social agency who can be adversely affected by particular kinds of intensive care and attention. Although psychiatrists, especially those more dynamically oriented, often work under the assumption that all persons can benefit from therapy—or at least, that it will not harm them—and although the plea for help is usually taken on pragmatic grounds as proof for the need for psychiatric assistance, it is important to consider the counterproposition—that certain kinds of assistance, however well-meaning, can be detrimental for certain patients. There are those, for example, for whom excessive focus on symptoms and life difficulties may reinforce an already hypochondrial pattern, induce or encourage further displays of illness behavior, and bring about reduced coping effectiveness. As we have already noted, illness is one of the few widely recognized and acceptable reasons for failing to meet social responsibilities and obligations and thus the sick role often carries advantages for those who wish to escape the difficulties of meeting social expectations without incurring disapproval. The improper use of the sick role and the willingness to encourage persons to assume the role of the patient without careful consideration of its implications involves serious dangers. The improper use of the sick role under some circumstances can reinforce "immature" and "irresponsible" patterns of behavior. Military psychiatrists have learned—and this is consistent with the observations of Beecher we discussed earlier—that under military conditions where persons often wish to evade responsibilities and dangers, the sick role may offer clear advantages. This is one of the reasons military organizations often make it so difficult to be sick, and similarly totalitarian governments have done so during periods of labor shortage. During the second world war, it was observed that when troops became upset under combat stress and were evacuated for treatment it was extremely difficult to return these men as functioning soldiers. When these men were brought back to the hospital, and when their problems were defined as having roots in their early years, the men had an acceptable reason for failure which could be viewed as beyond their control and it was difficult to mobilize them.[46] In contrast, during the Korean war, when such problems were defined as problems of mastery of common fears shared by many others, it was possible to encourage men to make instrumental efforts to cope with the extreme difficulties in their situation.[47]

The issue is not, of course, whether we should adopt a permissive approach to illness or on the other hand subjugate health organizations to other social institutions. From the perspective of a free medical system (that is, one where the doctor acts primarily as the patient's agent and on his behalf), the doctor-patient relationship is one where the doctor has considerable influence in affecting the patient's feeling state and behavior. As we have noted, patients often seek care when they are distressed; and there is a large amount of evidence that distressed persons are highly suggestible and open to influence.[22] Thus, the doctor's attitude toward the patient and his illness are important forces which can be used to support coping efforts, or they can encourage an elaboration of the disability.

There are factors which affect illness behavior perhaps less visibly but which strongly influence coping efforts and the nature of disability. It is now well recognized that particular hospital environments can have deleterious effects on the patient.[48,49] Patients who are cared for in environments which fail to stimulate them may deteriorate. Wing and Brown showed that in the case of schizophrenia, in socially poor hospitals, patients are more withdrawn and have more symptoms such as poverty of speech.[50,51] Similarly, Brown and his associates found that schizophrenic patients have poor outcome in family environments characterized by "high emotional involvement."[52] Through well planned programs encompassing community care and "social treatment," the advantages of more limited medical treatments and procedures can be realized without incurring inactivity, separation from social ties, loss of confidence and skills, and other liabilities associated with long-term patient roles.

As we noted at the beginning of this discussion, the problems of separating out "primary" biological from "secondary" psychological and social factors in conditions such as "institutionalism" are enormously complex, though perhaps easier with some physical diseases than with psychiatric disorders.[49,53] In research efforts, attempts to reliably separate these components is an important and necessary endeavor. In the practice of clinical medicine and psychiatry, however, concern with social and psychological disabilities may achieve results comparable, and under some circumstances superior, to those gained by directing attention to the "primary" disorder.

We often tend to forget that our language and the professional stances we take have a moral as well as a scientific and practical importance. And since our orientation toward patients implies a vocabulary of motives, it is not surprising that it has effects on their future motives and efforts. Over the years there has been an increasing tendency to view problems of living within a deterministic model of illness, and there is no question but that this tendency has served a valuable social function in perpetuating the humanitarian perspective which it encompassed. But as we increasingly recognize the social influences of the labelling process and of environmental contexts, it is important to consider how iatrogenic disability may be avoided without abandoning the human values to which medicine and psychiatry have made so important a contribution.

Notes

1. Mechanic, D. (1962). "The Concept of Illness Behavior." *Journal of Chronic Diseases,* **15:**189–194.

2. Mechanic, D. (1963). "Some Implications of Illness Behavior for Medical Sampling." *New England Journal of Medicine,* **269:**244–247.

3. White, K. L., et al. (1961). "The Ecology of Medical Care." *New England Journal of Medicine,* **265:**885–892.

4. Koos, E. (1954). *The Health of Regionsville: What the People Thought and Did About It.* New York: Columbia University Press.

5. Saunders, L. (1954). *Cultural Differences and Medical Care.* New York: Russell Sage Foundation.

6. Clark, M. (1959). *Health in the Mexican American Community.* Berkeley: University of California Press.

7. Zborowski, M. (1952). "Cultural Components in Responses to Pain." *Journal of Social Issues,* **8:**16–30.

8. Croog, S. H. (1961). "Ethnic Origins, Educational Level, and Responses to a Health Questionnaire." *Human Organization,* **20:**65–69.

9. Mechanic, D. (1963). "Religion, Religiosity and Illness Behavior." *Human Organization,* **22:**202–208.

10. Segal, B. "Scholars and Patients: Religion, Academic Performance and the Use of Medical Facilities by Male Undergraduates." Unpublished Paper. Department of Sociology, Dartmouth College.

11. Scheff, T. J., and A. Silverman (1966). "Users and Non-Users of a Student Psychiatric Clinic." *Journal of Health and Human Behavior,* **7:**114–121.

12. Segal, B., et al. (1965). "Emotional Adjustment, Social Organization and Psychiatric Treatment Rates." *American Sociological Review,* **30:**548–556.

13. Srole, L., et al. (1962). *Mental Health in the Metropolis.* New York: McGraw-Hill.

14. Linn, L. (1967). "Social Characteristics and Social Interaction in the Utilization of a Psychiatric Outpatient Clinic. *Journal of Health and Human Behavior,* **8:**3–14.

15. Suchman, E. (1964). "Sociomedical Variations Among Ethnic Groups." *American Journal of Sociology,* **70:**319–331; (1965), "Social Patterns and Medical Care," *Journal of Health and Human Behavior,* **6:**2–16.

16. Anderson, O. (1958). "Infant Mortality and Social and Cultural Factors: Historical Trends and Current Patterns. In E. G. Jaco (ed.), *Patients, Physicians, and Illness.* New York: Free Press.

17. Mechanic, D. (1964). "The Influence of Mothers on their Children's Health Attitudes and Behavior." *Pediatrics,* **33:**444–453.

18. Anderson, O. (1963). "The Utilization of Health Services." In H. Freeman et al. (eds.), *Handbook of Medical Sociology.* Englewood Cliffs: Prentice Hall.

19. Mechanic, D. (1965). "Perception of Parental Responses to Illness." *Journal of Health and Human Behavior,* **6:**253–257.

20. Sternbach, R. A., and B. Tursky (1965). "Ethnic Differences Among Housewives in Psychophysical and Skin Potential Responses to Electric Shock." *Psychophysiology,* **1:**241–246.

21. Beecher, H. (1959). *Measurement of Subjective Responses.* New York: Oxford University Press.

22. Frank, J. (1961). *Persuasion and Healing.* Baltimore: Johns Hopkins Press.

23. Speisman, J. C., et al. (1964). "Experimental Reduction of Stress Based on Ego-Defense Theory." *Journal of Abnormal Social Psychology,* **68:**367–380.

24. Freidman, S. B., et al. (1963). "Behavioral Observations on Parents Anticipating the Death of a Child." *Pediatrics,* **32:**610–625.

25. Freidman, S. B., et al. (1963). "Urinary 17-Hydroxycorticosteroid Levels in Parents of Children with Neoplastic Disease." *Psychosomatic Medicine,* **25:**364–376.

26. Wolff, H. (1953). *Stress and Disease.* Springfield, Ill: Thomas.

27. Hinkle, L. E., and H. G. Wolff (1957). "Health and the Social Environment: Experimental Investigations." In A. H. Leighton et al. (eds.), *Explorations in Social Psychiatry.* New York: Basic Books.

28. Roessler, R., and N. Greenfield (eds.) (1962). *Physiological Correlates of Psychological Disorder.* Madison, Wis.: University of Wisconsin Press.

29. Graham, D., et al. (1962). "Physiological Response to the Suggestion of Attitudes Specific for Hives and Hypertension." *Psychosomatic Medicine,* **24:**159–169.

30. Meyer, R. J., and R. J. Haggerty (1962). "Streptococcal Infections in Families." *Pediatrics,* **29:**539–544.

31. Balint, M. (1957). *The Doctor, His Patient, and the Illness.* New York: International Universities Press.

32. Mechanic, D., and E. H. Volkart (1961). "Stress, Illness Behavior and the Sick Role." *American Sociological Review,* **26:**51–58.

33. Schachter, S., and J. Singer (1962). "Cognitive, Social, and Physiological Determinants of Emotional State." *Psychological Review,* **69:**379–399.

34. Schachter, S. (1959). *The Psychology of Affiliation.* Palo Alto: Stanford University Press.

35. Phillips, D. (1965). "Self-Reliance and the Inclination to Adopt the Sick Role." *Social Forces,* **43:**555–563.

36. Goldsen, R. (1963). "Patient Delay in Seeking Cancer Diagnosis: Behavioral Aspects." *Journal of Chronic Diseases,* **16:**427–436.

37. Mechanic, D., and E. H. Volkart (1960). "Illness Behavior and Medical Diagnoses." *Journal of Health and Human Behavior,* **1:**86–94.

38. Mechanic, D. (1962). "Some Factors in Identifying and Defining Mental Illness." *Mental Hygiene,* **46:**66–74; (1966), The Sociology of Medicine, Viewpoints and Perspectives. *Journal of Health and Human Behavior,* **7:**237–248.

39. Zola, I. (1964). "Illness Behavior of the Working Class." In A. Shastak and W. Gomberg (eds.), *Studies of the American Worker.* Englewood Cliffs: Prentice Hall.

40. Parsons, T. (1951). *The Social System.* New York: Free Press.

41. Mechanic, D. (1959). "Illness and Social Disability: Some Problems in Analysis." *Pacific Sociological Review,* **2:**37–41.

42. Mechanic, D. (1966). "Community Psychiatry: Some Sociological Perspectives and Implications." In L. Roberts et al. (eds.), *Community Psychiatry*. Madison, Wis.: University of Wisconsin Press.

43. Szasz, T. S. (1962). "Bootlegging Humanistic Values Through Psychiatry." *Antioch Review*, **22**:341-349.

44. Field, M. (1957). *Doctor and Patient in Soviet Russia*. Cambridge: Harvard University Press.

45. Zola, I. (1963). "Problems of Communication, Diagnosis, and Patient Care." *Journal of Medical Education*, **10**:829-838.

46. Glass, A. J. (1953). "Psychotherapy in the Combat Zone." In *Symposium on Stress*. Washington: Army Medical Service Graduate School, Walter Reed Army Medical Hospital.

47. Group for the Advancement of Psychiatry (1960). *Preventive Psychiatry in the Armed Forces: With Some Implications for Civilian Use*. Report No. 47. New York.

48. Goffman, E. (1961). *Asylums:* New York: Doubleday-Anchor.

49. Wing, J. K. (1962). "Institutionalism in Mental Hospitals." *British Journal of Social Clinical Psychology*, **1**:38-51.

50. Wing, J. K., and G. W. Brown (1961). "Social Treatment of Chronic Schizophrenia: A Comparative-Survey of Three Mental Hospitals." *Journal of Mental Science*, **107**:847-861.

51. Brown, G. W., and J. K. Wing (1962). "A Comparative Clinical and Social Survey of Three Mental Hospitals." *The Sociological Review*, Monograph 5, Sociology and Medicine, Studies within the Framework of the British National Health Service, Keele.

52. Brown, G. W., et al. (1962). "Influence of Family Life on the Course of Schizophrenic Illness." *British Journal of Preventive Social Medicine*, **16**:55-68.

53. Brown, G. W., et al. (1966). *Schizophrenia and Social Care*. London: Oxford University Press.

CHAPTER XIII

Sociological Issues in Mental Health*

In recent years we have witnessed tremendous growth in government support for the provision of mental health services, manpower training, and mental health research. Although essential, the vast expenditure of funds for psychiatric research has provided limited information relevant to the effective operation of community mental health centers, and the tremendous growth of the community mental health movement has depended more on an ideological thrust than on evidence supporting the feasibility and effectiveness of using available mental health resources in community programs. Mental health politics being what they are, mental health workers had to take what they could get when they could get it. But it would be a tragic mistake if the community mental health movement came to believe its own rhetoric and substituted such propaganda for detailed investigation of the effectiveness of alternative systems of delivering mental health care.

Community mental health is based on a variety of assumptions and values which are not always explicit, and they penetrate many scientific psychiatric issues which are hotly debated and far from resolved. The community mental health movement operates on the assumption that by locating problems in living at an early stage in their development disability can be prevented, and that continuing gains are achieved through early treatment which retards chronic morbidity and disability.[1] Yet psychiatrists have not established that problems in living are part of the same continuum as the chronic psychoses, and there is considerable evidence to the contrary. With the growth of enthusiasm for community

---

* Adapted from a chapter that appeared in Bellak and Barten (eds.), *Progress in Community Mental Health*, 1969, New York: Grune and Stratton, by permission of the publisher.

mental health programs, evidence supporting the claim that the chronic psychoses are different from other life problems is frequently forgotten and, thus, a short review of such evidence is necessary here. First, rates of hospitalized psychoses are relatively similar among developed Western nations, and they do not appear to vary greatly from one period to another.[2] Second, despite radically changing policies used by psychiatrists within the armed services which resulted in substantial alterations in rates of admission for psychoneurotic conditions, there is impressive consistency in the rates of psychoses requiring hospital care.[3] These rates do not appreciably vary from peacetime to wartime, nor were they very different in World War II as compared with World War I. And there is various evidence showing no change in rates for psychotic breakdown under extreme combat conditions or exposure to bombing attacks. Third, there is no evidence that rates of psychotic breakdown increase in civilian populations exposed to bombing attacks or other major stresses.[4] Fourth, contrary to popular conceptions, there is no adequate evidence that urban living, the hectic pace of modern life, and the like, affect rates of psychotic breakdown. An excellent and carefully executed study of the rates of mental illness over a century in Massachusetts found no support for the contention that the occurrence of the psychoses was increasing in modern society.[5] I do not mean to suggest that conditions other than the psychoses may not lead to severe problems incapacitating the individual and his ability to carry out his social roles—and such conditions are clearly worthy of significant help. I do not believe, however, that we can function effectively if we work on the basis of assumptions which are not correct.

It is also far from clear that we have adequate knowledge to effectively locate morbidity conditions at an early point and to treat them effectively. Furthermore, there is some possibility that preventive programs as they are generated through community mental health clinics may involve a higher risk of iatrogenic illness than is desirable, and that such programs may encourage feelings of helplessness and dependence among clients and stimulate a closer correspondence between their symptoms and sense of self-identity. Finally, community programs inevitably raise the issue of the expansiveness of the mental health concept. Are mental health programs to be directed primarily at persons suffering from clear psychiatric syndromes, or do mental health problems include most of the ordinary problems of living that people encounter in their lives? Are such problems as delinquency or criminal behavior a part of the community mental health vision, or are they really most basically outside the psychiatric sphere? Are poverty, discrimination, employment difficulties, and educational deficiencies targets for community mental health action, or is community mental health more fruitfully restricted to more limited spheres? Indeed, we all know that there are many concepts of community mental health.[6]

Despite the lack of agreement on many issues, there appears to be considerable consensus that mental health centers will play an increasingly important role in mental health care. Health centers were originally seen as having three basic roles: (1) the treatment of acute mental illness; (2) the provision of care for mental patients either prior to admission to a hospital or after discharge from the hospital; and (3) mental health education.[7] With the changing character of mental hospitals—particularly the considerable shortening of hospital stay—the need for a wide variety of community services to help sustain mental patients in the community is apparent. Yet, several observers are already concerned that community mental health centers are committed less to this goal than to others and, very much like clinics that previously existed, are devoting their attention to less disabled clients. But the community mental health effort is still very much unformed, and many such clinics are searching for professional roles and perspectives that are related to community needs and an approach for a broad attack on the mental health problem. The major purpose of this chapter is to consider the difficulties of defining community needs and designing a program to meet them, as well as to explore various alternative approaches to the field of mental health rehabilitation.

Mental Health and Social Policy: Some Dilemmas

Since resources are never unlimited, decisions concerning the provision of mental health care must be based on some conception of priorities and some criteria for establishing these. Priorities always depend on values in one way or another. It appears that there are two paramount values that are ordinarily applied in thinking about the provision of mental health services. The first is a humanitarian one—the concept of "need"—which is based on the idea that the best services that can be offered should be made available to those who need them despite the cost, difficulty, or pressures on social resources. The second concept—the notion of "gain" —is based on the idea that services should be made available when it is clear that the result achieved is equal to the investment, relative to using resources for competing investments. Excessive emphasis on the concept of "gain" inevitably comes into conflict with humanitarian considerations, and it is clear that public policy usually involves some marriage, however uncomfortable, between the notions of "need" and "gain."

The concept of "need" can be defined in terms of sickness and disability. It appears reasonable to argue that need exists depending on the severity of the condition and the amount of handicap it causes. Thus, the more sick and disabled a person is, the more he requires help, and the greater is the responsibility of public programs to insure that these needs are somehow met. However, from the point of view of the concept of "gain," decisions should depend in part on the efficacy of alternative services and the success of varying forms of intervention. Vast investments in unproven and ineffective services may result in little gain other than conformity with the value of offering help and, indeed, some services may harm patients as well. But frequently we lack sufficient data to make an informed assessment of the most reasonable directions for public programs.

Although there is widespread agreement that chronic mental patients have great needs, mental health workers have been reluctant to provide services to such persons for they argue that their methods produce little gain. Instead, the bulk of their resources are devoted to patients with less severe problems and disabilities who they feel can be helped more readily. It is also commonly argued that services to the young and those with lesser disorders lead to prevention of future morbidity and disability, and that such preventive services provide a greater yield than those devoted to maintaining and supporting patients already chronically ill. This view, widely held by psychiatrists and mental health workers, results in part from a biased statement of the larger issue; for the issue is not which patients respond best to a therapeutic relationship and various forms of psychotherapy as they now exist, but rather what forms of intervention are most fruitful for patients with varying disabilities, and what are their relative levels of success.

The conceptions of mental illness underlying public policy are important because different views suggest varying approaches to classifying psychiatric conditions and different assumptions on which to base care. If we assume, for example, that psychological difficulties and problems in living are pervasive throughout the society and have always been so, and that those who suffer from psychiatric diseases such as schizophrenia are fundamentally different from the mass of those who have common psychological problems, we are in a very different position than if we make the opposite assumption. Most mental health workers are probably not fully clear on what their positions are, and many hold both concepts of mental illness simultaneously. Such persons reason that even if common problems of living do not have the same character as schizophrenia, they nevertheless constitute severe difficulties incapacitating the individual and his ability to carry out his social roles. And thus, it is argued, such problems are worthy of help however they are characterized. But schizophrenia and other chronic conditions will not necessarily be amenable to the same approaches as "problems in living," and thus the mental health clinic, if it is to be effective, and if it is to meet its original goals, must be organized so as to provide a highly diversified pattern of services.

In the long run we must await better answers to a wide variety of questions: What conditions and problems if they go untreated become chronic, and which ones are transitory? What are the effects of varying systems of intervention in dealing with particular disorders? What social services and policies limit disability and handicap, and which ones lead to an exacerbation of such problems? Do preventive psychiatric services present any substantial risk of increasing the number of iatrogenic disturbances or encouraging psychological hypochondriasis? How successful are preventive psychiatric services in insulating persons from future serious morbidity and disability? We must continue to ask such questions and to formulate them in a fashion that is amenable to empirical investigation. Public policy must continue to develop despite the uncertainty of knowledge, but such a policy must lack a sense of dogmatism and encompass encouragement for research and evaluation which may negate it.

The Patient and the Society: An Insoluble Dilemma

Mental illness may be viewed from several vantage points that are themselves in conflict. Most commonly, psychiatric difficulties are viewed either in terms of the psychological distress the person is experiencing or in terms of his social functioning. Although psychological comfort may contribute to adequate social functioning, these two aspects of adaptation are not necessarily facilitated by the same social conditions. Individuals and communities have long-range as well as short-range goals, and it frequently becomes necessary to incur psychological costs in the short run to achieve larger and more distant intentions.

There is no society in the history of civilization completely devoted to eliminating personal discomfort and pain, since some of the social conditions producing distress are consistent with important societal values and goals. Our most valued social institutions do much to produce psychological stress and, of course, contribute to social difficulties, personal distress, alienation, and a sense of failure. Implicit in the value structure of our society is the idea that the incentives for performance or the need for acquisition of skills require the cost of inducing some stress and personal pain in people's lives. Most societies operate on the premise that social stress provides incentives and facilitates the development of important instrumental goals. It is often possible to reduce personal distress by relieving persons of their obligations and responsibilities or doing more to alleviate their social conditions, but policy makers often consciously choose not to do so.

The moral dilemma community psychiatry must face relates to the relative emphasis to be placed on performance in comparison to the control of personal distress. Psychiatrists working for such institutions as the military operate under a policy which seeks to minimize the number of psychiatric casualties from the perspective of social performance; but, no doubt, this is achieved at some cost to the psychological comfort of the men who are dealt with. When a time dimension is built into perspectives on mental health difficulties, such problems become enormously complicated, and it becomes impossible to assess in scientific terms the value of one alternative in relation to others. These obviously will depend on the goals of individuals and groups and the extent to which societal pressures are necessary to achieve such goals. For example, if we facilitate the minimization of psychological distress at one stage in a person's life at some cost to his performance and the extent to which he develops new skills, we may find that at some later point in his life such inadequate skills constitute an important element of the person's life difficulties and personal distress. In contrast, if we neglect the issue of personal distress and place undue value on the development of performance skills, it is possible to "stress" a person to the extent that he is continuously miserable and refuses to function at all. In short, some balance must be sought in encouraging mastery of the environment on the one hand and concern for individual needs on the other, not only for humanitarian reasons but also to facilitate continuing performance and mastery.

The Problem of Demand: Illness Behavior and the Societal Reaction

As new contexts for psychiatric care develop, they are usually absorbed quickly into the community; and there appears to be little difficulty in finding a source of demand for such services. In part, such demand exists because there are many people who have unmet needs for psychiatric care, and they are responsive to the provision of new facilities. But we also know that the factors producing psychiatric difficulties may be very different from those which lead to social intervention and care.[8] Thus every clinician must appreciate the differences between the factors producing illness and disability and those bringing persons to the attention of psychiatric facilities. And every mental health organization must be concerned with encouraging greater congruency between the need for services and their provision.

Factors characterizing illness behavior and societal reactions to symptoms determine the public recognition of illness and the provision of psychiatric and social assistance. There is considerable evidence that many factors unrelated to the severity of illness and disability play some part in differentiating those who receive psychiatric assistance from those who do not. This is not to imply that the *character of the symptoms* themselves is unimportant. Much of the behavior of sick persons and other definers of illness is a direct product of the specific symptoms manifested: their intensity, the quality of discomfort they cause, their persistence, and the like. No matter how stoical a person is or how extreme his attitude toward illness may be, a fractured leg, a broken back, a severe psychosis, or any of a variety of other conditions is likely to bring him into care. Various studies of mental illness have shown, for example, that although there are vast differences in the willingness of significant others to tolerate bizarre and difficult behavior, few relatives appear willing to house a patient who is suicidal, homicidal, incontinent, hallucinatory, delusional, or disoriented.[9-11] Social definitions of illness are relevant because many important serious illnesses develop so that they are not particularly striking in their impact.

The foregoing would appear to be particularly relevant to the work of community mental health centers in that the populations they serve suffer for the most part from moderate disabilities, and whether care is or is not sought for such conditions is very much dependent on patterns of illness behavior and differing societal reactions (see Chapter 12).

In a British study[12] involving the use of child guidance facilities it was found that seeking care for children with specified problems was related to a variety of factors unrelated to the child's condition such as socioeconomic status, parental age, size and composition of the family, and other social factors. Also implicated in the process of help-seeking were the mental health of mothers and other parental responses. The mothers of clinic children were more likely to be anxious, depressed and easily upset by stress, felt less able to cope with their children, and they were more likely to discuss their problems and seek advice. In a follow-up study of the outcome of the children's conditions two years later, little difference in rates of improvement was observed in comparing the treated group with a matched group of children with similar conditions but untreated. Moreover, within the treatment group the amount of improvement observed was unrelated to the amount of treatment provided. Approximately two-thirds of the children in both groups had improved during the follow-up period. The investigators conclude that many so-called disturbances of behavior are no more than temporary exaggerations of widely distributed reaction patterns which tend to improve over time without treatment. They argue that clinicians have a tendency to attribute an exaggerated significance to single behavioral problems which may not have pathological significance and that the arrival of such children at help facilities is related to a variety of contingencies. The investigators further conclude that many problems of children cannot be regarded as morbid without knowledge of their frequency, duration, association with other kinds of behavior, and the settings within which such behavior occurs.

The foregoing is significant for workers in community health centers because, if they wish to utilize their resources in a meaningful way, they must attempt to discriminate between morbidity and the social forces which bring people to their attention. Although such clinics may wish to provide some form of service to any individual who seeks help, the character of this service might depend very substantially on the relative importance of the illness condition as compared with factors unrelated to morbidity which encouraged the person to seek help. Just as there are many persons in the general population who require care and treatment and who can benefit from it although they do not come to the attention of help facilities, so there are some who have developed an overdependence on the physician, psychiatrist, or social agency and who can be adversely affected by particular kinds of continued care and attention. Increasingly, psychiatrists are learning that often the sick role offers rather clear advantages under conditions where persons wish to evade responsibilities and dangers, and thus they are learning to use illness labels more carefully.[3]

Although it is impossible to provide a formula specifying the conditions under which the sick role could fruitfully be withheld, it may be valuable to at least describe a few areas where an illness label may be detrimental. It seems likely that careful scrutiny from this perspective is desirable in circumstances where situational stress plays an important part in the development of social and personal mastery, and where successful adaptation provides the conditions for further mastery and success. This would be particularly true where the sphere of action involved requires considerable effort and is personally threatening. Experience from the field of military psychiatry supports these observations. Often soldiers waver between their defined responsibilities in that role and their personal lack of commitment, fear of harm, and distaste for army life. It is, therefore, not surprising that in the past when disruption in behavior was defined as a psychiatric problem originating in the developmental history of the soldier, it became difficult to return soldiers to active duty. Once the army provided the soldier with an acceptable excuse for failure, the unattractiveness of army life was too great to lead to the mobilization of the necessary effort for coping with these harsh conditions.[13] From the point of view of a civilian clinic, an analogous population consists of persons undergoing various stressful role transitions: adolescents, the newly married and divorced, widows, retired persons, and the like. There is growing evidence that role transitions or major life changes often precede psychological distress and illness, and that these life changes are not themselves necessarily caused by the person.[14] In such circumstances the clinician must consider very carefully the consequences of allowing the person to explain his life situation within a psychiatric framework, as against the consequences resulting from alternative explanations and approaches to the client's problems.

Some Alternative Rehabilitation Approaches

Much of the work with mental patients in the past was based on a view of man as a recipient of developmental and environmental stimuli rather than one which views him as an active agent molding and affecting, to some extent, the conditions to which he will be exposed. Thus, much of our psychological vocabulary is phrased in terms of the intrapsychic reactions to environmental stress rather than in terms of active striving and social adaptation. Although all scientific activity must ultimately be based on a deterministic model of some form, social activity is a product of the manipulation and negotiation of symbols. The scope of the symbolic environment in a complex and dynamic society— and even in more simple ones—is so vast and so rich in complexity that man has considerable opportunity to affect the direction of his life. It seems, therefore, to be of some advantage to conceptually specify for psychiatric purposes the more active problem-solving aspects of human adaptation and their relationship to the larger social structure.

In considering the meaning of the concept of social and psychological "stress," it becomes evident that this term refers to neither "stimuli" nor "reactions" in themselves, but rather to a discrepancy between a problem or challenge and an individual's capacity to deal with or accommodate to it. This definition makes clear the importance of skill and performance components as well as psychological defenses, and for this reason I feel it useful to differentiate between the concepts of coping and defense.[15] Coping, as I use the term, refers to the instrumental behavior and problem-solving capacities of persons in meeting life demands and goals. It involves the application of skills, techniques, and knowledge that a person has acquired. The extent to which a person experiences discomfort in the first place is often a product of the inadequacy of such skill repertoires. In contrast to coping, the concept of defense (as I am using the term) refers to the manner in which a person manages his emotional and affective states when discomfort is aroused or anticipated. Most psychodynamic and psychological work in the mental health area deals with defense and not with coping. Implicit within the typical psychological approaches is the idea that the links between abilities and performance are obvious or irrelevant, and that only the psychodynamics of intrapsychic response remain problematic. This assumption, in my opinion, is an erroneous one, and much that is regarded as intrapsychic dynamics can be seen—perhaps more fruitfully—from a skills-abilities perspective. There has been an increasing interest in the behavioral sciences in considering the role of skill acquisition in processes which traditionally have not been regarded as having skill components. Although there is a substantial literature on skill components in criminal behavior and on the acquisition and use of illegal means,[16] it is only more recently that the skill component has been viewed as a consideration in drug use,[17,18] suicide,[19] being mentally ill,[20] and the like. Consistent with this have been studies such as the one by Schachter and Singer[21] which implies the importance of learning how to define internal arousal; and Schachter has attempted to explain conditions such as compulsive eating as a product of inadequate ability to differentiate hunger from other forms of physiological arousal.[22] In passing, I would like to note that the process of acquiring most of our skills for dealing with threats (most of which are symbolic and interpersonally organized) is usually indirect and informal; and the skills themselves may have no descriptive vocabularies to depict them. Thus these skills may be very unevenly acquired, and skill deficiencies may not be easily identified until extreme situations develop.

From the point of view of individuals who are faced with particular life crises, it is necessary to raise at least three central questions: Does he want to deal with the situation? (motivation); Can he deal with it if he wants to? (coping); And can he maintain his emotional equilibrium in the situation? (defense). Each of these dimensions has an equivalent dimension on the societal level. For convenience I shall refer to them as (1) incentive systems; (2) preparatory institutions; and (3) evaluative systems. By incentive systems I refer to societal values and the systems of rewards and punishments which organizations and communities develop that push activities in particular directions. Preparatory institutions refer to societal attempts to develop skills and competence among persons to prepare them to deal with societal needs, demands, and challenges. This includes not only schools and other formal learning experiences, but even more importantly the varieties of informal learning that are acquired through family living and peer association. By evaluative institutions, I refer to the approval and support or disapproval and disparagement resulting from particular courses of activity. I will elaborate on these concepts in the next chapter. One essential implication to note here, however, is that intervention techniques devoted to improving responses to life situations may occur at the societal level as well as at the individual level.

In general, clinicians who work with the psychiatrically disabled tend to emphasize the psychological barriers and techniques and give relatively lesser attention to the strategies or techniques through which persons deal with tasks and other people. This failure is implicit in the psychological bias and in the entire orientation to the patient. Instead of exploring the nature of the patient's life difficulties that lead him to seek care or others to insist that he be removed from his social situation, emphasis is given to early development and relationships. Too often therapy designed to change the patient is undertaken without giving careful consideration to the situation and problems to which he must return, the skills he will require, and the attitudes and feelings about his disabilities among significant others. Although much of an individual's ability to accomplish difficult tasks or to deal with the social environment realistically may not be amenable to intervention, it is not unreasonable to believe that mental health workers can help improve patients' coping effectiveness either by changing or modifying their level of instrumental efforts or by helping alter the social conditions under which they live so that their skills are more adequate and their problems less handicapping.

In considering therapeutic approaches within the context of the community health center, it is impossible to overemphasize the need for a flexible approach. Providing community care to persons returning from the mental hospital and to those with chronic disabilities presents very different problems to such programs than providing care to an adequately functioning neurotic patient whose problem is largely one of psychological discomfort. Since there has been a tendency on the part of community mental health programs to neglect the care of the more severe disabilities, I shall concentrate the discussion on this aspect of community mental health.

Continuing Community Care and Chronic Mental Illness

In recent years the most striking change in mental health needs has resulted from the changing use of psychiatric hospitalization. Many patients who in the past would have been retained in mental hospitals are now returned to the community after a relatively short stay. Most patients now leave the mental hospital within a year, and the average length of stay is no more than several weeks. The perceived importance of keeping the patient in the community rather than in the hospital is evident from the report of the Joint Commission on Mental Illness and the legislation that has followed the Commission's report. It was contended that:

The objective of modern treatment of persons with major mental illness is to enable the patient to maintain himself in the community in a normal manner. To do so, it is necessary: (1) to save the patient from the debilitating effects of institutionalism as much as possible, (2) if the patient requires hospitalization, to return him to home and community life as soon as possible, and (3) thereafter to maintain him in the community as long as possible. Therefore, aftercare and rehabilitation are essential parts of all service to mental patients, and the various methods of achieving rehabilitation should be integrated in all forms of service.[7]

Returning the patient to the community or retaining him within it is no panacea if the quality of the patient's life and social functioning cannot be improved. Given the great emphasis placed on "carrying one's own weight" in the American value system, it is not surprising that some persons view residence in the community as a "good" in itself, independent of the quality of the patient's life outside the hospital. But this poses the issue too simply. There are good sheltered institutional environments and some very bad community living contexts, and the conception that any community context is more therapeutic than any hospital context is absurd. The prevailing oversimplification is a consequence of the fact that most institutional contexts for the psychiatrically ill have been appalling from a therapeutic standpoint and inhumane from a social perspective. In our enthusiasm for new programs, however, we must also be aware that if patients are sufficiently aberrant and disturbed, their residence in the community poses innumerable difficulties for their families and others and may result in a general outcome inferior to good institutional care. Whatever one's standpoint on this issue, we must all realize that changing policies in the administration of mental health care have vastly increased the public's responsibility for providing services for the mentally ill, and the failure to provide such services is not only an injustice to the patient but to his family as well, since it is they who must now continue to cope with his disturbed behavior.

One would anticipate that the consequences of this shift in mental health policy have been so vast that researchers would be flocking to study them. It is disillusioning, indeed, to find how underdeveloped this research area is and how blindly decision-makers must grope in attempting to develop coherent policies and approaches. The most coherent study to date that promotes an informed public policy was one carried out by Pasamanick and his colleagues.[23] The major intent of the study was to determine under varying circumstances the relative value of hospital versus home treatment for schizophrenic patients. The investigators randomized 152 schizophrenic patients who were referred to a state hospital into three groups: (1) a drug home-care group; (2) a placebo home-care group; (3) a hospital-control group. Patients treated at home were visited regularly by public health nurses and were also seen, but less frequently, by a staff psychologist, social worker, and psychiatrist for evaluation purposes. The study was primarily concerned with a comparison of hospital treatment against home-care treatment by public health nurses. Patients were involved in the study for periods from 6 to 30 months, and the investigators found that 77 per cent of drug home-care patients remained continuously at home in contrast to 34 per cent of those receiving placebos. Using the hospital-control group as a base, they estimate that the 57 home patients receiving drugs saved over 4800 days of hospitalization, and the 41 patients in the placebo group saved over 1150 inpatient days. Even more impressive is the observation that after members of the hospital-treated control group returned to the community, they required rehospitalization more frequently than the patients who were treated at home on drugs from the very start.

Without disparaging the importance and significance of this study, it is essential to raise the question as to whether remaining at home constitutes an adequate or meaningful measure of rehabilitation. Patients were selected for the study when they were sent to the state hospital for treatment. The relatives of patients who were randomly selected for home treatment were informed that hospital treatment was unnecessary and that home care was more appropriate; moreover, "a due amount of persuasion" was used to convince the relative to accept the patient at home. The design of the study, thus, had two consequences which differentiated those treated in the hospital from those treated at home. First, the hospital defined itself as a less appropriate context for treating the symptoms and conditions of some patients and may have served to reinforce among relatives of home-care and hospital-care cases different frames of reference as to what symptoms justify hospitalization. Second, by restricting the hospitalization of patients in the home-care group, the hospital may have communicated a greater lack of willingness to help the relatives of this group during periods of crisis in contrast to the hospital-care group. It is not unreasonable to assume that once a person is refused help of a particular sort, he is less likely to request it on a second occasion, and this may explain the greater use of the hospital on subsequent occasions among patients in the hospital-treatment group. In sum, the design of the study program may have resulted in greater changes in "illness behavior" than in illness. It is my contention that the rehabilitation value of varying alternatives for treatment must be considered primarily in terms of social and psychological functioning.

Pasamanick and his colleagues provide data that reflect in one way or another the psychiatric and social functioning of patients who were evaluated after 6, 18, and 24 months. These data generally show considerable improvement in all groups by the sixth month with rather little improvement thereafter. In general, the rates of improvement observed during the first six months were no larger for one group than another, and thus these results provide little substance for the idea that one form of treatment has better long-range results than another. Thus, using the criterion of social functioning, there is no justification for extended hospital care over home care.

Finally, it is important to consider the social costs of retaining patients in the community. These can be assessed to some degree through data provided on various burdensome kinds of behavior. The investigators demonstrate that these difficult behaviors decrease substantially by the sixth month although they occurred very frequently during the initial study period. At the beginning of the study all three groups showed an equivalent level of family and community disturbance. When the patients were removed to the hospital the family and community were relieved of these difficulties, but when the patients stayed home these problems continued although they decreased through time. Unfortunately, the data from the study do not allow us to assess how rapidly the initial disturbances become alleviated; my colleagues and I are now in the process of carrying out a prospective study of released mental patients that will allow us to formulate a better answer to this question. It is clear from the Pasamanick study, however, that disturbing and troublesome behavior was relieved more quickly than inadequate role performance which does not show impressive improvement. In summary, an examination of the Pasamanick data indicates that there is considerable social cost in retaining schizophrenic patients in the community during the florid episodes of their illness, but by six months the costs are sufficiently low so as to make hospitalization unreasonable. However, we do not know how quickly within the initial six-month period the reduction in troublesome behavior occurs.

The data from the Pasamanick study support either of two treatment alternatives. First, if a policy of avoiding hospitalization is pursued with an emphasis on home care, maximal services and community aids must be applied quickly to help alleviate the strain on the patient and his family during the period when social costs are highest. This requires flexibility and the ability to mobilize rapidly in meeting social crises within the community. A second alternative is to depend on short hospitalizations during periods of florid symptomatology, followed by speedy releases, and accompanied by various services made available in the community. Decisions between these alternatives will, of course, depend on the individual circumstances of the case, the services actually available to relieve the patient and aid the family in home-care situations, and further knowledge which more specifically defines the costs and advantages of alternative approaches.

In our enthusiasm for new forms we should be careful not to underestimate the possible social costs in placing a greater burden than before on the family of the mental patient. There are some indications that the social costs involved may be very substantial, especially when community services are inadequate or highly fragmented. For example, the behavior of patients and the impact of their behavior on relatives and the community were studied in relation to 339 schizophrenic hospital patients who were returned to the community.[24] This English five-year follow-up study found that in the six months prior to interview 14 per cent of first admissions and 27 per cent of previously admitted patients showed behavior such as violence, threats, and destructiveness; 28 per cent and 45 per cent, respectively, had other symptoms of schizophrenia such as marked social withdrawal, slowness, posturing, and odd behavior. Finally, 41 per cent of the first admissions and 47 per cent of previous admissions had other symptoms such as headaches, phobias, depression, and the like. A significant proportion of relatives of these patients reported that the patient's illness was harmful to their health, affected the children adversely, created financial difficulties, and resulted in restrictions on leisure activities and the ability to entertain guests. Despite these problems approximately three-quarters of those who were living with a patient seemed to welcome him at home, and another 15 per cent were acceptant and tolerant.

One of the intentions of the investigators was to evaluate the effect of different hospital policies on patient care and rehabilitation outcome. They thus compared the patterns of hospitalization in three hospitals, one of which was known for its community care program. They found that outcome of patient care was much the same in the three hospitals. Patients spent less time in the hospital that was oriented toward the community, but since they were as sick as patients in the other hospitals, they were more likely to be unemployed when they were in the community and they were readmitted to the hospital more often. Since readmission usually occurred following a period of disturbed behavior and social crisis, such crises occurred more frequently in the hospital region that returned patients to the community more readily. Moreover, relatives of patients in this hospital reported more problems than relatives of patients in the other hospitals.

The data must of course be viewed in perspective. They pertain to the most disabled category of patients, and the results cannot be generalized to other psychiatric conditions which involve less social disturbance. Moreover, the adequacy of a community care program must depend on the adequacy and integration of the services available outside the hospital, and it was clear that the community services that were available were just not adequate to the task. This investigation demonstrates that the consequences of changing administrative policies must be evaluated in terms of the level of social functioning and social pathology, and not only in terms of administrative statistics.

In a related study Grad and Sainsbury[25] compared the effects on family life of two different types of services—a community care service and a hospital service. They were able to compare outcomes in two relatively comparable communities which had these different forms of service. The investigators measured the amount of burden incurred by relatives on referral of the patient and three to five weeks later. Approximately two-thirds of the families with severe burdens showed some relief of the original burden regardless of the nature of the service. Among patients presenting less severe burdens, improvement was somewhat higher in the hospital-centered service. In general, the investigators found little relationship between psychiatric symptoms related to burden and the extent to which they were relieved in the two services. They did find, however, that a patient with depression caused more hardship if treated in a community service rather than in a hospital service. There were other gains in having a hospital-based service; in this situation the closest relative felt less anxiety, and he suffered less interference with social and leisure activities.

In a report of a two-year follow-up study of the same patients,[26] Grad found that the hospital-based service was more effective in reducing anxiety and distress among patients' relatives and created less financial difficulties for the family. Moreover, families in the community care area were much more likely to have other problems as well two years later compared with those who had patients in the hospital-based service. Furthermore, younger men treated in the community service were much more likely than those treated in the hospital-based service to remain unemployed for the entire two-year period. Differences on social outcome are of large magnitude and bring into question the philosophy underlying a community-based service. On further investigation the researchers report that patients in the community-based service were treated more superficially than those in the hospital-based service. Grad notes the following in discussing the community-based service:

> . . . many social problems, especially those of a more subtle nature, were missed by the psychiatrists. First, their home visits were usually necessarily brief because of pressure of work; second, their interviews in accordance with their training and responsibilities and the families' expectations were patient-focused; third, the high social esteem in which doctors are held meant that family members would often either not presume to detain them by talking about their own troubles or feel relaxed enough in their presence to discuss those family trivia which often reveal social conflicts and stresses.

The study by Grad and Sainsbury provides a warning to us that changing administrative policies and modifying psychiatric procedures to a limited extent are not enough to launch a successful community care program. In our enthusiasm for change we would do well to heed this warning. Grad and Sainsbury have come to believe that the essential ingredient of relieving burden is to assure relatives that help is available and something could be done, and that this is a reasonable goal within either kind of service. This "sense of control," which Grad and Sainsbury imply, has been recognized in other areas of investigation as an important factor mediating stress response in difficult circumstances.[27] The investigators further suggest that for "certain types of patients" in "certain social circumstances" home care may leave the family with many more problems than hospital care. But since psychiatric patients are not a homogeneous group, it is necessary to learn in far greater detail what patients are most likely to flourish in home care and under what social and psychological circumstances. Moreover, it should be clear that if the public's responsibility is to be met, it is necessary not only to change administrative procedures, but to guarantee that adequate services are available to help relieve the consequences of such changes and to promote effective functioning of patients outside the hospital. We now turn to a consideration of some alternatives for doing this.

Some Considerations for Rehabilitation Programs

Since there is no agreement on modes of treatment for community care programs, the decision to provide a program in no sense specifies what is to be done. The various forms of psychotherapy stand at one extreme, and some visualize community care as nothing more than the extension of these therapies to new categories of people. More commonly, community care is visualized as a form of social work in which a trained practitioner helps the patient and his family "weather" crises by applying some knowledge of group and psychodynamic functioning, or where the practitioner serves as an ombudsman, helping to bail the patient and his family out of difficulty with a variety of official agencies. I suspect that all of these approaches supply a certain degree of support and help that mental patients do not ordinarily receive. But none of these approaches corresponds to the magnitude of disability these patients often experience, nor do they encourage patients to more actively strive to improve their capacities to cope with their environment. Let me make it clear that I would not want to belittle any source of support and sustenance offered to these patients, since the most elementary forms of such help are so frequently absent from their lives; and we know that even contact with unskilled but sympathetic workers can do much to keep the patient functioning in the community. But if we are to meet our responsibility to the mentally ill, we must aspire and achieve much more than this.

As we consider various alternatives for rehabilitation programs, an educational approach often seems better fitted to the needs of community care than do traditional medical approaches.[28] Successful functioning is due in large part to the way people learn to approach problems and to the practice obtained through experience and training. Patients frequently lack information, skills, and abilities that are important in satisfactorily adapting to community life. Although improving the patient's capacity to make a satisfactory adjustment to the community in no way constitutes a "cure," the acquisition of new and relevant skills can inspire hope, confidence, and involvement in other aspects of a treatment program as well. An educational approach to the patient focuses attention and emphasis on the patient's current level of social functioning and less on his past; it encourages more detailed, careful assessment of how the patient behaves in a variety of non-hospital contexts.

Successful social functioning depends on a person's ability to mobilize effort when such effort is necessary, on the manner in which efforts are organized and applied, on psychological and instrumental skills and abilities, and on supports in the social environment. Although social support is well developed within most community care programs, the other facets of social functioning have been relatively neglected.

The mobilization of effort, assuming some level of involvement, may be facilitated by developing personal and social controls which reinforce and encourage good "work habits." Traditionally, in the care of the mentally ill in America, patients defined as sufficiently sick to require institutional care were defined as too deteriorated to perform in work roles. Instead, patients were frequently allowed to sink into apathetic stupor while their work skills atrophied. Although in recent years the attitude toward the work of mental patients has become more reasonable, persons receiving hospital care continue to be regarded as too sick to pursue meaningful task activities; and there is a very limited scope of meaningful activity available to the patient in such treatment contexts. Yet, the ability to continue performing meaningful tasks while under treatment can do much to raise the patient's confidence in himself and to encourage persistence in coping efforts. The assumption that mental illness is totally incapacitating is reinforced by programs that fail to keep active those aspects of social functioning that can be sustained.

The problem of the organization of effort involves the manner in which persons anticipate situations, how they seek information about them, the extent of planning, preparation, and rehearsal in a psychological and social sense, the testing of problem solutions, the consideration and preparation of alternative courses of action should the situation require it, and the allocation of time and effort. When one begins to look at this problem with mental patients, it is astonishing how poorly their efforts are organized. In general psychiatric practice the ineffectual organization of effort often is seen as a by-product of the patient's condition and not a basic component of it. From the viewpoint of intervention, however, attack on some of these problems of organization may produce rather valuable results for the patient's self-confidence and mental state generally.

One of the difficulties that all psychiatric programs face involves the inability to obtain a comprehensive view of how the patient behaves in a variety of meaningful social contexts. Since mental health workers are unable to follow the patient closely within the community, they must depend either on informants or information gleaned from observations of the patient's behavior in the clinical context. But the clinical context is a highly artificial one and may produce problems of coping which may be very much unrelated to those that confront the patient in the community. To the extent that clinical contexts can be constructed so that they are more characteristic of "life," the more realistic are the potentialities for assessing the patient accurately and providing a program fitted to his needs. To return to the work example, it would be valuable if mental health centers could construct work contexts which approximate community work contexts more realistically.[29] This has been achieved to some extent in various European countries which allow for the provision of more realistic contexts for evaluation and instruction and where hospitals have been able to contract meaningful work of substantial variety.[30]

In one sense the ideal clinic might be viewed as a school where the educational program, like a good tutorial, takes into account the social, educational, and psychological needs of the student. From at least one perspective mental patients suffer from inadequate and misguided socialization experiences in that they have failed to acquire the psychological and coping skills necessary for reasonable social adjustment. Such failures may be the product of inherited capacities, brain damage, impoverished childhood circumstances, inadequate training for dealing with stress, or a variety of other reasons. The source of the difficulty, however, is not as important as whether it is remediable with an appropriate program.

One can visualize various advantages in using an educational model in contrast to a medical one. Successful social functioning requires some ability to act as one's own agent, and one of the disadvantages of the medical model is the tremendous dependence the patient develops on physicians, nurses, social workers, and other mental health workers. An educational model is more likely to encourage higher expectations concerning personal responsibility and initiative; and its goals become specific in contrast to the diffuseness of general psychiatric approaches. Moreover, the educational model is a familiar model in our society. One of the persistent problems faced in the expansion of mental health care to new populations is how to reach working-class people. Although esteem for education may not be equally shared by all social strata, this model is one which persons from all social segments know and have experienced; and increasingly working-class people who aspire to a better life for themselves and their children have defined education as an essential means. There is some reason to believe that such a model is more appealing to working-class patients who feel more comfortable with this approach than with modern psychodynamics. Moreover, patients share in the educational process to a greater extent than in traditional medical approaches, and they are more likely to accept the goals toward which they are moving. Although patients also share in psychodynamic therapies, the goals tend to be more diffuse and appear less relevant to the specific problems patients face. The active role of the client toward well-defined and understandable goals within the educational model has great potential for stimulating a sense of control over one's life, self-confidence, competence, and encouraging activity toward self-improvement.

The educational model in contrast to a medical model may be particularly useful in that it makes the difficulty of patients appear more reasonable to the uninformed and minimizes the stigma attached to the patient's difficulty. Despite a vast educational campaign the concept of mental illness still carries the connotation of insanity, and a large proportion of patients receiving treatment in mental hospitals still deny that they suffer from "mental illness." In placing such emphasis on the normal potentialities of the mental patient, the educational approach may serve to decrease social distance between treatment personnel and patients, and between mental health contexts and community. There are various suggestions that others find mental patients more acceptable when their problems are described in interpersonal terms (as problems of living and interpersonal relations) in contrast to "illnesses of the mind." In the long run, of course, little is achieved by changing the labels we use in contrast to changing our practices. Obviously, the proper organization of an educationally oriented rehabilitation program would depend on the attitudes and approaches of mental health workers. To the extent that they nurture patients' dependency responses, encourage sick role reactions, and serve patients rather than motivate them to serve themselves, educational efforts will be limited. An educational approach must start with the assumption that mental patients either have or can develop the capacities to meet their own needs; through sympathetic attention, encouragement of motivation, and the scheduling and reinforcement of mastery experience it may be possible to set the stage more effectively for patients' improvement in social and psychological functioning.

The foregoing considerations of an educational approach in dealing with disabled patients are based on the assumption that much of the psychological discomfort that persons experience results from failure in social functioning. If skills and mastery can be developed so that persons can respond more appropriately to difficult events in their environment, the experience of successful performance and mastery will in itself help resolve much of the personal suffering and distress characteristic of many mental patients. That such general comments as these do not apply to every patient or exclude taking advantage of psychoactive drugs should require no elaboration. One of the greatest defects of current efforts in mental health rehabilitation is the administrative assumption that the same model of care can encompass a broad and diverse spectrum of social and psychological disability. If mental health clinics are to deal seriously with the magnitude of the problems they face, they must develop diversified and flexible services that more realistically approach the varied needs of their clients.

In conclusion, we can do well to note once again the tremendous uncertainty and profound disagreements that characterize thinking in the mental health field. In no real sense do we agree on the nature or character of mental disorder—its nosologies, its etiologies, efficacy of alternative forms of intervention, and other important matters. In seeking pragmatic solutions to help the unfortunate and alleviate suffering, none of us is in a position to preach dogma.

Notes

1. Felix, R. H. (1967). *Mental Illness—Progress and Prospects*. New York: Columbia University Press.

2. Wing, J. (1967). "The Modern Management of Schizophrenia." In H. Freeman and

J. Farndale (eds.), *New Aspects of the Mental Health Service*. New York: Pergamon Press.

3. Group for the Advancement of Psychiatry (1960). *Preventive Psychiatry in the Armed Forces: With Some Implications for Civilian Use*. Report No. 47. Topeka, Kansas.

4. Reid, D. (1959). "Precipitating Proximal Factors in the Occurrence of Mental Disorders: Epidemiological Evidence." In *Causes of Mental Disorders: A Review of Epidemiological Knowledge*. New York: Milbank Memorial Fund.

5. Goldhamer, H., and A. W. Marshall (1953). *Psychosis and Civilization: Two Studies in the Frequency of Mental Disease*. New York: Free Press.

6. Roberts, L. M., S. L. Halleck, and M. B. Loeb (eds.) (1966). *Community Psychiatry*. Madison, Wis.: University of Wisconsin Press.

7. Joint Commission on Mental Illness and Health (1961). *Action for Mental Health*. New York: Science Editions.

8. Mechanic, D. (1966). "Response Factors in Illness: The Study of Illness Behavior." *Social Psychiatry*, 1:11–20.

9. Angrist, S., M. Lefton, S. Dinitz, and B. Pasamanick (1963). "Tolerance of Deviant Behavior, Posthospital Performance Levels, and Rehospitalization." *Proceedings of the Third World Congress on Psychiatry*, 237–241.

10. Dinitz, S., S. Angrist, M. Lefton, and B. Pasamanick (1961). "The Posthospital Psychological Functioning of Former Mental Hospital Patients." *Mental Hygiene*, 45:579–588.

11. Freeman, H., and O. Simmons (1963). *The Mental Patient Comes Home*. New York: Wiley.

12. Shepherd, M., A. N. Oppenheim, and S. Mitchell (1966). "Childhood Behavior Disorders and the Child-Guidance Clinic: An Epidemiological Study." *Journal of Child Psychology and Psychiatry*, 7:39–52.

13. Glass, A. J. (1958). "Observations Upon the Epidemiology of Mental Illness in Troops During Warfare." *Symposium on Preventive and Social Psychiatry*. Washington: U. S. Government Printing Office.

14. Brown, G. W., and J. L. P. Birley (1968). "Social Changes and the Onset of Schizophrenia." *Journal of Health and Social Behavior*, 9:203–214.

15. Mechanic, D. (1962). *Students Under Stress: A Study in the Social Psychology of Adaptation*. New York: Free Press.

16. Cloward, R. A., and L. E. Ohlin (1960). *Delinquency and Opportunity*. New York: Free Press.

17. Becker, H. S. (1963). *Outsiders: Studies in the Sociology of Deviance*. New York: Free Press.

18. Becker, H. S. (1967). "History, Culture and Subjective Experience: An Exploration of the Social Bases of Drug-Induced Experiences." *Journal of Health and Social Behavior*, 8:163–176.

19. Wilkins, J. (1967). "The Locus of Anomie in Suicide." Paper presented at the 62nd Annual Meeting of the American Sociological Association.

20. Scheff, T. (1966). *Being Mentally Ill: A Sociological Theory*. Chicago: Aldine.

21. Schachter, S., and J. Singer (1962). "Cognitive Social and Physiological Determinants of Emotional State." *Psychological Review*, 69:379–399.

22. Schachter, S. (1967). "Cognitive Effects on Bodily Functioning: Studies of Obesity and Overeating." In D. C. Glass and C. Pfaffman (eds.), *Biology and Behavior: Neurophysiology and Emotion*. New York: Rockefeller University Press and Russell Sage Foundation.

23. Pasamanick, B., F. R. Scarpitti, and S. Dinitz (1967). *Schizophrenics in the Community*. New York: Appleton, Century, Crofts.

24. Brown, G. W., M. Bone, B. Dalison, and J. K. Wing (1966). *Schizophrenia and Social Care*. London: Oxford University Press.

25. Grad, J., and P. Sainsbury (1966). "Evaluating the Community Psychiatric Service in Chicester: Results." *Milbank Memorial Fund Quarterly*, **44**:246–277.

26. Grad, J. (1968). "A Two-Year Follow-Up." In R. H. Williams and L. D. Ozarin (eds.), *Community Mental Health: An International Perspective*. San Francisco: Jossey-Bass.

27. Lazarus, R. S. (1966). *Psychological Stress and The Coping Process*. New York: McGraw-Hill.

28. Mechanic, D. (1967). "Therapeutic Intervention: Issues in the Care of the Mentally Ill." *American Journal of Orthopsychiatry*, **37**:703–718.

29. Neuhaus, E. *Rehabilitating the Emotionally Disturbed*. Long Island, N.Y.: The Rehabilitation Institute.

30. Furman, S. (1965). *Community Mental Health Services in Northern Europe*. PHS Publication No. 1407. Washington: U. S. Government Printing Office.

CHAPTER XIV

Social and Psychological Factors Affecting Disease Processes*

It is widely believed that social and psychological factors affect the occurrence and outcome of disease processes. This generalization in itself has limited significance for it provides no clear guidance to the clinician as to how he might manage his patient to achieve a higher probability of success in treatment or rehabilitation. For such knowledge to be useful, it is necessary to indicate what *specific* social and psychological factors influence what *specific* disease processes under what *specific* circumstances. To aim for less than this is to engage in exercises that neither affect our understanding of disease processes or the successful management of patients.

The concept of multiple etiology is one which has a long history. More often than not it has shielded ignorance and lack of understanding of the processes leading to disease states. It has served as the ultimate rationalization for the ignorance of the doctor and the public educator, for in maintaining that everything is important in disease processes he escapes the necessary task of specifying what is crucial and what is ancillary. Behavioral knowledge is useful to the physician because it presumably increases the information available to him in making particular decisions, and we operate under the assumption that such added knowledge increases the probability of a correct determination and decreases the probability of error. If, indeed, behavioral factors are important in disease processes, understanding of how such variables operate may improve the doctor's predictive capacities.

From a clinical point of view, it is also necessary to separate behavioral and other knowledge which informs the doctor's perspective and that

---

* Adapted from a paper presented at the Symposium on Behavioral Aspects of Disease Etiology, University of Kentucky Medical Center, April, 1969.

which increases his scope of action. If we find, for example, that particular persons are more prone to disease than others, we may or may not have the capacities or techniques to successfully modify traits associated with disease. The knowledge of the relationship between smoking and lung cancer and the assumed relationship between exercise and coronary heart disease does not necessarily lead the doctor to effective action, since the ability to modify habit patterns developed over a long period of time is highly limited. He may, however, have more success in other realms where the habit pattern leading to or exacerbating disease is less central to the patient's behavioral pattern and therefore more amenable to modification.

Disease, of course, is always the outcome of a complex interaction between conditions of the host and conditions of the environment to which he is exposed. It is frequently pragmatic, however, for the researcher and clinician to assume a more simple relationship between agents in the environment and disease processes, since these agents are frequently effective causes and are amenable to control. Persons exposed to the same external agent such as a bacillus or pollen may react differently, and this raises intellectual if not clinical issues; but often the soundest approach is to combat the agent itself. The most common diseases, however, which now pose problems for public health are those in which it is more difficult to isolate effective causes that can be manipulated through medical measures. While investigators continue to seek specific factors contributing to coronary heart disease, cancer, arthritis, schizophrenia, and chronic diseases in general, it appears that these diseases will not conform as simply as many infectious diseases to approaches based on specific etiology. Moreover, many of the major problems affecting chronic disease and producing morbidity and mortality among young people are clearly problems that have a very large behavioral or environmental component —accidents (particularly motor vehicle accidents), suicide, alcoholism and related drug problems, mental illness and psychological disorders, venereal disease, obesity, and the like.

To illustrate some of the complex considerations that pertain to these fields, let us consider motor vehicle accidents. Motor vehicle accidents result in more than 50,000 deaths a year and several hundred thousands of injuries. Such accidents are the main contributor to physical trauma, constitute the major cause of death among young people, and result in vast consumption of our total medical resources. Motor vehicle accidents can be approached from at least three perspectives: (1) the structure of the environment and conditions affecting it; (2) aspects of the vehicle; and (3) aspects of the host. From an environmental point of view, the occurrence of motor vehicle accidents depends very substantially on the nature of road systems and the manner in which they are organized, the control of traffic, the visibility and rationality of communications to drivers, lighting, and the like. The occurrence of accidents and consequences resulting from them may depend on such considerations as the layout of highways, whether they are divided or not, the magnitude and pace of traffic, road markings, the quality of basic materials used on the center and side railings, and so on. External social and environmental conditions also may be important such as the quality of policing, road maintenance, and weather conditions.

The second element—the vehicle itself—has received considerable discussion in recent years,[1-3] and I do not want to belabor the issues. Here there are two basic categories: (1) the qualities of the vehicle which allow it to cope with emergency conditions such as its ability to maneuver, braking capacity, ability to take a skid, and tendency to overturn. More in the background are such questions as quality control of the basic design, the willingness of companies to build in safety features, and cultural and commercial attitudes toward safety. (2) A second aspect of the vehicle from a health point of view is the ability of the vehicle to contain passengers without injury in the event of an accident. We have made substantial progress in this area in recent years with breakaway engines, seat belts, safety glass, the elimination of knobs and handles that can injure, and the like. Much more can be accomplished along these lines.

Then, of course, there is the host himself. Although we think a great deal about such matters as reaction time, safe as compared with unsafe drivers fall within quite a range in the rapidity of their reaction times. Much more basic to safety are the attitudes and habits of the driver. Here we know that males have a higher rate of accidents than females. This conceivably is spurious in that males are more likely to drive their vehicles and drive many more miles than females of comparable age. But there is some reason to believe that bold attitudes toward driving— and aggressive driving in particular—are more prevalent among males. One of the most important factors in the occurrence of accidents, particularly single-vehicle accidents, is alcohol,[4] and the higher prevalence of drinking among males as compared with females also contributes to the male excess in motor vehicle accidents. There is increasing study of the relationship between psychological attitudes and aggressive driving, and some suggestion that anger and emotional distress lead to more erratic and dangerous driving.[5] Although systematic studies of attitudes as they relate to accidents have not been frequent, there are suggestions that the automobile is an instrument serving psychological as well as travel needs, and may even become expressive of manliness, daring, and other forms of cultural expression valued by some members of the population.

If we take a broader view of motor vehicle accidents, it becomes clear how closely they are tied to our economic and social values. Indeed, we can probably significantly control accidents by refusing to license particularly high-risk groups of the population, such as young men under age 20 or 25. This would clearly clash with the interests of auto manufacturers, our way of life, and the aspirations in our society of all young people to have and drive cars; and such measures would not be feasible politically. Or as an alternative, we might take a punitive view toward persons who violate norms of road safety—intoxicated drivers, speeders, and those who drive defective vehicles—but we will not because such action violates strong cultural viewpoints and interests. Clearly, there are many approaches to motor vehicle accidents. Some of the most effective approaches are not used because they clash with cultural values, economic interests, and attitudes of the public.

Our automobile culture as a "way of life" has health effects well beyond the immediate cost of accidents. Automobiles are a major contributor to pollution of the environment with its associated effects on health and life. An automobile-oriented society, such as our own, has many indirect effects on the health and life of people, since it affects the planning of cities, the movement of people, the relocation of homes, and habit patterns generally. The construction of highways is a major cause of the involuntary relocation of persons from their homes, and indeed the public commitment to such construction has vast effects on the nature of other public commitments which would and could enhance the life and health of people. If one considers, for example, such a car-infested city as Los Angeles, we see that the city itself is organized around its freeway systems, and that the failure to develop an adequate mode of public transportation is largely the product of the individual's commitment to his automobile. Health consequences flow from such decisions. For example, one of the major grievances of those without cars in the Watts area of Los Angeles was the lack of access to transportation to medical and hospital facilities, and this was one factor resulting in failure to receive adequate medical assistance. Or, to consider another example, it seems clear that habit patterns built around the use of and dependence on cars have affected the amount of usual daily exercise characteristic of many persons in the population and indirectly may contribute to heart disease, diabetes, obesity, and so on.

In choosing accidents for the purpose of illustrating some of my points, I want to emphasize that the factors I am describing are not atypical relative to other health problems we face; but in the more typical case seen by the internist, the behavioral factors may not be so obvious and, therefore, may not appear to be so relevant. Although most doctors recognize that a large proportion of patients seeking their advice and help have psychosocial problems and that this may affect visiting patterns, it is often assumed that those who are really "sick" do not. This assumption permeates all of medical practice and has very substantial effects on the quality of patient care. Querido and his colleagues in Holland,[6] for example, studied 1630 patients suffering from a variety of medical conditions in a general hospital in Amsterdam. They found a significant difference in the chance of recovery between patients who had to cope with problems apart from their physical illness and those who did not. The investigators found that 69 per cent of their 1630 patients had a favorable clinical prognosis on the basis of medical factors alone. But only three-fifths of these patients actually did well. The investigators found that patients who did poorly could be characterized as suffering from psychological distress. Duff and Hollingshead,[7] in an intensive study of the care received by 161 patients in a teaching hospital associated with one of the most eminent medical schools in the United States, found considerable failure on the part of doctors to appreciate psychological factors in illness, and that these failures had adverse effects on the quality of medical care. These investigators estimate, on the basis of their study, that less than one half of the diagnoses on the medical service studied were accurate, and a large proportion of the medical errors made were due to the failure to understand the psychological and social condition of patients. They also estimated that doctors appreciated the mental status of the patients they dealt with in only one-tenth of the cases. Although these estimates are somewhat arbitrary and can be disputed, the study illustrates how the mental state of patients affected the course of their illnesses and the degree of disability following hospitalization.

The tendency for subjective factors to be evident at the same time that physical factors are apparent is characteristic of all illness, and this has considerable significance in understanding the sick. Whether, indeed, the "psychological" and the "physical" are just two different languages to describe the same events, as Graham[8] has argued, or whether they interact in some complex but poorly understood way need not deter us here. It is plain, however, that subjective factors are part of illness and its outcome. Whether in considering a reaction like pain on the one hand, or a more elaborate syndrome like disability on the other, one finds time and time again that the phenomenon of illness itself varies when different subjective states are present. As Beecher[9] and many other investigators of pain have demonstrated,[10] there is no dependable relationship between the number of pain endings stimulated or the extent of their stimulation, and the resultant experience of pain. Moreover, the degree of pain experienced is related to changing definitions of the meaning and consequences of pain. Similarly, in illness, it is apparent that the manner in which symptoms are defined and meanings attributed to them have a pervasive effect in many instances on the condition of the patient and the physical, psychological, and social dysfunction evident.

The manner in which subjective and physical factors may become related is indicated by the work of Imboden and his colleagues[11] in their study of various infectious diseases. In brief, they found that patients with psychological vulnerabilities may organize their difficulties in relation to a physical illness such as influenza, and that their disabilities may become chronic although there is no further evidence of the infectious condition. These patients tend to identify the physical illness as the cause of their distress and to view the problem as one requiring physical in contrast to psychological treatment. A tendency on the part of the physician to neglect the complexity of such chronic disorders and to treat only the symptomatic aspects may contribute to reinforcing the patient's definition of his illness.

The role the doctor plays in the organization of the patient's illness has been sensitively described by Michael Balint,[12] and it is clear that subtle negotiation takes place in the relationship between doctor and patient as to what the distress is and to what it may be attributed. It is not infrequent in many of the complex syndromes that doctors deal with for the patient to realize that subjective factors are an important part of his difficulty, and he himself may only half-believe the somatic framework he gives to his symptoms when he presents them to a physician. However, when the physician accepts without question the physical framework, and neglects emotional aspects of the illness, what was presented tentatively and with doubt becomes reinforced and organized and may readily lead to greater distress and further neglect of the patient's true life situation.

The Role of Cultural and Social Values in Disease

Men seek health so that they can avoid personal distress, perform their life tasks, and pursue their goals. But men's goals and aspirations and the consequences of achieving them create new problems of illness and new threats to life. As Rene Dubos[13] has noted:

[Man's] self-imposed striving for ever-new distant goals makes his fate even more unpredictable than those of other living things. For this reason health and happiness cannot be absolute and permanent values, however careful the social and medical planning. Biological success in all its manifestations is a measure of fitness, and fitness requires never-ending efforts of adaptation to the total environment, which is ever changing.

The problems men have are mainly the product of the aims they promote and the goals they aspire to achieve. Perhaps, in some hypothetical state, men can be satisfied with what they have and lead healthful lives, avoiding risks and life patterns dangerous to their health. But such a life strikes many as being dull and unpleasant, and men seek new challenges and cultivate risk. An important issue for medicine, therefore, concerns the manner in which men face challenging and trying circumstances, the modes by which they attempt to reverse or accommodate to them, and the price they pay for their efforts. For illness is largely a response to ways of life and a product of man's strivings and aspirations. Although there has been a great deal of concern with the concept of "stress" in medicine, there has not been widespread appreciation that stress is not an event but rather a relationship between problems and challenges and men's capacities to deal with or accommodate to them.[14] "Stress" pertains not only to events perceived as threatening or harmful but also to more positively defined events such as promotions, which may strain the homeostatic balance of the body and take their toll on the person's biological system.

In recent years there has been a variety of studies that provide evidence for the contention that the cumulation of life stresses or major changes in one's life often precedes the occurrence or exacerbation of illness states. Many of the earlier studies in this area had major methodological defects that made their meaning ambiguous, but the results have persisted even as study designs have become more adequate. There is evidence, for example, that the impact of such life changes is evident even if one controls carefully for the possibility that the occurrence of illness or its early stages contributed to the occurrence of the life problems themselves.[15] Overall, the meaning of these studies and the dynamics they imply are not very clear. However, we must not fail to note that the life aspirations of people, the nature of the struggles they take on or those which befall them, and the character of their life situations have an important impact on when they become ill, the rapidity of their recoveries, the reoccurrence of their symptoms, and the kinds of adjustment they make to their illnesses. To neglect such factors in the treatment of people is to neglect the art and essence of medicine.

The importance of stress in illness is an issue still characterized by considerable uncertainty and disagreement.[16] Research efforts in the field of psychosomatic medicine vary widely in their designs and general adequacy, and in the case of most diseases there are conflicting and contradictory findings concerning the role of stress as an etiological agent. Work in the psychosomatic area is based on the awareness that all psychological and social experience is associated with changing states of man's physiology and biology. Although no one would doubt such relations, it is a more difficult matter to demonstrate that feeling states and social events produce specific bodily dysfunctions or increase susceptibility to a variety of diseases.

As a sociologist, I do not feel that it is my role here to describe the issues or perspectives that concern investigators in the psychosomatic field. Nor do I feel that it is my role, particularly, to review the evidence supporting the claim that social and psychological factors are important in particular diseases. I will stand by my original contention that it is essential that such knowledge be specific and imply particular actions in the care of particular patients as well as add to the general perspective of the doctor. Before I complete my discussion, therefore, I shall try to provide some illustrations of the kinds of studies I feel contribute to this goal. But as a social scientist, I feel it is necessary to put the issues of psychosomatic medicine in a larger perspective on the assumption that when persons' capacities or life resources become discrepant with the demands they must face in their daily lives, or with their aspirations and needs, illness and social disruption become more likely.

The Social Context of Stress

The extent to which individuals experience distress and feelings of danger and inadequacy is dependent on the nature of their social networks, the kinds of demands to which they are exposed, the goals to which they aspire, and the types of preparation and experience they have to deal with these conditions and changing circumstances. Merton,[17] for example, has argued that social structures exert definite pressures upon particular people or subgroups which influence them in the direction of particular deviant adaptations. He believes that when an incongruency develops between cultural norms and goals and people's capacities to behave in accordance with them a state of anomie exists. Individuals who learn cultural goals and values, but who fail to acquire the means to fulfill these either because of their location in society or for some other reason, adapt to these anomic conditions in a variety of ways, some of which are more socially destructive than others.

In viewing "distress" from a social point of view, it becomes essential not only to consider personal strivings, strengths, and inadequacies but also the manner in which these are shaped by the social structure of a community or its social networks. Psychological distress need not be socially caused; indeed, much distress originates from biological defects. But social contexts give significance to the character of symptoms, and the definitions, reactions, and meanings assigned by associates do much to either retard or exacerbate their significance. In examining an individual in light of any particular set of life tasks, there are at least three central considerations that must be applied in evaluating the likelihood that he can successfully execute them; I shall label them instrumentality, motivation, and socioemotional state. Instrumentality refers to the individual's skills and capacities relative to the task; the enactment of these skills is more commonly known as coping. The person's socioemotional state, including his feelings of self-confidence and self-esteem, I call defense. In evaluating a person's response to any task, we must consider his willingness to assume it, his capacities to do so, and the feelings the task arouses and his abilities to deal with these feelings. Each of the dimensions described has community counterparts, which I refer to as preparatory institutions, incentive systems, and evaluative systems. By preparatory institutions, I mean any community attempt to develop skills and competence among people to prepare them to deal with social demands and challenges. Included here are not only schools and formal learning experiences but also the many varieties of informal learning that are acquired through parents and peers, and through normal social interaction. By incentive systems, I refer to community values and the developed systems of rewards and punishments which families, organizations, and communities promote in order to push activities in particular directions. These incentive systems can be powerful, indeed, and can encourage persons to aspire beyond their capacities or to limit their aspirations and goals. By evaluative systems, I refer to the approval and encouragement or disapproval and disparagement resulting from pursuing particular activities.

There is an obvious link between the three personal dimensions I have described—coping, defense, and motivation—and the three community dimensions—preparatory institutions, evaluative systems, and incentive systems. Levels of skill and competence are very much dependent on the nature and organization of preparatory systems; social support and favorable evaluation ordinarily facilitate defensive processes, while opposition and disapproval frequently increase the magnitude of personal distress; and motivation is correlated in various ways with incentive systems. Although I would not like to push the analogy too far, the model can be applied to physical as well as behavioral events. For example, coronaries frequently occur among men who undertake activities, such as shoveling snow, which far exceed their accustomed level of exercise. The sedentary life of such men often fails to allow them to develop the physical capacities to undertake such jobs without risk of personal injury. In one sense, their bodies are unprepared for the tasks they assume because of the lack of continuity in exercise or practice. Such men frequently lack the motiva-

THE SOCIAL CONTEXT OF STRESS   255

tion to maintain a state of physical fitness not only because their jobs and way of life involve little exercise, but also because there is little incentive for exercise within the social milieu in which they function. Finally, there is little difficulty in such persons justifying their sedentary activities (defense) as there are few negative sanctions for failing to maintain physical fitness, and much of the culture and technology apparent in our society supports and encourages further inactivity through a variety of labor-saving devices such as motorized mowers, snow removers, and the like. Even on one's afternoon of exercise, one is not "quite in" unless he has a motorized golf cart. And with the advent of electric toothbrushes and electric knives, even these common sources of exercise are becoming difficult to maintain. And as our cities adapt to the automobile, it is increasingly more difficult to bicycle or walk without risking injury, if not from the automobiles, from the wastes they emit as they speed by.

Clinicians must recognize that psychological discomfort is often a product of insecurity or failure in coping with life tasks. The more developed a person's coping skills, the less likely it is that when faced with a challenge he will suffer lack of confidence and discomfort. In short, the adequacy of preparation is a major determinant of the experience of stress. Persons in different groups experience different events as challenging because they have had the benefit of different preparatory and incentive systems and they, therefore, have differing skills and aspirations. Illustrations of each of these points are in order.

In studies of combat situations it has become clear that combat preparation and experience play an important part in combat effectiveness. It is fairly obvious, for example, that the success of astronauts in space experiments is dependent on a long and technically complicated training experience during which plans are made for varying possibilities and contingencies, and the astronauts themselves are prepared to deal with these problems well before they are encountered.[18] General combat training is less complicated and complete, and thus the soldiers' training and experience must take place, in part, under actual combat conditions. Studies have shown that when new recruits enter combat, there is an initial period in which coping skills must be acquired if the soldier is to function effectively. He must learn to distinguish between friendly and enemy battle noises; he must learn to judge the caliber and closeness of artillery projectiles; he must be able to spot snipers, to conceal himself effectively, and so on.[19] These are not matters of psychological defense; they involve the learning of specific skills. The absence of such skills is related to unnecessary fear and anxiety. For example, when soldiers first enter combat they are frequently scared by noises of enemy firing, although the firing is too far away to constitute any threat to them. As they learn to distinguish the meaning of battle noises, their "stress" responses become more specific to enemy fire which actually threatens them.

In a study of stress response among graduate students involved in Ph.D. preliminary examinations, I analyzed the ways in which students met this challenge and the factors associated with different responses to the same threat.[14] First, it became clear that how students viewed these important examinations was related to their personal aspirations and the stake they had in their education. Older students and those more committed to a professional career were under much greater stress than others. This study, as well as others, shows that when people feel unprepared to meet a situation they experience strong feelings of discomfort and disruption in mood. Such feelings of inadequacy may result from lack of appropriate knowledge and skills, the uncertainty and ambiguity involved in the situation, or from particular traits of the person such as low self-confidence. Students who had strong skills and preparation were more likely to feel confident than those who did not. Incidents that students were involved in made salient that other students knew materials that they were unaware of and these incidents often stimulated intense anxiety.

The realities of life are, of course, often complicated. We know that people with similar skills and preparation actually may perform very differently. It is well known that assessments made during training do not necessarily predict successful performance in the real situation. It appears that in situations where motivation is high, the task difficult, and ultimate performance clouded by uncertainties, a high level of discomfort may be aroused despite the person's competence. Thus, the person's socioemotional defenses become important in dealing with the situation. A high level of discomfort interferes with the application of skills requiring effort and ability. To the extent that a person can control his emotional state, the coping process is facilitated. Thus how well he performs will depend on the techniques and intrapsychic mechanisms by which he contains his emotional state. Whether his defense restricts, distorts, or falsifies reality has no important meaning in and of itself. The relative usefulness and adequacy of defense processes depend on the way defense affects coping. The primary function of psychological defense is to facilitate the coping process. There are boundaries within which psychological defense must function if it is to be effective. Defense processes cannot be so out of line with social definitions of appropriateness that they lead to negative social evaluation and withdrawal of social support. From the perspective of long-range adaptation, defense processes cannot be so restrictive that they lead the person to avoid taking advantage of preparatory opportunities. Defense is never an end in itself; defense processes divorced from coping or those that hinder the coping process are usually viewed as evidence of emotional disturbance.

I can illustrate this point with the study of Ph.D. students taking examinations referred to earlier. Some students who found the examinations anxiety-provoking attempted to deal with their discomfort by avoiding other students and department affairs generally. Although such avoidance relieved their anxiety, it also prevented access to information important to their preparation and, thus, they were handicapped in various ways. The most effective way of dealing with such anxiety appeared to involve selective exposure to the department and other students with temporary avoidance during periods of intense anxiety and discomfort.

The adequacy of individual adaptation is closely linked to societal characteristics. Preparatory systems in a particular community may be more or less congruent with characteristic problems that people in this society are likely to face, and they impart more or less competence to deal with these difficulties. In formal educational areas this relationship is obvious; educational institutions are always revising their curriculum toward greater compatibility with the state of knowledge in particular areas. This does not necessarily insure that formal education will be geared to societal needs and challenges, but at least this matter is open to a reasonable assessment. But the adequacy of preparatory institutions in less formal areas is much more difficult to assess and the discrepancies more difficult to correct. Are our preparatory institutions sufficient for allowing people to adjust satisfactorily to a rapidly changing, mobile, and heterogeneous community? Are people being adequately prepared to cope with a greater amount of leisure time? Are workers prepared adequately for early retirement without ultimate feelings of uselessness and despair? Obviously, improving preparatory institutions in these areas is much more difficult than bringing formal training in mathematics or social studies up to date.

Because typical difficulties and challenges in social life differ from one culture to another, and change over time, the accommodation of preparatory institutions to these changes must be an ongoing process. Similarly, societal incentive and evaluative systems structure and channel motivation and adaptive processes. They affect not only what the person wants to do but, perhaps even more important, the means he can use in dealing with particular challenges. In any social system it is likely that incentive and preparatory systems are highly related. Skills are provided for doing things that are valued; but frequently the areas that receive emphasis are not necessarily those that pose the greatest challenges to human adaptive capacities and health maintenance.

Communities may fail to provide adequate preparatory resources for many reasons. Frequently the cost seems too high. Also, since typical challenges and difficulties change over time, the preparatory systems have to be relatively flexible and adaptive. But frequently preparatory systems become heavily bureaucratized, and as a consequence they may develop strong resistance to change in that particular bureaucratic goals and special interests are valued more highly than societal instrumental goals.

Societal incentive and evaluative systems also affect preparatory institutions in that they help define the areas of proper concern for training programs. The technology for controlling family size is clearly available; whether a community trains persons to use the technology effectively and provides access to the technology (as in the case of contraceptive devices) depends on social values and the distribution of particular organized groups in the community. It is an unfortunate fact of life that frequently the technology necessary to solve social problems violates the interests or values of particular social groups in the community. When poverty programs stimulate persons in deprived areas to assert their rights and to protest, invariably this has consequences for social groups who have something to gain from the status quo. In short, evaluative institutions influence in important ways what kinds of preparatory attempts are politically feasible.

Effective coping depends on several types of preparation, and much that we have to know to get along in life is not taught in any direct or formal way. A person has to acquire not only task skills but must as well learn general approaches to problems that occur with some frequency.[20] These inevitably involve such skills as anticipation, information seeking, anticipatory problem solving, rehearsal, task organization, and so on. They include ability to pace activities, preparation of alternative strategies, sensitivity to task and interpersonal cues, and ability to anticipate reactions in the environment.

It is important to consider the difference between skills learned through formal teaching of a direct kind and those which are derived in an incidental fashion through experience. Even within the most concentrated and explicit educational programs significant failures in imparting skills occur. In contrast, in those situations where learning is covert and perhaps unintentional it is likely that the number of failures and errors is very large, and skills may be imparted very unevenly. For example, interpersonal skills are for the most part indirectly learned. More frequently than not the skill is subtle and not recognized at the verbal level as a skill. Yet such interpersonal skills in a complex bureaucratic society are central to effectiveness on both an occupational and a personal level. Interestingly, an adequate vocabulary to describe such skills has not been developed although such descriptions can be gleaned from various social psychological studies.[21,22] The language used to describe behavior is for the most part a language of emotions and personality traits, and it is difficult to find designations that are descriptive of the way people "handle," "manipulate," or "deal with" other people.

The Problem of Motivation

It is not realistic to attempt to specify why some people are motivated to deal with challenges while others are not. Except for involuntary situations where persons are given little alternative, the mobilization of effort depends on the personal history of the actor, his aspirations, and the way he comes to view a challenge. Motivation, of course, is also influenced by the societal incentive and evaluative systems. But even within the context of high motivation some persons find themselves able to apply effort to a task, while others of similar aspirations seem unable to persevere. It begs the question to argue that differences in behavior in such situations are a consequence of differences in "motivation." Even where life and death are concerned, there are vast differences in people's staying power and persistence in meeting adversities. There are two basic alternatives in studying such differences. First, we can make some attempt to understand the personalities of the actors involved, and through analyses of their developmental histories attempt to account for their successes and failures. This mode of investigation thus far has been less than fully productive. To explain failures in coping by attributing traits to the personality—inadequacy, rigidity, authoritarianism, lack of achievement motivation and so on—tells us little about why such people fail to function successfully. The other alternative, which has not really been exploited, is to study the way people organize and prepare to deal with difficult tasks and how they go about doing this. We really know very little about the ways successful people construct problem solutions and approach difficult situations. There is great variability among people in the extent to which they experience life as a combination of inevitable and accidental events, and the extent to which they actively seek out alternatives, make choices, and facilitate their own welfare by anticipatory planning. We know that many people regard themselves as relatively powerless to influence and control events, while others have a strong sense of their own potency in affecting their fate and are active in controlling their alternatives and outcomes. We need a much better understanding of these life stances in relation to particular challenges.

At one time or another we have all probably met individuals who appear to be highly motivated but who are unable to expend effort on any long-range task, because when they get down to the task the achievement appears insignificant and the effort too great for the anticipated results. These people tend to be characterized by high motivation which becomes dissipated on the confrontation of tasks. Although such persons probably have different "personality structures" than those who apply themselves more easily, it might be fruitful to approach such performance differences not in terms of the personal histories of such individuals but rather in terms of how they differentially approach trying tasks. For if we study the way different people approach trying tasks, it becomes possible to locate the coping devices that facilitate persistence and tenaciousness as well as to examine the personality and social characteristics that may influence these.

In some of our own exploratory research on populations that could be characterized as "poor copers," we have been impressed by how frequently these respondents accept their inability to have any control over their situations. They appear to recognize few alternatives and to have few plans or strategies for taking on some of the problems which characterized their lives. This acceptance of "fate" may be regarded as one form of adaptive behavior, since such respondents who gave us the impression of "having given up," were less tense and anxious than those who were struggling actively against extremely difficult problems. It would be important to know to what extent "giving up" is a product of seeing no alternatives for approaching life problems and to what extent it is attributable to other factors.

The physician never treats his patient in a vacuum. He must always be cognizant of the real demands the patient must face not only because of his aspirations and goals but also because those in the community with which he may live most intimately have expectations that are trying to his capacities and inclinations. These expectations, of course, are not unchangeable, but they do not change easily. Medical care if it is to be effective must be restricted to some extent. It may be unreasonable to expect the physician to define as a major goal the enhancement of the patient's instrumental skills but neither can he function effectively if he neglects such concerns. Obviously, the doctor must, to some extent, have an educational role. Patients with irreversible disease and disability require some training to live with their conditions, and often the doctor is the appropriate teacher as in the case of handling the diabetic or coronary patient. Similarly, given all of the sources of men's goals, it is unreasonable to expect health institutions to have any large impact on community incentive systems and the risks men choose to take or avoid. It is primarily in the area of offering socioemotional understanding, support, and simple instruction that many doctors have failed in tasks inherent in the practice of medicine.

The suggestive powers of the physician are very substantial, and doctors and other health workers are in a position to very much reduce the distress their patients feel by small gestures and behaviors that show an awareness and concern for the patient. Egbert and his colleagues,[23] for example, selected a random group of patients undergoing surgery and gave them simple information, encouragement, and instruction concerning their impending surgery and means of alleviating postoperative pain. The researchers, however, were not involved in the medical care of the patients studied, and they did not participate in decisions concerning them. An independent evaluation of the postoperative period and the length of stay of patients in the experimental and control groups showed that this communication and instruction made a real difference. This is consistent with the research of Janis[24] which demonstrated that preoperative fear was correlated with postoperative reactions among surgical patients.

In a similar experimental study by Skipper and Leonard,[25] children admitted to a hospital for tonsillectomy were randomized into experimental and control groups. These groups differed in that in the experimental group patients and their mothers were admitted to the hospital by a specially trained nurse who "attempted to create an atmosphere which would facilitate the communication of information to the mother, maximize freedom to verbalize her fear, anxiety and special problems, and to ask any and all questions which were on her mind. The information given to the mother tried to paint an accurate picture of the reality of the situation. Mothers were told what routine events to expect and when they were likely to occur—including the actual time schedule for the operation." The investigators found that the emotional support reduced the mothers' stress and changed their definition of the hospital situation which, in turn, had a beneficial effect on their children. Children in the experimental group experienced smaller changes in blood pressure, temperature, and other physiological measures; they were less likely to suffer from postoperative emesis and made a better adaptation to the hospital; and they made a more rapid recovery following hospitalization, displaying less fears, less crying, and less disturbed sleep than children in the control group.

In short, a little support and instruction can have large benefits. More frequently than not, those who endorse the idea that the doctor should provide sympathy and support to the patient do so on the belief that this is a noble and human thing to do. It is less appreciated, however, that establishing such relationships with patients facilitates the informational

process between doctor and patient, and contributes in an important way
to the management of the patient and his progress toward recovery. Social
and behavioral knowledge are not "good" in themselves; such knowledge
is important because the successful diagnosis and treatment of patients
require some adequate assessment of the factors contributing to the
patient's illness and those that will contribute toward his recovery. To
neglect, therefore, important facts that have a bearing on these processes,
because they are social or psychological in contrast to biological, increases
errors in prediction on the part of the physician and lack of efficacy in the
management of his patients.

Notes

1. Nader, R. (1965). *Unsafe at Any Speed: The Designed-in Dangers of the American Automobile.* New York: Grossman.
2. Haddon, W., Jr., et al. (eds.) (1964). *Accident Research: Methods and Approaches.* New York: Harper and Row.
3. Selzer, M., et al. (eds.) (1967). *The Prevention of Highway Injury.* Ann Arbor: Highway Safety Research Institute, University of Michigan.
4. Haddon, W., Jr., and V. Bradess (1964). "Alcohol in the Single Vehicle Fatal Accident, Experience of Westchester County, New York." In W. Haddon, Jr., et al. (eds.), *Accident Research: Methods and Approaches.* New York: Harper and Row.
5. Selzer, M. (1969). "Alcoholism, Mental Illness, and Stress in 96 Drivers Causing Fatal Accidents." *Behavioral Science,* **14:**1–10.
6. Querido, A. (1959). "An Investigation into the Clinical, Social, and Mental Factors Determining the Results of Hospital Treatment." *British Journal of Preventive and Social Medicine,* **13:**33–49.
7. Duff, R. S., and A. Hollingshead (1968). *Sickness and Society.* New York: Harper.
8. Graham, D. (1967). "Health, Disease, and the Mind-Body Problem: Linguistic Parallelism." *Psychosomatic Medicine,* **29:**52–71.
9. Beecher, H. (1959). *Measurement of Subjective Responses.* New York: Oxford University Press.
10. Sternbach, R. (1968). *Pain: A Psychophysiological Analysis.* New York: Academic Press.
11. Imboden, J. B., et al. (1961). "Symptomatic Recovery from Medical Disorders." *Journal of the American Medical Association,* **178:**1182–1184.
12. Balint, M. (1957). *The Doctor, His Patient, and the Illness.* New York: International Universities Press.
13. Dubos, R. (1959). *Mirage of Health.* New York: Harper.
14. Mechanic, D. (1962). *Students Under Stress.* New York: Free Press.
15. Brown, G., and J. L. T. Birley (1968). "Crises and Life Changes and the Onset of Schizophrenia." *Journal of Health and Social Behavior,* **9:**203–214.
16. Mechanic, D. (1968). *Medical Sociology: A Selective View.* New York: Free Press.

17. Merton, R. (1957). *Social Theory and Social Structure*. New York: Free Press.

18. Ruff, G. E., and J. Korchin (1964). "Psychological Responses of the Mercury Astro-nauts to Stress." In G. H. Grosser et al. (eds.), *The Threat of Impending Disaster*. Cambridge: MIT Press.

19. Kern, R. P. (1966). *A Conceptual Model of Behavior Under Stress*. Technical Report 66-12. George Washington University Human Resources Research Office.

20. Mechanic, D. (1967). "Therapeutic Intervention: Issues in the Care of the Mentally Ill." *American Journal of Orthopsychiatry*, **37**:703–718.

21. Jones, E. (1964). *Ingratiation*. New York: Appleton, Century, Crofts.

22. Argyle, M., and A. Kendon (1967). "The Experimental Analysis of Social Per-formance." In L. Berkowitz (ed.), *Advances in Experimental Social Psychology*. New York: Academic Press.

23. Egbert, L. D., et al. (1964). "Reduction of Post-Operative Pain by Encouragement and Instruction of Patients." *New England Journal of Medicine,* **270**:825–827.

24. Janis, I. (1958). *Psychological Stress*. New York: Wiley.

25. Skipper, J. K., Jr., and R. C. Leonard (1968). "Children, Stress, and Hospitalization: A Field Experiment." *Journal of Health and Social Behavior,* **9**:275–287.

CHAPTER XV

Social Considerations in Medical Education: Points of Convergence between Medicine and Behavioral Science*

In recent years there has been growing interest in behavioral science among medical educators. This interest has been encouraged by the acute realization that medical institutions and the American society in general are undergoing rapid technological and social change, and that the problems of accommodation between medical and other social institutions are increasingly difficult. Interest has also been encouraged by the changing structure of disease patterns in American society and the growing relative importance of chronic, psychosomatic, and psychosocial problems. It is now commonplace to reflect on how the changing age-structure, the shorter workweek with increased leisure, increased geographic mobility, urban concentration and the like affect the kinds of problems the physician is called upon to deal with and the services he is expected to render. Associated with these changes are the tremendous changes in medicine itself: changing modes of rendering care, the growth of new forms of payment and practice organization, increased specialization and the decline of the general practitioner, increased cooperation and coordination between physicians and other health professions, and many others.

The purpose of this essay is to discuss some of the points at which consideration of the behavioral sciences may contribute to medicine. The basic premise is that if behavioral science is to be important in medical

---

* Adapted from a paper, coauthored by Margaret Newton, published in the *Journal of Chronic Diseases*, 1965, **18**:291–301, with permission of Pergamon Press.

education, it must be taught to the prospective physician in a fashion which makes clear how such social considerations make him a better practitioner. Also, before behavioral science can be accepted fully as an intrinsic aspect of medical education, the relevance of such teaching for medical practice must be demonstrated. With the growth of medical knowledge and increasing specialization and the pressures for accelerated programs and elective periods, there is deepening concern among medical educators as to how to best apportion the medical curriculum among competing subjects so that the medical student acquires the basic medical sciences and clinical techniques. Thus, in introducing any new area into the medical curriculum, the relevant question is not whether such learning may be valuable, but rather its relative value as compared with competing demands.

Perhaps this is not the time to be skeptical. But skepticism is realistic in that most medical schools view behavioral science and social considerations as relatively unimportant as compared with traditional medical sciences, except perhaps for departments of psychiatry and community medicine which themselves are often low in the medical status hierarchy. It should be clear that if behavioral science is to be accepted generally as basic to medicine, pediatrics, and other medical disciplines, demonstration is required that such teaching makes a difference in the kind and quality of physician produced by medical schools.

Thus, it seems important to discuss specifically the points at which convergence between behavioral science and medicine exists, and where behavioral science teaching is particularly likely to make a difference in the quality of medical practice. In this paper we shall draw largely on those areas where collaboration in teaching and research appear most fruitful.

Basic to both medicine and behavioral science is the statistical model as it relates to disease processes, patient selection, and medical decision-making. Probability theory is not only essential in understanding the course of disease, but also it is implicit in every treatment situation. *All medical decisions involve the weighing of probabilities.* Behavioral science enters the picture of disease and its treatment in that social, cultural, and psychological factors affect the probabilities of certain occurrences. Failure, therefore, to utilize such information produces certain biases in the predictions made in treatment situations. The points at which behavioral science can be most useful to the physician, consequently, are those where such considerations help him reduce bias or error in prediction. One of the major contentions of this paper is that if medical decisions are to be fully rational, they must take into consideration not only the salient medical facts but also the manner in which organizational contingencies have molded and, perhaps, even biased these facts. Thus, attention must also be focused on patient selection, the manner of eliciting medical information, and the prevalent medical and value assumptions affecting practice.

Patient Selection

The physician usually trained in medical schools, university hospitals, and various kinds of general hospitals sees a variety of patients with different diseases who have become patients through a process of selection, dependent not only on the severity of symptoms but also upon various social and cultural influences.[1] He is not usually attuned to the question of what kind of population his patients come from and what factors other than illness brought them under his scrutiny. White, Williams, and Greenberg[2] have estimated, on the basis of various data from the United States and Britain, that of an adult population of 1000 patients, 750 persons are likely to report one or more illnesses per month, 250 are likely to consult a physician, 9 patients are likely to be admitted to a hospital, 5 patients are likely to be referred to another doctor, and 1 patient is likely to find himself at a university medical center. Miller, Court, Walton, and Knox[3] in their study of 847 children during their first five years in Newcastle-upon-Tyne, recorded 8467 significant incidents of illness of which 42 per cent were untreated. They report that untreated illness was not insignificant in that it included 1 in 5 attacks of bronchitis and pneumonia during the first year, and 2 of every 3 attacks of vomiting and diarrhea during the five-year period. Mechanic,[4] in analyzing data relevant to a college student population, demonstrated that patients in various diagnostic categories constituted persons who were overrepresented in respect to particular social variables which suggested biases in how patients with certain diseases became subjects for treatment.

These and various other studies suggest that there are various selective forces which influence how clinical populations arrive from a population at risk. They point very clearly to the importance of considering patterns of *illness behavior* (i.e., the ways in which different symptoms may be variously perceived, evaluated, or acted—or not acted—upon by different kinds of persons) in understanding why some persons suffering from particular diseases come under medical scrutiny while others fail to seek care. Thus, studies of social variables may serve as a focus for understanding patient-selection bias and its implications for medical care and medical investigation. They also serve to initiate discussion of the significance of *presenting symptoms* as an aspect of the treatment process. Relatively unimportant symptoms may be presented to the physician to justify a medical visit, while the major motivation for the visit becomes evident only after careful and skillful questioning.[5] Physicians are frequently faced with symptoms which are relatively trivial from a medical standpoint, and which occur with very high prevalence among untreated populations. The fact that the patient presents a relatively simple and common symptom may be one indication of other problems in the patient's life which motivate the medical visit. To the extent that the physician directs himself only to manifest symptoms or views the patient as a hypochondriac, he fails to deal with the larger context of human *dis-ease*.

Patient selection and the catalog of ordinary human complaints that every practising physician hears also have implications for the effectiveness of medical education. As Huntley[6] points out, there may be vast discrepancies between the practice that a typical physician must deal with and the kind of practice for which he is prepared. In short, patient selection has implications for medical care, medical research, and medical education.

Eliciting Medical Information

One of the most essential aspects of a medical examination is an adequate medical history. Although textbooks on medical diagnosis carefully discuss medical history-taking, they rarely utilize systematic research on interviewer effects and interview bias. Nor is the structure of questions, their order, and reliability discussed in a fashion which makes use of empirical studies of the interview. Cochrane and his associates[7] have demonstrated a considerable range of disagreement among competent physicians in the histories they elicit from patients even in fairly standardized interviews. Cobb and Rosenbaum[8] have shown differences in symptom data elicited by physicians and nonmedical interviewers with regard to joint pain, morning stiffness, and joint swelling. Various investigators studying general practitioners[9,10] have been dismayed at the quality of the examination and history-taking procedure. All of these investigations suggest the importance of systematic study and teaching in this area.

In recent years interview bias has received considerable attention among survey analysts and other behavioral scientists. It is now widely recognized, for example, that slight wording variations in questions may elicit different response distributions; and at least one model of constructing attitude scales involves asking a similar question with slight variations in order to locate an individual's score on a particular attitude dimension as precisely as possible.[11] A great deal of research has been completed on the interview, the survey, and the questionnaire. Although it is sometimes difficult to generalize to the medical situation, which is unique in a variety of ways, consideration of such research does encourage more systematic work on the medical interview itself,[12] and existing studies can clearly sensitize the student to the various ways in which error may be introduced in the process of eliciting medical information. Hyman,[13] in an excellent introduction and summary of empirical research concerning the interview situation, discusses interviewer effects, respondent reactions, situational determinants of interviewer effect, interviewer effects under normal operating conditions, and the reduction and control of error. His approach is largely an empirical one, and data are presented that clearly show various ways in which bias may be introduced.

Careful attention to the medical interview—in addition to its apparent practicalities—is important also as an approach to the doctor–patient relationship as a social system. In 1935 Henderson[14] made a plea for the consideration of influence processes between doctor and patient, and its importance for medical practice. Various persons involved in research on medical care and medical education have continued to view the doctor–patient relationship as an important focus for analysis and concern. Freidson,[15,16] for example, has discussed the mutual influence of doctor and patient in solo and group practice, and Bloom[17,18] sees this as the focus for the behavioral scientist's major contribution to the medical setting.

How the social system aspects of the doctor–patient relationship can best be communicated to physicians is a matter of strategy. But we would contend that it must be taught within a framework meaningful for the doctor's practice; and careful evaluation of the medical interview is an excellent focus for developing an understanding of the nuances of the doctor–patient relationship. The consideration of the physician's biasing effects in the medical interview involves by necessity a consideration of doctor–patient transactions. The advantage of introducing social system considerations at this juncture is that its importance and practicality are clearly evident, as in the case of frequent failures in communication resulting in nonconformity with prescribed treatment.

Consideration of Assumptions Underlying Medical Errors

Some errors are unavoidable; but they often occur because of carelessness, ignorance, and haste. Such errors are usually not difficult to identify by the experienced physician or in a medical auditing procedure. There are, however, a variety of possible errors which may result from the clinician's location in the patient-care system, and various implicit assumptions he holds. This type of error is usually more difficult to isolate and correct.

It has already been suggested that the physician finds his contacts with patients preceded by various selective influences. It is, thus, extremely difficult to generalize from such groups to larger populations at risk. The importance of the fact that different observer perspectives yield different impressions underlies the significance of controlled clinical trials and epidemiological methodology.[19] Even the most carefully controlled doubleblind, clinical trials involve difficult problems of inference and interpretation;[20] failure to view medical practice from a statistical as well as a clinical perspective is likely to give the physician an erroneous conception of the natural course of disease processes.

Another possible source of error may stem from the physician's assumptions of the risks involved in various aspects of medical decision-making. Scheff[21] nicely illustrates this problem in his discussion of decision rules physicians use in deciding to treat or not to treat a patient. He argues that physicians usually adopt a conservative decision rule. He writes:

> Do physicians and the general public consider that rejecting the hypothesis of illness when it is true, or accepting it when it is false, the error that is most important to avoid? It seems fairly clear that the rule in medicine may be stated as: "When in doubt, continue to suspect illness." . . . most physicians learn early in their training that it is far more culpable to dismiss a sick patient than to retain a well one. This rule is so pervasive and fundamental that it goes unstated in textbooks on diagnosis.[21]

Scheff goes on to point out that there are various disease entities where the decision rule to continue to search for illness when disease is not apparent may be of greater harm to the patient than the possible risks of failing to provide treatment. Although various aspects of Scheff's viewpoint can be debated, his basic point is clearly important. The excellent physician must learn to weigh carefully the risks of diagnosis and treatment (whatever they may involve) with the anticipated risks of failure to pursue diagnosis and treatment. Such evaluations must involve not only medical considerations (such as the probability that a drug will prove useful as weighted against possible adverse effects) but also social considerations (the positive and unfortunate consequences of treatment for the patient in social, psychological, and economic terms). Of course, this is not an easy thing to do well; and every physician does it to some extent. But often the difference between an excellent and mediocre practitioner is his skill in making such difficult determinations.

A model which urges consideration of the probability of positive and adverse effects of various treatment alternatives and nontreatment is important also in light of the growing emphasis on computer technology and the likely significance of computer systems as future aids in medical diagnosis.[22-25] By sensitizing the prospective physician explicitly to the various components of medical decision-making, not only do we encourage sophistication about such processes, but also he becomes better prepared to understand and accept new technical aids in medical diagnosis and medical care based on similar logic.

Consideration of the Context of Medical Error and Variabilities in Practice

There are a number of studies and discussions concerning medical error,[26-29] and such papers should be valuable in familiarizing medical students with the many contexts in which such errors occur and possible means of avoiding them. Johnson[30] has discussed some of the perceptual factors which may affect observation and the possible role of considerations of observer errors in medical education. Most of the emphasis on medical error, however, concerns the personal, perceptual, and informational aspects of making medical judgments.

In addition to these types of factors, there are various organizational influences that may encourage particular forms of error in the optimal utilization of available medical resources. As Kilpatrick[26] observes, it is perhaps wiser not to think of errors *per se*, but rather of variabilities in medical practice. In this way, discussion is less threatening and physicians are more willing to participate in relevant investigations. The major question to be posed is this: Given various medical, laboratory, and hospital resources, how may they be utilized to produce optimal patient care? Thus, investigations can be posed in terms of how various resources are utilized under different prevailing forms of medical organization. Variabilities in practice, thus, call for careful investigation, evaluation, and discussion in medical education.

Assuming, for example, that the effective transmission of medical innovations is essential in good medical practice, *the social factors that hinder transmission* of information and *adoption* of new techniques can become sources of medical error. Coleman, Menzel and Katz[31-33] have carefully studied the social processes that differentiated physicians in four cities in terms of how quickly they adopted a relatively important new drug placed on the market. They found considerable variability depending on the physician's exposure to certain information media and his relationships with his colleagues.

To take a somewhat different example, we can utilize some of the data reported by Myers[34] on the use of antibacterial drugs in cases of simple and complicated inguinal hernia in various hospitals. He comments that:

It is well known that simple or uncomplicated inguinal hernia is one condition which should not be complicated by infection after herniorrhaphy, if the patients are properly selected and prepared for operation and if adequate surgical asepsis is observed during operation. Therefore, there is no need for antibacterials to be given routinely for prevention of infection following herniorrhaphy. Consequently, the indiscriminate use of these dangerous drugs is one indication of the quality of care of such patients.[34]

Myers finds a tremendous range of use of antibacterials in herniorraphy in data from 24 community hospitals, varying from 9.2 per cent to 100 per cent of all cases. What is particularly interesting is that he finds antibacterials used in 38.2 per cent of all simple cases, but not used in 47.8 per cent of all complicated cases. He further reports that 84 per cent of the patients with simple hernias who received antibacterials received them specifically for prophylactic use; what is particularly surprising is that the percentage receiving antibacterials for prophylactic use in complicated hernia ("in which the possibility of infection is greater") was almost identical. He concludes that inadequate clinical practices exist in the great teaching hospitals as well as the smaller hospitals, and that "regular, valid, and informative evaluations of the quality of care" are required. The factors underlying such variabilities, as described by Myers, appear to be more than personal factors since hospital patterns clearly emerge.

As the studies previously discussed suggest, the conditions of patient care are affected not only by the physician's competence and the quality of his training, but also by the organization of medical care. Although organization is often discussed in terms of moral imperatives, what is really needed is careful consideration of how various means of organizing medical care produce different pressures for physicians and patients. Freidson,[35] for example, in an analysis of the organizational contexts of 'solo' and 'group' practice, has pointed to the different degrees of influence patients and colleagues may have relative to the physician. He argues that physicians in group practice have greater protection against patient demands, and thus it is less difficult to practice good medicine at least in the respect that the physician can do what is medically indicated. However, he notes that the same organizational factors that produce the conditions for high professional quality may produce a certain rigidity in dealing with patient demands which can be disruptive to the doctor–patient relationship.

The financial arrangements for providing medical care also obviously affect decisions. It is well known that rates of hospitalization increase among persons carrying hospital insurance; although under comprehensive health insurance plans like the Health Insurance Plan of New York, rates of hospitalization and surgery appear to be less than among similar populations covered by less comprehensive Blue-Cross and Blue-Shield plans.[36-38] There are also some indications that lower rates of inpatient utilization occur under capitation plans as compared with fee-for-service plans, although at least one study suggests that the form of payment is not an important variable in the populations studied.[39]

In future years there will be increasing information available concerning the consequences of organizing and financing medical and hospital care in various ways. Data concerned with utilization, recommended hospitalization, and surgery are susceptible to varying interpretations. It is difficult, for example, to specify what is an optimal utilization rate for a particular population.[40] Although such uncertainties in interpretation exist, these data can be extremely useful for medical education. Obviously, various interpretations of the same data should be considered as well as the methodological aspects of the study which may be related to the reported results. But it should also be clear that decisions can be evaluated in terms of the criteria and procedures used by the physician in making his decision. In addition, discussion of such data serves two broad purposes in medical education: it exposes the prospective physician to the organizational contingencies of his decisions; and it stimulates consideration and understanding of the advantages and problems of various organizational schemes for providing medical services and patient care.

What we wish to emphasize is that medical variabilities must be viewed within their largest context. The medical student must be attuned not only to his own mistakes and their possible consequences, but also he should have some understanding of the context of practice as it influences his alternatives and decisions.

The Role of Values in Medicine

Values play an important part in medicine as in any other human endeavor, and it is particularly important that the physician recognize the points at which values influence medical decision-making. Values come into play in medical practice in two ways. Most simply, the physician's values may influence who receives treatment,[41,42] the extent of treatment, how drugs are prescribed (generic vs. brand names), how medical procedures involving moral implications are dealt with (e.g., contraceptives), whether support is given to claims of disability, legal contests, etc.[43] More complex and subtle are those situations where medical decisions that are seemingly objective have moral, psychological, and social consequences for the patient's future. Thus, decisions about hospitalizatior may be influenced not only by the patient's illness and his finances but also considerations of the physician's convenience, the need for teaching material in some hospitals, etc. Although most physicians realize that delays in treatment and diagnosis or unnecessary periods of hospitalization often may have serious consequences for the patient in terms of his employment, family, or educational situation, one often wonders about how much more could be done to alleviate such consequences.

The typical physician is constantly faced with such dilemmas which involve values. To what extent should he seek to search for a definite diagnosis when the probability of finding a serious disease is low at increasing costs to patients with varying ability to finance such care? How long should a physician make "heroic" efforts to keep patients with "hopeless" outcomes alive—at great economic and social cost to others in his family?[44] How should the physical risks of a "radical" as compared with a more "conservative" approach to a particular illness be weighted against the social, psychological, and economic costs of these procedures for the patient? How much should the physician tell the patient? These and many other questions of a similar kind are frequently faced by the practicing physician.

There are no simple answers to such questions. Not only do we know very little about what physicians as a group do in such situations, but also such matters are often outside the limits of polite discussion. Careful consideration of these issues as part of medical education will not provide answers, but it will make students more conscious of what it is they will be doing and the ramifications of the problems they will be faced with. To the extent that such matters become conscious, the physician is more likely to separate such judgments in his own mind from more specific medical judgments and, therefore, is more likely to allow patients to share in such judgments.

Some Further Comments Relevant to Medical Education

We have considered five examples of areas where medical and behavioral science can collaborate fruitfully. In conclusion we shall consider some general points relevant to medical practice and medical education.

Patient care (which is usually used to refer to the quality of care rendered to a particular patient) is often viewed independently of medical care (the manner in which patient care is provided to various areas, groups, and persons). It is perhaps meaningful to view the quality of care a particular physician provides a particular patient independent of the larger medical system as a whole. But it should be clear that the organization of medical care in any community influences the kind and quality of services rendered, as well as the distribution of care. In this sense, at least, patient and medical care are inseparable. Thus concern with the quality of care must take into consideration how organizational influences affect it.

By medical organization we mean more than the formal means of rendering care. Medical care also includes the informal relationships among medical practitioners: the manner in which referrals occur, the forms of achieving status among colleagues, and the informal and subtle pressures that influence how a doctor practices.[45-51]

Medical educators are often amazed and concerned about the considerable deviation from good medical procedures taught by them, among practicing physicians.[52] Often they seek to understand how they have 'failed' so badly in developing certain high standards. Practicing physicians, in contrast, often feel that the medical faculty fail to understand them and regard them as second-class citizens. In the opinions of some, it is easy for medical faculty to talk about the complete work-up, the comprehensive history, and family and community considerations since educators often do not find themselves faced with offices full of demanding patients, and other pressures of a full-time general practice.

A dialogue of reciprocal indignation serves no useful purpose. There is some merit in the idea that medical schools should concern themselves to a greater extent with problems that the typical physician is likely to face in practice. To teach standards of high quality that are difficult to make operative within the usual practice is not likely to encourage quality care. There is some merit in medical schools approaching the problem of high quality care with greater recognition and understanding of the pressures faced by the community practitioner.

This realization is becoming more widespread in respect to the context of medical education. There is now greater awareness that students tend to respond to the realities of the demands placed upon them as compared with the values expressed by the faculty.[53,54] If family and community medicine, for example, are to become viable aspects of medical education, they must be more than expressions of concern; they must involve a working program in which the faculty are themselves involved.

Conclusion

Although more good medical care in a technical-scientific sense is available to more people than ever before (who are increasing their level of utilization) many of the economic, social, and organizational aspects of medical practice have become extremely complex. The success of medical practice at the community level is largely dependent on the organization of facilities, the distribution of services, and the effective utilization of practitioners. Moreover, as patients become more able to purchase medical services, and become more impressed with the medical products, they increasingly bring a variety of new complaints.

The physician operates within certain organizational, economic, and social forms. These boundaries of practice present many opportunities for good patient care; they also impose limits on what the physician can do. The physician—if he is to be effective—must understand and be able to utilize the advantages that complex medical organization provides and, similarly, he must be vigilant so that he recognizes and takes into account the forces within social life and medical practice that may interfere with adequate diagnosis and care.

If the physician is to be a fine doctor in the most comprehensive sense, he must be trained to recognize social and psychological influences that affect his patients and influence the care he provides. Medical care—no matter how technically competent—is trivial unless the patient benefits. Thus, the physician's role obligates him to concern himself not only with the proper diagnosis and regimen, but also with the conditions that allow these to be translated into patient improvement.

In this paper we have suggested various examples of how a behavioral science perspective better allows the physician to perform his role. Perhaps one could choose many better examples than those presented here. The most important point, however, should be clear: social and psychological variables affect the probability of medically relevant occurrences, and thus must be taken into account in predicting and controlling such occurrences. Similarly, medical education would be more effective if medical educators took into account not only what is desirable but also the social and organizational contexts which allow medically desirable practices to be successfully maintained.

In sum, medical educators must go beyond the attempt to teach the medical student lofty values and ideals. They must supplement such teaching by promoting the conditions of practice and patient care that allow lofty values to be implemented in practice.

Notes

1. Mechanic, D. (1962). "Concept of Illness Behavior." *Journal of Chronic Diseases,* **15:**189–194.
2. White, K. L., T. F. Williams, and B. G. Greenberg (1961). "The Ecology of Medical Care." *New England Journal of Medicine,* **265:**885–892.
3. Miller, F. J., S. D. Court, W. S. Walton, and E. G. Knox (1960). *Growing Up in Newcastle-upon-Tyne.* London: Oxford University Press.
4. Mechanic, D. (1963). "Illness Behavior and Medical Sampling." *New England Journal of Medicine,* **269:**244–247.
5. Balint, M. (1957). *The Doctor, His Patient, and the Illness.* New York: International Universities Press.
6. Huntley, R. (1963). "Epidemiology of Family Practice." *Journal of the American Medical Association,* **185:**175–178.
7. Cochrane, A. L., et al. (1951). "Observer Errors in Taking Medical Histories." *Lancet,* **1:**1007–1009.
8. Cobb, S., and J. Rosenbaum (1956). "A Comparison of Specific Symptom Data Obtained by Nonmedical Interviews and by Physicians." *Journal of Chronic Diseases,* **4:**245–252.
9. Peterson, O. L., et al. (1956). "Analytical Study of North Carolina General Practice." *Journal of Medical Education, Part II,* **31:**1–165.
10. Clute, K. F. (1963). *The General Practitioner. Study of Medical Education and Practice in Ontario and Nova Scotia.* Toronto: University of Toronto Press.
11. Torgerson, W. S. (1958). *Theory and Methods of Scaling.* New York: Wiley.
12. Feldman, J. J. (1960). "The Household Interview Survey as a Technique for the Collection of Morbidity Data." *Journal of Chronic Diseases,* **11:**535–537.
13. Hyman, H. H. (1954). *Interviewing in Social Research.* Chicago: University of Chicago Press.
14. Henderson, L. J. (1935). "The Patient and Physician as a Social System." *New England Journal of Medicine,* **212:**819–823.
15. Freidson, E. (1960). "Client Control and Medical Practice." *American Journal of Sociology,* **65:**374–382.
16. Freidson, E. (1961). *Patients' Views of Medical Practice.* New York: Russell Sage Foundation.
17. Bloom, S. (1959). "The Role of the Sociologist in Medical Education." *Journal of Medical Education,* **34:**667–673.
18. Bloom, S. (1963). *The Doctor and His Patient.* New York: Russell Sage Foundation.
19. Witts, L. J. (ed.) (1959). *Medical Surveys and Clinical Trials.* London: Oxford University Press.
20. Lasagna, L. (1955). "The Controlled Clinical Trial: Theory and Practice." *Journal of Chronic Diseases,* **1:**353–367.
21. Scheff, T. J. (1963). "Decision Rules, Types of Error, and their Consequences in Medical Diagnosis." *Behavioral Science,* **8:**97–107.

22. Lusted, L. B., and R. S. Ledley (1960). "Mathematical Models in Medical Diagnoses." *Journal of Medical Education,* **35**:214–222.

23. Lusted, L. B., and R. S. Ledley (1959). "Reasoning Foundations of Medical Diagnosis." *Science,* **130**:9–21.

24. Lusted, L. B., and R. S. Ledley (1962). "Medical Diagnosis and Modern Decision Making." *Math Problems in the Biological Sciences,* **14**:117–158.

25. Lusted, L. B. (1962). "The Proper Province of Automatic Data Processing in Medicine." *Annals of Internal Medicine,* **57**:855–857.

26. Kilpatrick, G. S. (1963). "Observer Error in Medicine." *Journal of Medical Education,* **38**:38–43.

27. Garland, L. H. (1959). "Studies of the Accuracy of Diagnostic Procedures." *American Journal of Roentgenology,* **82**:25–38.

28. Fletcher, C. M. (1952). "The Clinical Diagnosis of Pulmonary Emphysema." *Proceedings of the Royal Society of Medicine,* **45**:577–584.

29. Bakwin, H. (1945). "Pseudodoxia Pediatrica." *New England Journal of Medicine,* **232**:691–697.

30. Johnson, M. D. (1955). "Observer Error: Its Bearing on Teaching." *Lancet,* **2**:422–424.

31. Coleman, J., H. Menzel, and E. Katz (1959). "Social Processes in Physicians' Adoption of a New Drug." *Journal of Chronic Diseases,* **9**:1–19.

32. Coleman, J., E. Katz, and H. Menzel (1957). "The Diffusion of an Innovation Among Physicians." *Sociometry,* **20**:253–270.

33. Menzel, H. (1960). "Innovation, Integration, and Marginality." *American Sociological Review,* **25**:704–713.

34. Myers, R. S. (1961). "Quality of Patient Care—Measurable or Immeasurable." *Journal of Medical Education,* **36**:776–784.

35. Freidson, E. (1963). "Medical Care and the Public." *Annals of the American Academy of Political and Social Science,* **346**:57–66.

36. Anderson, O., and J. Feldman (1956). *Family Medical Costs and Voluntary Health Insurance: A Nationwide Survey.* New York: McGraw-Hill.

37. Densen, P., et al. (1960). "Prepaid Medical Care and Hospital Utilization in a Dual Choice Situation." *American Journal of Public Health,* **50**:1710–1726.

38. Anderson, O., and P. B. Sheatsley (1959). *Comprehensive Medical Insurance—A Study of Costs, Use, and Attitudes Under Two Plans.* Health Information Foundation Research Series No. 9. New York: Health Information Foundation.

39. Densen, P., et al. (1962). "Prepaid Medical Care and Hospital Utilization." *Hospitals,* **36**:62–65.

40. Health Information Foundation (1961). "Hospital Use by Diagnosis: A Study in Contrasts." *Progressive Health Service,* Vol. 10, No. 1.

41. Hollingshead, A., and F. C. Redlich (1958). *Social Class and Mental Illness.* New York: Wiley.

42. Myers, J. K., and L. Schaffer (1954). "Social Stratification and Psychiatric Practice." *American Sociological Review,* **19**:307–310.

43. Szasz, T. S. (1962). "Bootlegging Humanistic Values Through Psychiatry." *Antioch Review,* **22**:341–349.

44. Fletcher, J. (1960). "The Patient's Right to Die." *Harper's,* **221**:139–143.

45. Hall, O. (1946). "The Informal Organization of the Medical Profession." *Canadian Journal of Economics and Political Science,* **12**:30–44.
46. Hall, O. (1948). "The Stages of a Medical Career." *American Journal of Sociology,* **53**:327–336.
47. Bowers, A. D. (1963). "General Practice—Analysis and Some Suggestions." *New England Journal of Medicine,* **269**:667–673.
48. Silver, G. (1963). "The Hospital and Social Medicine." *New England Journal of Medicine,* **269**:504–508.
49. Silver, G. (1963). "Family Practice: Resuscitation or Reform." *Journal of the American Medical Association,* **185**:188–191.
50. Haggerty, R. J. (1963). "Etiology of Decline in General Practice." *Journal of the American Medical Association,* **185**:179–182.
51. White, R. L. (1963). "Family Medicine, Academic Medicine, and the University's Responsibility." *Journal of the American Medical Association,* **185**:192–196.
52. Miller, G. E. (1963). "The Continuing Education of the Physician." *New England Journal of Medicine,* **269**:295–299.
53. Becker, H. S., et al. (1961). *Boys in White: Student Culture in Medical School.* Chicago: University of Chicago Press.
54. Mechanic, D. (1962). *Students Under Stress: A Study in the Social Psychology of Adaptation.* New York: Free Press.

PART FIVE

DIRECTIONS IN THE FUTURE OF HEALTH CARE

Problems in the Future Organization of Medical Practice*

Despite vast and growing expenditures for medical care in the United States, there is an emerging consensus among observers that a state of crisis exists. The deficiencies in our present system of delivering health care services have become more visible as a consequence of difficulties in the successful implementation of Medicare and Medicaid.[1] These programs have focused attention on such issues as growing inflation in medical care costs; the inefficiency in the organization of medical care services; special problems in meeting the health needs of particular groups such as the poor and persons in rural areas; difficulties in administering the work of doctors and other professionals; scarcity of special facilities such as nursing homes that meet adequate standards; and the enormity of administrative details involved in these programs.

It is now widely appreciated that continued expansion of funds for medical care services—without associated incentives for major changes in the organization and delivery of medical care—will contribute to significant inflation in the health area and is unlikely to succeed in meeting population needs for health care. In light of this, it is ironic that more recent discussions of national health insurance have for the most part failed to address themselves to the significant organizational problems that any large new program can be expected to encounter. Most of the discussion has focused on the cost of alternative financing mechanisms and the scope of coverage without detailed concern for the components of health service or how they might best be provided.[2–5]

The present crisis offers an excellent opportunity for the development of new incentives for improvement in the delivery of health services.[6] In

* Adapted from a paper published in *Law and Contemporary Problems*, 1970, **35**:233–251, which appeared in the Symposium on Health Care, Part 1.

this concluding essay I begin by describing some of the major difficulties presently existing in the health care system and the problems that proposals for national health insurance must realistically confront. The failures of the Medicare and Medicaid programs are attributable to the fact that they have persistently side-stepped these issues on the assumption that the provision of money alone could overcome significant failures in the organization of health care. These programs, thus, have duplicated and exacerbated the persistent deficiencies, inefficiencies, and absurdities of the current organization of medical care in America.[1,7] The problems are complex and particularly difficult from a political standpoint. As painful as these problems may be, the presently deteriorating situation offers little alternative but to pursue constructive change or to court disaster. The wide appreciation of this fact in government, among various third parties, and even within the health professions themselves offers some hope that constructive change is indeed possible.

A Summary of the Present State of Affairs

The delivery of health care at the present time is plagued by failures in organization, lack of planning, and poor coordination among the components of care. The substantial demand for medical services characteristic of an affluent population offers physicians abundant opportunities for selling their services, however organized; and under these conditions it is not surprising that many doctors seek practice circumstances that maximize their autonomy and professional discretion and fulfill their conditions for personally satisfying work. This is a ubiquitous human tendency, and doctors cannot be faulted any more than others in our society for making the choices that are most congruent with their personal aspirations.

Hospitals, the major workplace of doctors, have undergone tremendous expansion of their facilities and technologies and have experienced growth in both the size and complexity of their manpower pool.[8] Still dependent on doctors for patients to occupy their beds, however, hospitals have been cautious and reluctant to make new demands on physicians despite enormous difficulties in efficient operation and associated financial problems. Indeed, hospitals often have been influenced substantially in their decision making by the need to provide facilities and organizational forms attractive to their medical staff so as to retain them. In short, the operation of hospitals and medical care in general is influenced largely by the physician's definition of his needs, his professional responsibility, his concepts of autonomy, and his life style. Any serious attempt to understand the organization of medical care requires detailed attention to the doctor's perspective.

The Physician's Perspective. Although the health industry encompasses well over three million workers, the 340,000 doctors define and control the basic pattern of organization of health services. This hegemony stems from a variety of factors: their specialized training and prestige, their central role in health care, the tremendous demand for their services, and their resulting independence. As Freidson has noted, the key to medical authority is that the doctor not only controls his own work but has the ability and centrality to control the work of other occupations as well.[9]

The physician's perspective is one that defines medical work in terms of responsibility to *individual patients*,[10,11] and the typical doctor wishes to provide optimal care without suffering infringements on his personal autonomy. In this sense doctors, like other professionals, strive to retain control over their work and the choice of the location, scope, and pace of their activities. For the most part, doctors do not regard it as their personal responsibility to see that medical care is available to all in need although many doctors would agree with such aspirations. The doctor sees his responsibilities fulfilled if he provides conscientious care to his patients, and he seeks to do so under conditions that fulfill his personal needs as well. Thus, unlike the student of medical care, he is not likely to review his effectiveness or contribution in terms of the greatest good for the greatest number. The consequences of this type of selectivity are an uneven distribution of doctors, an unbalanced division of medical functions, and a variety of inequalities in the delivery of medical care services to the population.

Government programs in health care have rarely demanded that doctors demonstrate responsibility in the charges for their services or in the manner in which they use hospitals, nor have hospital administrators been sufficiently secure in their own power to attempt to institute rigorous controls. In the typical private fee-for-service context, doctors can sell their services as long as there is sufficient demand and the patient is willing to pay, but patients' concerns about costs and their varying ability to pay impose a degree of control. As an increasing part of the medical care bill has been paid by intermediaries rather than the patients themselves, neither doctor nor patient has been pressed or inclined to resist rising costs.[12] Costs have thus mounted on every front, technology has expanded in an inefficient and unbalanced fashion, and relatively small inroads have been made in equalizing accessibility to good medical care.

It is worth noting that fiscal responsibility will require controls over the way doctors work, and insurance mechanisms by themselves are unlikely to have major impact. There are several studies that suggest that extended coverage of medical care outside the hospital by itself is unlikely to significantly affect rates of hospitalization or the use of particular medical procedures.[13] However, experience in prepaid group practices suggests that when prepaid mechanisms are linked with various incentives for the physician to limit utilization, rates of hospital utilization can be significantly reduced.[14,15] The difficult issues to decide are what rate of utilization is really appropriate for various populations, and what are the boundaries of under- and over-utilization.[16] Although it is important that unnecessary utilization and medical work be curtailed, it is equally urgent to insure that those who need particular forms of care receive it.

Another element of the physician's perspective is his growing concern with technology and scientific practice. In recent years there has been a phenomenal expansion of personnel and facilities to support the growth of medicine as a scientific enterprise, and no responsible person would debate the many advantages that have accompanied this growth. But the technical growth of medicine has not been fully balanced, and too many doctors have substituted excessive technical pursuits for understanding and communicating with their patients. Just as one can fail to use appropriate laboratory tests or other diagnostic procedures, so too can one overuse or misuse them. Accompanying the growth of technology has been an uncritical acceptance that has led to the tendency toward confusing the technical means of medicine with its practice, which has many humanistic concerns.[17] This emphasis on technology has also encouraged proliferation and duplication of complex technical arrangements to deal with particular disease conditions. Overinvestment in such technologies is not only costly and inefficient but also results in less effective care than would be given if investment were concentrated in fewer specialized facilities operated by adequate numbers of highly specialized personnel who would have a sufficient work load to maintain and develop their special skills.[18]

The physician's perspective has been encouraged in large part by developments in medical schools in recent decades. With the establishment and expansion of the National Institutes of Health, vast funds for research became available to medical schools, making possible rapid expansion of their facilities and research faculty. As a consequence, a strong technological and research emphasis was encouraged, influencing the character of medical education itself. Many new medical faculty were largely researchers working in highly specialized areas and conscious of new technological developments, and frequently they were not concerned with the more wholistic problems of medical care.[11,19,20] The models such faculty presented for students were ones encouraging emulation of specialized roles, and, since these were often the men to whom the largest rewards flowed, it is not surprising that they have had a profound influence on the image and orientation of medical students.

This is not to say that much of value did not flow from these developments, and there is no question but that specialization and technical development are prerequisites for the effective development of medical care. But the way in which these developments occurred created major imbalances in the medical school, and much of the early emphasis on the cultivation of the arts of patient care gave way to an excessive reliance on the laboratory and the technics of medicine. The fact that medical care is a set of attitudes and approaches as well as a set of technical procedures was frequently lost in this enthusiasm for expanding scientific developments.

One of the ironies of these developments was the fact that the community practice of medical care changed very little. Graduates of medical schools found it more difficult than ever before to translate what they had learned in the teaching hospital to the practice of medicine as it existed in the community, and one mode in which they adapted—with the encouragement of their medical professors—was to specialize in some segment of medical work.* Through specialization it became possible to practice in accordance with modern standards and to keep up with rapidly changing knowledge in one's own field. These trends have established the conditions for the current difficulties in providing primary medical care.

The failure of the community organization of medicine to adapt in the face of changing technology can be attributed to a variety of factors. Perhaps most important was the comfort that older doctors felt with existing arrangements and their fear of organized practice as an intrusion on their professional life style. The status quo was vigorously supported by organized medicine and the doctors it represented, and there were few forces in the medical profession who were inclined to challenge this powerful group. Small but important adaptations took place, as reflected in the growth of group practice, the pooling of resources among doctors for managerial purposes, and the further development of experiments with prepaid group practice. But the main current of medicine was in large part unaffected. Much of the growing public concern with the state of affairs was mitigated by the growth of voluntary health insurance, which was able satisfactorily to absorb the more educated and affluent segments of the population whose dissatisfaction could have posed the

---

* The family physician potential relative to the population declined from 94 to 50 per 100,000 population between 1931 and 1965. See R. Fein, 1967, *The Doctor Shortage: An Economic Diagnosis.* Washington, D. C.: The Brookings Institution.

greatest threat to the status quo. Groups not covered by such insurance were insufficiently organized or vocal to pose a serious threat to prevailing patterns. Still, despite this ability of organized medicine to deal with any political threat, the dominant solo practice orientation of medical practice was strained and began to weaken. This weakening process can be expected to continue as the major foundations of solo practice are further undermined by technical developments and the growing complexity of treatment and rehabilitation, and new incentives encouraging more organized practice.

The Present Crisis in the Geographic Distribution of Medical Care. A crisis constitutes a situation of challenge, the response to which determines the future fate of the system.* The crisis in medicine may be described as one where certain expectations have developed, and the issue remains as to whether the existing system can respond in an adequate way to the demands it encounters. Standards for a viable system of medical care in our emerging society probably include (1) the availability of basic medical services to those in need regardless of social position; (2) coordination and integration of the elements of health services, including primary outpatient care, hospital care, and rehabilitation services; (3) attention not only to diagnosis and treatment of disease but also responsiveness to the personal and social circumstances affecting the patient; and (4) a commitment to the concept not only that medical care should be delivered in relation to need but that preference should be given to those modes of medical activity having the greatest impact on the health of the population. It should be evident that these generalizations are easily stated while their implementation may involve judgments that are enormously complex. Considerable gaps in our knowledge exist, but reasonable priorities can be established, on the basis of current understanding, that would facilitate a more rational approach to health services delivery than presently exists.

Geographic Maldistribution of Physicians. Health facilities and health manpower are distributed geographically in an uneven fashion. This maldistribution of physicians is the most significant problem because the physician constitutes the first formal link between the community and the health services system and is responsible for supervising the efforts of other health workers as well. The distribution of physicians has followed general population trends in that physicians concentrate in urban areas and have moved with the middle class from inner city to suburb. The

* This point is nicely developed by Kissick in his discussion of potentialities resulting from new legislative developments (W. L. Kissick, 1970, "Health-Policy Directions for the 1970's." *New England Journal of Medicine,* **282**:1343–1354).

unavailability of physicians is thus felt most acutely in rural areas and small towns, and in the inner core of cities where the most impoverished segments of the population reside.

A variety of factors accounts for the distribution of physicians. Like other professionals, doctors seek to live in areas that provide educational and cultural opportunities, and where they can earn a comfortable living within pleasant surroundings. Many doctors find it more comfortable and less trying to work with patients who share their cultural definitions and understandings. Moreover, as noted earlier, medical training in the context of the teaching hospital encourages a pattern of practice that requires the technology of a hospital and considerable colleague cooperation. The isolation of practice in underdoctored areas outside close proximity to an adequate hospital and colleagues is frustrating to the physician who feels he cannot implement the level of scientific training he received. Many rural practices would isolate him from a colleague network, more complex diagnostic and treatment aids, and the ancillary assistance available in more densely populated areas. Practice in impoverished areas also involves other frustrations, such as a high prevalence of drug addiction and alcoholism which may threaten the doctor, shortages of assisting personnel and resources, and the complexity of social and economic problems that affect the care of patients.

Other problems predominate in the effective use of ancillary health occupations.[7,8] These occupations are dominated by women workers, who either remain in the work force for a short time or who are irregular in their work patterns. Labor turnover in these occupations is very high, in part the product of marriage and child rearing, but also due to low wages, barriers to job mobility, and the inflexibility of health institutions in adapting to a part-time labor force.

It should be clear that any program for providing adequate medical care on a national level must be attentive to the problems of distributing manpower in relation to the prevalence of need in the population, although it is also evident that present trends push in the opposite direction. As the shortage of medical manpower worsens* and the population's

---

* There has been a growing debate as to whether a doctor shortage exists. From a purely technical point of view, assuming rational organization and an instrumental approach to medical care, the position taken by Ginzberg and Ostow, Note 7, and McNerney, Note 12, that the shortage has been overemphasized has some merit. However, there is little evidence to support the assumption that the system can be made to operate efficiently under prevailing political conditions or can be made sufficiently responsive to consumer demand for more personalized care. (D. Mechanic, 1970, Book Review of Ginzberg and Ostow, *Science,* **168**:1563–1564). Thus, Fein's estimates of a serious doctor shortage appear more realistic (R. Fein, 1967, *The Doctor Shortage: An Economic Diagnosis.* Washington, D. C.: The Brookings Institution).

unmet demand for medical services increases, there are even fewer pressures on physicians to locate their practices in areas where their services are most needed, since they can sustain themselves without difficulty in most areas and can choose locations that offer optimal satisfactions. Thus, as more government funds flow into medical care services, present trends will be exacerbated rather than relieved. Any significant relocation or redistribution of medical manpower and resources will have to result from pressures brought about by explicit new public policies.

If one works on the assumption that our society is unprepared to seek redistribution of physicians through coercive mechanisms—and this is obviously the case—then it is most fruitful to consider intermediate solutions involving new incentives for redistribution. But by their very nature, noncoercive incentives are likely to have relatively little force. If such incentives are to have influence, they must be implemented in some coordinated way so that they buttress one another and so that their total impact constitutes a real basis for change. A program for a national redistribution of physicians must include attention to such matters as the recruitment of medical students, the content of medical education, the conditions for an adequate level of practice in underdoctored areas, and economic incentives for change. Each of these will be considered below in some detail.

Recruitment of Medical Students and Medical Education. Medical schools now find themselves in a significant financial crisis because of growing inflation and the cutbacks in federal grant funds. Most medical schools have expanded their research efforts substantially in recent decades without concomitant increases in their enrollment. With the contraction of federal funds, medical schools are finding it difficult to support their current efforts, and are reluctant to make major commitments under prevailing conditions to further respond to the nation's need for physicians. They look to the federal government for relief from their difficulties.

Inevitably the federal government will have to develop more effective mechanisms for sustaining the operation of medical schools, which constitute an essential national resource. It would be wise, however, to use the incentives that financing carries to insure the graduation of more doctors and this appears to be the prevailing thinking. For example, a condition for substantial federal funds can be expansion of medical class size; or the formula by which medical schools receive support can be geared to an evaluation of the extent to which individual medical schools are contributing their share of graduates to the total pool of physicians. Such incentives must not be crudely applied, and must take into account the distinctive qualities of particular medical schools that have achieved excellence in other areas; but, over-all, some application of the principle of "the carrot that has become a stick" seems a reasonable means of inducing action directed toward meeting public needs.

Associated with this, it would be useful to establish a National Fellowship Program for Medical Students which provides full costs and a living stipend. Such fellowships could be tied to an agreement on the part of the recipient to practice in federally designated underdoctored areas for stated periods of time. The determination of underdoctored areas can be made by committees including representatives of the medical profession, government officials, and others. The costs of medical education are sufficiently large so that medical students are disproportionately recruited from a small segment of the population. A national fellowship program is likely to bring about a wider recruitment of students from varying socioeconomic levels and ethnic groups, and such students may have different values and orientations from those now recruited.

Even given these policies, it is not clear that the incentives are sufficient for encouraging medical students to commit themselves to work in needy areas. One way to substantially increase the value of this incentive is to tie admission to at least some portion of medical school places to the national fellowship program. Since many more qualified students than there are places for wish to attend medical school,* it would be reasonable to allocate places, at least in part, in terms of students' commitment to the nation's health care needs. To insure that competent students in such a national fellowship program receive medical school places, the formula for financing medical schools should be tied to the willingness of medical schools to reserve a certain proportion of medical school places for national fellows.† Recipients should meet standards sufficiently high to anticipate success in medical school, but they need not be the highest ranking students in competitive terms. Since this recommendation violates a strongly held value in universities—that admission should be geared solely to the academic qualifications of the candidate—some elaboration is required. Medicine is an applied profession, and its work must be evaluated in terms of its direct service to the

---

* In 1970–71, there were 24,987 first-year applicants to American medical schools for approximately 11,500 school places (W. F. Dube, et al., "Study of U. S. Medical School Applicants, 1970–71." *Journal of Medical Education,* **46:**837–857). Many qualified students were not admitted, and many other students with comparable credentials do not apply because of the difficulty of obtaining admission.

† Loan forgiveness programs tied to service commitments have had mixed effects (H. P. Mason, "Effectiveness of Student Aid Programs Tied to a Service Commitment." *Journal of Medical Education,* **46:**575–583). Apparently, the Illinois Student Loan Program has provided reserved medical school places to students willing to commit themselves to rural practice with good success.

public. Although the highest academic standard may be required for medical research and medical school teaching, the work of a good doctor involves many qualities other than academic ones. The willingness of the physician to serve those in need or the kinds of attitudes he assumes toward patients may be more important than small differentials in grades or performance on the Medical College Admissions Test. It is reasonable to select medical students from a pool of eligibles established on the basis of aptitude for medical studies. Choice within the pool, however, would depend on criteria other than modest differences in past academic performance. Indeed, studies of the physician's performance show little relationship between scholastic performance—once the basic minimum level had been reached—and the effectiveness of the doctor in performing his functions.[21] I should add that there is a long history of universities' and medical schools' taking other criteria into account—as in the preference given to children of doctors or children of alumni—and all that is really advocated here is that such preferential treatment reflect public needs and public goals in contrast to private ones.

Also, much greater balance is necessary in medical education between developing technical proficiency on the part of students and teaching how these skills can be translated into effective medical care in the community. The realities of community practice vary from those of the teaching hospital, and doctors must learn how to provide effective medical care within the real constraints they are likely to encounter in community contexts. The growing tendency of medical schools to assume greater primary care responsibilities provides the opportunity to develop practice laboratories in which young doctors may learn to practice a high level of technical medicine in a fashion responsive to the needs of patients and the community. The medical student should become acquainted with the potentialities and difficulties of practice under varying organizational arrangements; and if medical schools can provide viable models for general community care, doctors may be more inclined to take on these types of practice following their training.

Medical Organization in Underdoctored Areas. Just as it is necessary for medical schools to develop varying models of practice for educational purposes, so it is also necessary that underdoctored areas develop the resources and other conditions conducive to a good and satisfying medical practice. Many of the remaining doctors in rural areas and in the inner city are disproportionately old, and they are not being replaced by younger doctors,[22] who aspire to practice a higher level of medicine than is often possible in many such areas. What is often lacking is a medical structure and supporting services that facilitate the doctor's efforts and that allow him to use effectively the skills he has learned. Government subsidy for the development of such supporting facilities could be extremely important in attracting doctors to such practice.

It is possible to develop exciting and effective opportunities for practicing a high level of medical care with room for considerable experimentation and innovation. The necessary organizational development would include the concentration of physicians, nurses, and other health workers in facilities providing good preventive, diagnostic, and treatment services. A variety of models already exists for developing regional health facilities, community health centers, mobile teams associated with regional complexes, and the like, and there is no dearth of experience around the world that provides perspectives on both the potentialities and the difficulties of varying approaches.* There are many different approaches that can be taken, and probably in each case the strategies should be geared to the special problems of the area and to the facilities already available. Given the tremendous difficulties in providing medical services to underdoctored areas, it is reasonable for government to give high priority to the development of a viable health structure that would be attractive to medical manpower and that would make optimal use of paraprofessional workers. Government must, however, be attentive to the dangers of having such structures defined as providing a lesser level of medicine than is available to other population groups.

Development of Economic Incentives. The use of economic incentives for achieving redistribution of physicians has been used formally in some countries and informally in our own. In Britain,[23] for example, general practitioners establishing practices in undoctored areas receive additional income above their usual remuneration, and under some circumstances they are assured a particular income level. Various communities in the United States have offered physicians free practice facilities, guaranteed incomes, and a variety of other attractive incentives. For the most part, such incentives are not particularly effective without other changes in the conditions of practice. In England, economic incentives are buttressed by closing certain overdoctored areas to new practices, which at least serves to insure some minimal redistribution. However, these restrictions involved areas encompassing only seven per cent of the total population in 1968,[24] and in large part doctors are free to practice where they choose.

Although it is unlikely that the United States would restrict doctors from practicing in areas of their choice, as a matter of public policy it

---

* For interesting contrasts of some varying approaches see J. Fry, 1969, *Medicine in Three Societies: A Comparison of Medical Care in the USSR, USA and UK.* New York: Elsevier; M. Roemer, 1969, *The Organization of Medical Care Under Social Security.* Geneva, Switzerland: International Labour Office; and E. Weinerman, 1969, *Social Medicine in Eastern Europe.* Cambridge: Harvard University Press.

would not be difficult to develop a tax policy that gives tax advantage to those who choose to practice where they are most needed. Such incentives by themselves—unless extremely large—would probably make no substantial difference but when linked with other reforms might constitute significant elements of an over-all plan.

There are, of course, other mechanisms available to restrict practice choice. Various states could control the establishment of new practices through their licensing function, although this would entail a perhaps undesirable change of the licensure program from one of competence certification to a kind of public utility regulation. Similarly, it is conceivable that the control over the granting of hospital privileges could serve as a mechanism that discourages doctors from practicing in relatively overdoctored areas. Given the general scarcity of doctors, however, it is difficult to see what political forces could bring about such use of the hospitals' powers.

Developing a Mechanism for Implementing Priorities in Medical Care Delivery

Medical care is diffuse by its very nature, combining technical operations with a variety of human concerns. The total package is difficult to define, and it is even more difficult to determine whether some part of it is worth paying for in an amount sufficient to cover its cost. Yet we know that the typical practice of medicine includes considerable use of medical and technical procedures that are dangerous and costly beyond any conceivable value to the patient. Since it is not difficult to find conflicting opinions concerning the management of almost any disease,* the field of the doctor's work is characterized by considerable murkiness which interferes with the establishment of priorities. Yet it seems perfectly reasonable that those who pay the bill ought to have some basis for determining what is worthy of payment, and that procedures not worth their cost, either in general or in particular circumstances, ought to be discouraged in a time of general scarcity of medical resources. A precedent for professional evaluation of effectiveness exists in the evaluations made by scientific committees of the National Academy of Science-National Research Council of the efficacy and safety of various therapeutic agents.

How, for example, does one justify a rate of more than 600 tonsillec-

---

* For a fascinating discussion among sophisticated experts concerning opposing approaches to the treatment of such common conditions as hypertension, ulcers, emphysema, rheumatoid arthritis, and other diseases, see F. Ingelfinger, *et al.* (eds.), 1966, *Controversy in Internal Medicine.* Philadelphia: W. B. Saunders.

tomies per 100,000 population performed in the United States in 1965,[25] when the medical literature contains carefully controlled studies demonstrating the procedure to be both potentially dangerous to the patient and medically worthless except in very limited situations? Further,[26] how does one justify a program of medical care insurance or financing that pays for such procedures and that may have the effect of increasing their prevalence* Since we know that particular dubious procedures are performed with great frequency, would it not be reasonable to require some demonstration of the need for such procedures before public funds are expended? Of course, in endeavors where clinical judgment of particular circumstances is important, it may be prudent to adopt a liberal definition of effectiveness and worth, but review of procedures frequently misused is likely to conserve funds and improve the over-all quality of medical activity. The fact of review itself is likely to make doctors more conscious of the implications of their decisions and more cautious in the use of unnecessary procedures that involve risks of harm.

The idea of review is one that professionals find unattractive, and I have no doubt that my remarks on the topic will be upsetting to many physicians. It will be argued that such review is cumbersome, time-consuming, and inefficient, and a disincentive to necessary work and innovation in treatment. I should note that prereview exists within various social security systems in the world, and has been used effectively to control unnecessary work by physicians and dentists within these systems.[27] I believe that these mechanisms deserve careful attention and research, and that some modification of them might have something to contribute within the context of our existing system of medical care. I might add that review of certain procedures has been quite common in the United States, most notably in the case of abortions before the current climate of change set in.[28]

In considering the definition of appropriate and inappropriate procedures and those worthy of public support, several distinctions must be kept in mind. Many medical activities are ameliorative and supportive, and the extent to which such services are sought and used is heavily dependent on consumer decisions. Other procedures and activities depend largely on the doctor's judgment. Still others occupy a hazy middle ground involving negotiations between patient and physician, and considerable client control may be evident in pushing the physician toward a particular course of treatment.[29] There are a variety of options available in developing mechanisms for reviewing or sharing the cost of services whose

* As Bunker, Note 25, shows, the rate of such procedures in the United States is double the rate in England and Wales.

utilization is effectively determined by the consumer. Experience in other countries suggests that the viability of any particular mechanism of control of such costs depends on the habits and attitudes of the population involved and that it is difficult to generalize about such experience from one country to another.[27]

Financial barriers to medical care affect rates of utilization. Many doctors feel that the total elimination of cost to the patient stimulates trivial and inappropriate consultations, although the evidence in the British case does not disclose an excessive rate of utilization when such barriers are removed.[30] The intermediate solution adopted in Sweden requires a small percentage of the fee to be paid by the consumer, and this may cut down frivolous consultations without creating significant cost barriers to needed medical care, since full benefits are available for those who cannot afford to pay. The Swedish case is difficult to evaluate since there is a considerable shortage of general physicians; and the difficulty of obtaining an appointment with a doctor and long waiting periods in seeing him probably pose a much more significant barrier to utilization.[31] Outpatient care constitutes the least expensive type of medical service, and a strong case can be made that patients ought to be encouraged to seek medical assistance whenever they feel the need, and that the doctor and other health workers ought to use such occasions, when the problem is not serious, for establishing an educational and preventive care relationship.

The most costly element of medical care is hospital care, and admission is fully dependent on the consent of the physician. Prepaid care may be organized in such a way that primary services are readily available, but there is relatively little incentive for the doctor to hospitalize the patient or to perform unnecessary medical and surgical procedures.[32] In contrast, many of the payment schemes, including Medicare and Medicaid, provide strong incentives for unnecessary hospital care, and abuse is particularly likely when medical services are operating at less than full capacity.[1] In weighing relative costs it appears clear that excessive utilization, if it is to occur, is most appropriate and least harmful at the primary care level and most expensive and risky at the hospital level. Moreover, since a medical decision is a prerequisite for hospital care, it is primarily in this area that effective controls that achieve the goals toward which they are intended can be realistically implemented.

Government programs ought not to pay for expensive procedures that informed medical opinion defines as having little worth. In the past physicians have opposed the extension of benefits for chiropractic services, but perhaps some medical procedures ought also to be looked at in the same light. Some procedures that have value in some circumstances but involve large costs and large potential risks to patients and are known to have a high prevalence of misuse might benefit from prereview by an appropriate medical committee before the work is undertaken and payment authorized. Still other procedures involving less danger and cost but considerable abuse might be controlled through periodic informational audits. It is not my purpose to suggest how such mechanisms should operate, but it seems reasonable to anticipate that satisfactory procedures can be developed that would protect the patient and the public purse more appropriately without infringing significantly on the doctor's clinical freedom. Whatever these mechanisms are, they should be developed and administered largely by physicians, and should reflect informed professional opinion. There are problems in specifying what is and is not necessary, and such decisions will often depend on the facts of the individual case. However, abusive practices are not too difficult to locate, and the need for added controls is indicated by the growing evidence that a small proportion of doctors can seriously threaten the viability of a major program.*

Developing Criteria for Evaluating the Effectiveness of Health Care Programs

How we know a good medical product when we see one and how we identify alternatives worthy of development are larger problems than they may appear. Relatively little effort has been devoted to identifying and refining criteria by which to evaluate competing programs of medical care, and few rigorous measures exist. In this final part of the discussion I shall briefly suggest some major dimensions in comparing alternative forms of delivering medical care. Among the criteria used from one discussion to another are the following: relative mortality and morbidity; patient satisfaction; professional satisfaction; cost; stimulation of new investments; coordination and integration of elements of care; recruitment and retention of personnel; quality of special services (such as mental health services); capacity for innovation and adaptation; accessibility of services; effectiveness of manpower distribution; quality of controls over professional work; incentives for abuse of services; and

* See Lewis and Keairnes, Note 13. They note that "Two to 3 per cent of the physician population can create a 'leak' in the system through which an inordinate amount of dollars can pour without any improvement in the overall quality and quantity of health care rendered to society." This is based on their own study where they found that 8.7 per cent of the physicians received 44 per cent of all special-benefit dollars.

continuity of care. Many of these criteria are misunderstood and applied carelessly, and a brief discussion of some of these criteria is in order.

One of the ways in which comparisons are most frequently attempted between different programs is to compare relative mortality and morbidity rates.[33] Although the quality of medical care has some relationship to infant and adult mortality, for the most part differences in rates reflect variations in the quality of life and the environment and cannot be traced directly to the provision of medical services.* Any comparison on mortality must be sensitive to the characteristics of the populations served, and must take account of variations in other factors conducive to illness and death among the populations being compared. Sensitive use of mortality data can be valuable. For example, if it can be demonstrated that a particular system of medical services working with a population of measurably greater difficulty achieves rates that are superior to those achieved with more privileged populations, such information is particularly suggestive. But rates even specific to particular procedures must be inspected carefully since favorable rates may reflect the unwillingness of a medical service to take difficult problems where risks of mortality or chronicity are very high. Superficial examination will show, for example, that midwives and home delivery arrangements yield lower infant deaths than special obstetrical units in hospitals. It is clear, however, that these services work with different types of risks, and intepreting the outcome without attention to the inputs contributes little to our understanding.

Morbidity is more difficult to measure, and relative rates of morbidity may reflect the availability of medical services for identification and diagnosis of disease. Specific morbidity evaluations may be useful, as in comparisons between iatrogenic reactions, the rate of occurrence of preventable conditions among persons under care, and the like. But even these services work with different types of risks, and interpreting the out-to some extent on the ambitiousness of the cases which doctors are willing to tackle. Careful comparative work is possible and extremely useful, but it is not easily done.

A common criterion by which the success of health service systems is evaluated is the degree to which the consumer feels his needs are successfully met and is satisfied with the care he receives. Various studies show that consumers place high value on the skill of their physician and his interest in them. It is primarily the latter which can be evaluated by the

---

* For a review of factors affecting infant mortality, see D. Mechanic, 1968, *Medical Sociology: A Selective View*. New York: Free Press. See also S. Shapiro, *et al.*, 1968, *Infant, Perinatal, Maternal, and Childhood Mortality in the United States*. Cambridge: Harvard University Press.

consumer, and judgments of the quality of care by consumers often reflect the doctor's personality, his accessibility, and his attention to the patient's wishes. Patients are frequently not in a position to understand the quality of care potentially available to them, and often form their judgments on the basis of past experience with physicians. In general, patients report considerable satisfaction with their personal medical care, although they are much readier to criticize the system of care in general. Also, one frequently finds significant differences in satisfaction among varying segments of the population reflecting their varying orientations, the actual services available to them, and so on. Some dissatisfaction arises among consumers when doctors are less amenable to client control, as in prepaid group practice, but the doctor's orientation to his colleagues' standards under such circumstances may be conducive to higher quality medical care.[34]

Since patients often are reluctant to report dissatisfaction with their own physicians, one can benefit by measuring dissatisfaction of consumers indirectly. The rising rate of malpractice suits in American medicine probably reflects in part the growing impersonality of the relationships between doctors and their clients.[35,36] When close personal relationships exist, persons are loath to bring suit even when the doctor has made significant errors; when the relationship is weak, frustration may readily lead to legal action. Other possible criteria of dissatisfaction include the rate of use of facilities outside the patient's medical care system, as occurs when patients in prepaid plans seek additional private care[29,37] and when consumers in the National Health Service, for example, seek private care.[38] All such rates are influenced as well by factors other than satisfaction and must be used sensitively and cautiously, but they can alert us to the aspects of organization that arouse consumer dissatisfaction and breakdowns in medical service. Although consumer satisfaction is not the central goal of medical care, the development of significant dissatisfaction is a serious threat to the continuity of medical care and its overall effectiveness.

A particular pattern of medical care can also be frustrating and dissatisfying to the doctor and other professionals, but frequently doctor and patient satisfactions are not related to the same factors. Ideally, the patient would like his personal doctor available to him at any time in need, willing to visit his home, and responsive to his wishes; but many doctors prefer relief from total responsibility, are reluctant to make house calls, and feel their decisions should reflect their professional judgment and not patient pressures. Many factors influence professional satisfaction, including the doctor's remuneration, the conditions of work, his status in the community, and his autonomy.[39–41] Doctors have considerable political power which they use to protect the conditions they value, and any viable system of organization must insure to some extent the conditions doctors prefer. Alienation of the physician is disruptive to the smooth functioning of a medical care program and, under conditions of manpower shortage, may lead to work mobility. Doctors around the world are becoming more militant in expressing their interests, and the threat of doctor strikes is increasing. Moreover, there is tremendous elasticity in the amount and the quality of the work a physician can do, and it is important that incentives for effort and excellence be maintained.*

The competition for medical manpower is sufficiently fierce among varying programs within the United States and among nations that the imposition of controls and changes in the organization of practice must take into account the recruitment and retention of personnel. Organizational change must be based to some extent on the conditions that are likely to attract and retain professional resources, and this is particularly true when programs must compete for scarce manpower with alternative programs. A dilemma may present itself in that mechanisms that may be conducive to more effective health care, such as the imposition of controls on professional work or the making of care more easily accessible (which also increases the possibilities for abuse), may be perceived as creating unattractive conditions for professional work, and programs instituting such mechanisms may have difficulties in attracting sufficient doctors.

All organizational systems, as they grow in complexity and differentiation, have problems in integration and coordination. Considerable resources must be devoted to maintaining communication, the flow of information, and a clear set of goals. Medicine is no different, and considerable attention is required for maintaining the continuity of care. The ability to use special services such as physical rehabilitation, mental health, and the like effectively as part of the total flow of services contributes in important ways to the overall care effort.

Since there are always limited resources in the real world, and health must compete with other priorities for the resources available, the question of cost is always paramount. Different forms of organization provide varying outputs at similar costs, and we obviously must strive to get as much for our investment as we can. But there are other aspects of the issue as well. Different forms of organization may have differential capacities to attract investment for development and innovation, and, to

---

* For an interesting argument on this point see R. M. Bailey, 1970, "Philosophy, Faith, Fact and Fiction in the Production of Medical Services." *Inquiry*, 7:37–53.

the extent that health is defined as a priority deserving greater attention, the ability of health care plans to grow in an effective way may be worth a certain degree of inefficiency and confusion.* In any case, capacity for innovation and investment potential are extremely difficult indicators to measure; as listed evaluation criteria, they at least alert us to issues that we should not ignore.

As we look toward the future of health organization in America, there is much that lacks focus. Many of the issues at stake are intricately linked, and their piecemeal discussion by its very nature is deficient. Without some clear concept of the over-all system and its priorities, it is difficult to specify the necessary manpower needs, the way in which different forms of manpower will interrelate, the kinds of physical facilities necessary, the types of new paraprofessionals that can fill gaps, and many other items of importance. If we work with the concept of a "personal doctor," then one set of priorities seems reasonable; but if we work with concepts of hospital-based primary practice, health centers, or more organized health teams, then quite another approach seems to be of greatest advantage.

In the final analysis, the development of the health services system will very largely depend on the political dialogue and on various kinds of political compromises taking into account government expenditures, political power, existing economic interests, and professional organization. Therefore, it is the height of fancy to believe that we can prescribe entirely new models of delivering health services that will replace the existing system. Even the limited proposals presented in this paper would be enormously difficult to implement, and the future pattern of health services in the United States will be largely woven out of already existing elements and traditions. Change will evolve with new events and new pressures, and we will do well if we can use such conditions in the next few years to develop new competing structures for those professionals who are dissatisfied with present alternatives and for those population groups who are relatively disenfranchised under the current organization of health care. Taking a somewhat longer perspective, it is clear that as universal entitlement emerges vast changes in the provision, distribution, and administration of health care services will be required. We would do well to learn what we can from the experiences of others who have faced similar problems and to assure that whatever structure emerges offers alternatives to those with varying needs and inclinations. For, above

* For an argument along these lines see O. Anderson, 1963, "Health Services Systems in the United States and other Countries." *New England Journal of Medicine,* **269**:896–900.

all, we must remain aware that health care is most basically a distinctively human institution and in the last analysis its success must be measured not by its technical virtues or its scientific precision but rather by its capacities to meet needs and sustain men in enhancing their own goals as they define them.

Notes

1. Staff of Senate Committee on Finance, 91st Congress, Second Session (1970). Medicare and Medicaid: Problems Issues and Alternatives. Washington D. C.: U. S. Government Printing Office.

2. Waldman, S. (1969). Tax Credits for Private Health Insurance: Estimates of Eligibility and Cost Under Five Alternative Proposals. Staff Paper No. 3. Washington D. C.: Social Security Administration.

3. Cohen, W. J. (1970). National Health Insurance: Problems and Prospects. Michael Davis Lecture. Chicago: Center for Health Administration Studies, University of Chicago.

4. Griffiths, M. W. (1970). "Health Care for all Americans." AFL-CIO Federationist.

5. Falk, I. S. (1969). "Beyond Medicare." *American Journal Public Health,* **59**:608–619.

6. Kissick, W. L. (1970). "Health-Policy Directions for the 1970's." *New England Journal of Medicine,* **282**:1343–1354.

7. Ginzberg, E., and M. Ostow (1969). *Men, Money and Medicine.* New York: Columbia University Press.

8. Greenfield, H. (1969). *Allied Health Manpower: Trends and Prospects.* New York: Columbia University Press.

9. Freidson, E. (1970). *Profession of Medicine.* New York: Dodd-Mead.

10. Becker, H., *et al.* (1961). *Boys in White: Student Culture in a Medical School.* Chicago: University of Chicago Press.

11. Miller, S. (1970). *Prescription for Leadership: Training for the Medical Elite.* Chicago: Aldine.

12. McNerney, W. J. (1970). "Why Does Medical Care Cost So Much?" *New England Journal of Medicine,* **282**:1458–1466.

13. Lewis, C. E., and H. W. Keairnes (1970). "Controlling Costs of Medical Care by Expanding Insurance Coverage." *New England Journal of Medicine,* **282**:1405–1412.

14. Densen, P., *et al.* (1960). "Prepaid Medical Care and Hospital Utilization in a Dual Choice Situation." *American Journal of Public Health,* **50**:1710–1726.

15. Perrott, G. S. (1966). "Federal Employees' Health Benefits Program: Utilization of Hospital Services." *American Journal of Public Health,* **56**:57–64.

16. Health Information Foundation (1961). "Hospital Use by Diagnosis: A Study in Contrasts." *Progress in Health Services,* Vol. 10, no. 1.

17. Mechanic, D. (1967). "Changing Structure of Medical Practice." *Law and Contemporary Problems,* **32**:707–730.

18. Ratner, H. (1962). Medicine. Santa Barbara: Center for the Study of Democratic Institutions.

19. Mumford, E. (1970). *Interns: From Students to Physicians.* Cambridge: Harvard University Press.

20. Richmond, J. (1969). *Currents in American Medicine.* Cambridge: Harvard University Press.

21. Peterson, O. L., *et al.* (1956). "Analytic Study of North Carolina General Practice." *Journal of Medical Education,* 31:1–165.

22. Sidel, V. W. (1969). "Can More Physicians be Attracted to Ghetto Practice?" In J. Norman (ed.), *Medicine in the Ghetto.* New York: Appleton, Century, Crofts.

23. Stevens, R. (1966). *Medical Practice in Modern England.* New Haven: Yale University Press.

24. Department of Health and Social Security (1969). *1968 Annual Report.* Cmnd. No. 4100. London: Her Majesty's Stationery Office.

25. Bunker, J. P. (1970). "Surgical Manpower: A Comparison of Operations and Surgeons in the U. S. and in England and Wales." *New England Journal of Medicine,* 282:135–144.

26. Bolande, R. P. (1969). "Ritualistic Surgery—Circumcision and Tonsillectomy." *New England Journal of Medicine,* 280:591–596.

27. Glaser, W. (1970). *Paying the Doctor: Systems of Remuneration and Their Effects.* Baltimore: Johns Hopkins Press.

28. Lader, L. (1966). *Abortion.* Indianapolis: Bobbs-Merrill.

29. Freidson, E. (1961). *Patients' Views of Medical Practice:* New York: Russell Sage Foundation.

30. Cartwright, A. (1967). *Patients and Their Doctors: A Study of General Practice.* London: Routledge and Kegan Paul.

31. Anderson, R., *et al.* (1970). Medical Care Use in Sweden and the U. S.: A Comparative Analysis of Systems and Behavior. Research Series No. 27. Chicago: Center for Health Administration Studies, University of Chicago.

32. Saward, E. (1969). "The Relevance of Prepaid Group Practice to the Effective Delivery of Health Services." Washington D. C.: U. S. Dept. H.E.W., Office of Group Practice Development.

33. Rutstein, D. (1967). *The Coming Revolution in Medicine.* Cambridge: MIT Press.

34. Freidson, E. (1963). "Medical Care and the Public: Case Study of a Medical Group." *The Annals of the American Academy of Political and Social Science,* 346:57–66.

35. Staff of Subcommittee on Executive Reorganization of the Senate Committee on Government Operations, 90th Congress (1969). Medical Malpractice: The Patient vs. The Physician. Washington D. C.: U. S. Government Printing Office.

36. Blum, R. (1960). *The Management of the Doctor-Patient Relationship.* New York: McGraw-Hill.

37. Silver, G. (1963). *Family Medical Practice.* Cambridge: Harvard University Press.

38. Mencher, S. (1967). *Private Practice in Britain: The Relationship of Private Medical Care to the National Health Service.* Occasional Papers on Social Administration No. 24. London: Bell and Sons.

39. Mechanic, D. (1968). "General Medical Practice in England and Wales: Its Organization and Future." *New England Journal of Medicine,* 279:680–689.

40. Mechanic, D. (1970). "Practice Orientations Among General Medical Practitioners in England and Wales." *Medical Care,* **8:**15–25.

41. Mechanic, D. (1970). "Correlates of Frustration Among British General Practitioners." *Journal of Health and Social Behavior,* **11:**87–104.

Index

303